WOUNDS OF WAR

How the VA Delivers Health, Healing, and Hope to the Nation's Veterans

SUZANNE GORDON

ILR PRESS
AN IMPRINT OF
CORNELL UNIVERSITY PRESS
ITHACA AND LONDON

First published 2018 by Cornell University Press

Printed in the United States of America

Library of Congress Cataloging-in-Publication Data

Names: Gordon, Suzanne, 1945– author.
Title: Wounds of war : how the VA delivers health, healing, and hope to
   the nation's veterans / Suzanne Gordon.
Description: Ithaca, New York : ILR Press, an imprint of Cornell
   University Press, 2018. | Series: The culture and politics of health
   care work | Includes bibliographical references and index.
Identifiers: LCCN 2018018474 (print) | LCCN 2018018810 (ebook) |
   ISBN 9781501730832 (epub/mobi) | ISBN 9781501730849 (pdf) |
   ISBN 9781501730825 | ISBN 9781501730825 (cloth : alk. paper)
Subjects: LCSH: United States. Veterans Health Administration. |
   Veterans—Medical care—United States.
Classification: LCC UB369 (ebook) | LCC UB369 .W678 2018 (print)
LC record available at https://lccn.loc.gov/2018018474

Contents

To my daughters Alex and Jessica Early
My most beloved advocates of patients and their caregivers

A volume in the series

THE CULTURE AND POLITICS OF HEALTH CARE WORK

Edited by Suzanne Gordon and Sioban Nelson

For a list of books in the series, visit our website at cornellpress.cornell.edu.

WOUNDS OF WAR

ACKNOWLEDGMENTS

This book had many sources of inspiration, and I owe its publication to an entire battalion of friends, colleagues, VHA caregivers, veterans, and, of course, family members. It's not possible for me to list here by name everyone I spoke with for this book, so the "shout out" below is for those interviewed not once but multiple times. Many people have helped me better understand the specific nature of veterans' health care and the difficulties involved in delivering it. Others have helped me put current issues into historical context, or navigate the maze of congressional politics and policy making, especially in the chaotic environment of Washington, DC, since January 2017.

I want to express my gratitude to all the VA caregivers and staff, and veterans and their family members who shared their time and insights with me, or who allowed me to follow them as they worked or went to appointments. Some people who have helped me prefer to remain unnamed.

I am particularly indebted to Rajiv Jain, Rebecca Shunk, Bernie Sanders, and Philip Fiermonte, who encouraged me to pursue my idea of a book on VA health care. As then chairman of the Senate Veterans Affairs Committee, Bernie helped pave the way with the VA Central Office. I could never have parsed the complex issues of VA eligibility without the expertise of Steve Robertson, then serving in Bernie's Senate office in Washington. I also want to thank Katie Van Haste, Sanders's staff member in Vermont, for her continuing assistance, and Larry Cohen for his friendship and encouragement. I cannot do enough to express my gratitude to Bill Outlaw, who helped me get critical introductions to VHA staff across the country. And I want to thank Maureen McCarthy for her constant support.

Judi Cheary provided invaluable guidance and support in San Francisco, as did Russell Lemle, whose insights have been hugely important to me. A special thank you also to Bonnie Graham in San Francisco, and Cecelia McVey and Michael Charness in Boston. My cousin Andrew Budson generously shared his experiences caring for veterans for many years and doing related research on veterans' memory problems. And my cousin Nan Schnitzler also helped with work in Boston. Tom Kirchberg has my perpetual gratitude for his critical support, as do Harold Kudler, John McQuaid, and Tom Neylan. Ditto to Brett Copeland.

Phillip Longman and Kenneth Kizer always made time for my endless questions and acted as a critical sounding board for refining my ideas. Robert Kuttner, Eliza Carney, Gabrielle Gurley, and the whole *American Prospect* team helped me cover the VA "beat" for them while this book was being written. At *Washington Monthly*, Paul Glastris and Phillip Longman similarly encouraged and published my ongoing work. Randy Shaw at Beyond Chron consistently championed and published my work. The *Prospect*, the *Monthly*, and Beyond Chron provided an alternative perspective on veterans' affairs often missing from the mainstream media. Indeed, these three publications are some of the only ones that actually take the time to accurately report on the VHA. Veterans should thank them all.

In the course of my doing this book and a previous one, Michael Blecker at Swords to Plowshares became an invaluable Bay Area ally, whose patience I tried during many a long conversation. Bradford Adams and Kate Richardson at Swords and Rick Weidman at Vietnam Veterans of America helped me better understand the variety and specificity of veterans' health care problems. I also value my long conversations with

Peter Dickinson at the Disabled American Veterans. Thank you also to Joy Ilem, Garry Augustine, and Adrian Atizado at the DAV, especially for an award that really spurred me on. Amy Webb at AMVETS was always available, for fact checking and information sharing. At the American Legion, Lou Celli gave me and Phillip Longman a much-appreciated opportunity to prepare a report for Legion members on what is at risk if the VHA is privatized.

VHA public affairs staff throughout the country made it possible to observe health care delivery at the local level. I want to thank Matthew Coulson in San Francisco; Michael Hill Thomas in Palo Alto; Cynthia Butler in San Diego; Tara Ricks in Sacramento; Pamela Redmond in West Haven, Connecticut; Palas Wahl in Boston; Naman Horn in White River Junction, Vermont; David Martinez and Charles Ramey in Las Vegas; Paul Coupaud in Phoenix; Patricia Tiernan-Matthews in Honolulu; and Willie Logan in Memphis. As undersecretary for health at the VA, Dr. David Shulkin helped open many doors for me at local facilities. In return, I did my best, in this book and elsewhere, to promote *Best Care Everywhere*, his limited-edition collection of VHA success stories.

At the AFGE, Marilyn Park, Ian Hoffmann, and Sara Kuntzler deserve very special recognition for their research and unstinting fight against VA privatization. Ditto Will Fisher at VoteVets.

I want to give special thanks to the veterans who have shared their experiences with me. First comes my old friend Louis Kern, who shared very painful accounts of his military service and reflections on it. (Thank you Kathleen Burke, for introducing me to your husband Lou!) Paul Cox and Denny Riley have been essential to this project, along with Diane Reppun, David Antoon, Kevin Miller, Josh Oakley, Dan Luker, and Buzz Davis. My Richmond neighbors Steve Kittle and David Moore let me go to their VHA appointments; I met Rick Karp while sitting in on David's appointment with him. Thank you also to VHA physicians Dirk Woods, Poormina Goyal, and Ron Chueng. Many thanks to the pseudonymous Mojo and Robert Wallace (you know who you are in so many ways).

Other people at the VHA whose help was invaluable include Jason Kelley, Andy Pomerantz, Rebecca Brienza, Karen Seal, Tauheed Zaman, Jennifer Manuel, Bill Collins, Jeff Kixmiller, Sasha Best, Liza Katz, Keith Armstrong, Brandina Jersky, Joe Ruzek, Erin Finley, Anne Fabiny, Michael Drexler, Jim Lewis, Cathy Coppilillo, and my friend Kate McPhaul.

I also want to thank House Democratic leader Nancy Pelosi and her staff, Congressman Beto O'Rourke and his staff, and Josh Weitz at Congressman Mark Takano's office for their time and attention to veterans' issues. In health care policy and patient safety circles, I drew on the support of Don Berwick, Gordie Schiff, and Mardge Cohen. Thank you also to Charlyn Johns and Ken Watterson at the Dallas Veterans Resource Center.

At Cornell University Press, I am once again so grateful to the amazing team who got this book in print so quickly. First my coeditor and longtime friend Sioban Nelson and our equally dear colleague and friend Fran Benson, editor extraordinaire. I want to thank Dean Smith for his support, as well as Martyn Beeny for publishing—in a great hurry—*The Battle for Veterans' Healthcare* and for supporting this book. I also want to thank, once again, Ange Romeo Hall, Nathan Gemignani, and Jonathan Hall. Although they are not at Cornell, Matt Rothschild and Denise Logsdon provided crucial editorial assistance. Their quick response to my pressing, sometimes panicked, questions and concerns kept this book on the fast track. Thank you to my dearest agent Anne Borchardt.

Finally, there is my husband, Steve Early, who did much near-deadline editing as well. I especially remember the morning we both woke up at seven, not very rested because we had spent the night, tossing and turning, over what to title and subtitle this book. Our daughters Alexandra and Jessica Early have been my personal correspondents from the front lines of our fractured health care system.

It was a proud moment when Jessica became a nurse and then went to work, caring for veterans, at the VHA in West Haven, Connecticut. As a staff member for Rights & Democracy in Vermont, she advocated for universal health coverage. Every conversation with Alex, about her work as an organizer and advocate for nursing home staff represented by the National Union of Healthcare Workers, contains some new reminder of patient safety or staffing problems in for-profit nursing home chains.

Hopefully in their lifetimes, if not mine, the United States will join the rest of the industrialized world in guaranteeing that everyone in our country has access to quality care, as VHA patients do today.

Abbreviations

CBOC Community-Based Outpatient Clinic
DAV   Disabled American Veterans
DoD   Department of Defense
IAVA Iraq and Afghanistan Veterans of America
MOS   military occupational specialty
MRSA methicillin-resistant *Staphylococcus aureus*
MST   military sexual trauma
OEF   Operation Enduring Freedom
OIF   Operation Iraqi Freedom
OND   Operation New Dawn
PACT Patient Aligned Care Team
PTSD post-traumatic stress disorder
TBI   traumatic brain injury
VA   Department of Veterans Affairs (often used to refer to VHA)
VBA   Veterans Benefit Administration (part of VA)
VFW   Veterans of Foreign Wars

VHA   Veterans Health Administration (part of VA)
VISN   Veterans Integrated Service Networks
VistA   Veterans Information Systems and Technology Architecture
VSO   veterans' service organization

WOUNDS OF WAR

INTRODUCTION

What Kind of Care for Veterans?

The View from Fort Miley

It's a chilly day in late August 2015 at the facility known as Fort Miley, a medical center in San Francisco operated by the Veterans Health Administration (VHA), the largest agency in our US Department of Veterans Affairs (VA).[1]

Many of Fort Miley's cream-colored, art deco buildings provide sweeping views of the Pacific. Its hospital complex also offers one-stop shopping for Northern California veterans who need primary or specialist care, audiology or optometry services, mental health or substance abuse counseling, or many other services.

While researching this book, I've spent many hours at Fort Miley. I originally came to explore how the VHA, a publicly funded national health care system more European in form than our fragmented, market-driven private-sector model, serves its patients. During visits here and other veterans' hospitals across the country, I've looked at innovations in clinical care, teaching, and research (the three primary missions of the VHA). I've asked veterans about the quality of care they receive and observed how VHA doctors, nurses, social workers, and other staff deliver their care.

My own journalistic mission shifted somewhat, as more members of Congress—encouraged by conservative activists, like the Koch brothers—began to push for privatization of VHA functions. The ongoing debate about the future of our nation's largest health care system directly affects nine million veterans eligible for care because they are low-income or have a medical problem that is military-service related. So I began asking additional questions in my patient interviews. Do veterans prefer getting services directly from the VHA? Or has their experience, if any, with out-sourced care available since 2014 through the Veterans Choice program made them converts to the private hospitals and physicians favored by the Koch brothers, congressional Republicans, some Democrats, and President Trump?

The answers I usually get may surprise some readers, whose perception of publicly funded veterans' health care has been much influenced by largely negative mainstream media coverage of the VHA in recent years. Today, for example, I stop for coffee in the Fort Miley canteen after spending the morning observing the work of VHA "telehealth" specialists, who assist veterans in rural California unable to make the trip to San Francisco. I'm waiting to attend a class on "mindfulness meditation" for veterans suffering from PTSD. It's close to noon, and the cafeteria begins to fill up with veterans, their family members, and VHA employees. A stocky man in his forties, looking for an empty table and finding none, stops by mine. He points to a vacant seat and asks, "Do you mind if I sit down?"

"Please do," I respond. As he sits down, I glance at his lunch.

"No, I am not sharing with you," he jokes.

As we chat, I tell him that I am writing a book about veterans' health care. He quickly introduces himself and launches into an unsolicited testimonial to the VHA. His name is Rick Martinez,[2] and he tells me a story that will become very familiar as I conduct hundreds of conversations and formal interviews with veterans like him.

Martinez spent twenty years in the Marines. After he retired, he developed mental health problems and was eventually diagnosed with manic depression. Like so many men and women whose stories are told in this book, Martinez initially avoided seeking treatment, a reflex finely honed while on active duty. In the Marine Corps, he explained, "they discourage you from going to the medic or doctor. It's hard for us to get help because the majority of us don't want to be wimpy. 'I went to war—I don't need help' is the attitude. If I tell people I'm having trouble, I'll be processed out."

In civilian life Martinez could no longer "hang on to my brothers and charge on," he says. He began to drink a lot, didn't want to get out of bed, and experienced paranoid episodes. He now gets professional help at the VHA's downtown San Francisco clinic and also sees a psychiatrist at Fort Miley, who prescribes and checks on his various medications. At City College of San Francisco, where he is studying sociology and film, Martinez regularly visits the Veterans' Resource Center, where a social worker named Keith Armstrong has been "really helpful."

Talking with these staff members about his personal problems is still not easy for him. "I don't want to keep rehashing things. If I keep rehashing everything, it can get overwhelming," he tells me. But as a self-described "proactive" patient, Martinez gives his VHA helpers high marks for being good listeners and respectful of his own opinions. "I watch Dr. Oz," he says. "I ask questions. If I am not satisfied, I ask why. My doctor listens to me if I bring up my concerns." Martinez urges me to contact Armstrong at the Veterans' Resource Center, where he and others have been able to find camaraderie and community on campus, thanks to the VA.

As Martinez gets up to leave, a veteran at the next table leans over and tells me he's been listening to our conversation and would like to talk to me as well. Older than Martinez, fifty-nine-year-old Phillip Davis* has a craggy face, trim beard, and short gray hair. Davis served for twenty-three years in the Marines, most of that time as a platoon sergeant, a role in which he was a tough taskmaster. "A lot of people didn't like me," he says.

During the first Gulf War, his unit was scheduled for deployment but did not end up seeing combat. Like Martinez, Davis found transitioning to civilian life a hard adjustment. In the military, he says, things run smoothly. People do as they're told. If they don't, there are consequences. There are no consequences for civilians, he believes.

Later in his career, Davis suffered a noncombat injury to his back. That condition, plus PTSD, led him to Fort Miley. He confesses to having anger management issues. Medical center security was once called when he snapped and shouted at a young VHA doctor during a routine appointment. Despite that incident, he is grateful for VHA assistance with his physical and mental health problems. His wife also feels strongly supported by the VHA, he says.

While I'm still chatting with Davis, a third veteran, who has overheard our conversation, walks by and hands me a paper napkin with his phone number written on it and a scribbled note asking me to call him later. When I do, I learn that he, like one hundred thousand other VA employees, is a veteran himself. He just wants me to know that he would have found it very difficult to get employment outside the VHA and is grateful for being able to serve his fellow veterans.

As I walk out of the canteen to attend the mindfulness meditation class, I pass various waiting rooms, in which I see patients exchanging stories about their time in the military and their time at the VA. Sometimes people sit in silence, but most of the time the VA's corridors and waiting rooms are a bustle of human connections.

As a journalist and researcher who has spent the past thirty-five years writing about health care and observing clinicians and health care workers mostly in the private sector (and, as a patient, has received health care services for the past seventy-two years), I have spent a lot of time in hospital waiting rooms and cafeterias. In all those years, what I have noticed is people sitting in isolation. At VHA hospitals and clinics, patients actually talk to each other and support each other, providing a sense of camaraderie that is a facsimile of what they had in the military.

My visit to Fort Miley that day was just one of many I made between 2014 and 2018 while working on this book about veterans' health care and confronting how the Veterans Health Administration deals with the many wounds of war from which veterans suffer, whether they have been in combat or spent years or months preparing for it. In 2014 I decided to explore the kinds of care—and innovations in care—that can be delivered in a genuine national health care system. Rather than return to Canada, or the UK, or Australia, New Zealand, or Europe, where I have visited and even worked over the years, I decided to stick closer to home and see what our own homegrown national health care system has produced. In the course of my research, I spent months in different VHA facilities all over the country observing primary care providers and geriatricians, palliative care and hospice specialists, mental health practitioners, rehabilitation professionals, designers of prosthetic devices, pioneers in team training and patient safety, and researchers, among many others.

I have interviewed veterans of all ages, as well as their family members. I have watched veterans enter the system and be cared for after—sometimes years after—they separate from the military. I have watched older veterans as geriatric and palliative care specialists help them go through the pain and suffering of terminal illness and negotiate their last days of life with grace and comfort. (As someone who has long written about our society's failure to provide compassionate care at the end of life, I found these encounters some of the most moving I had while writing this book.)

In San Diego I visited the ASPIRE Center, a special VA program devoted to reducing homelessness among Iraq and Afghanistan veterans.

At a VA clinic in Martinez, California, I met younger men and women who served in these same wars but experienced traumatic brain injuries and suffer from severe post-traumatic stress disorder. They are now participating in an innovative program to help them live fuller lives.

I met young women, badly scarred by the experience of sexual assault in the military, who because of VHA outreach efforts directed at female veterans are now getting treated, in Sacramento or San Antonio or Boston, for military sexual trauma.

On the streets of San Francisco, I followed a VA social worker who was searching among the homeless who now crowd our cities to find veterans who could get housing and health care from the VHA.

I followed VA staff as they helped veterans in trouble with the law navigate the system of veterans' courts designed to help them avoid incarceration if they seek treatment for the alcohol and drug abuse problems or mental health issues contributing to their arrest records.

In upstate New York, I sat with VA employees who staff the agency's veterans' crisis hotline as they listened to call after call from distraught family members who worried that a loved one was about to take his life. And I watched as the suicide prevention team cautiously investigated where the veteran might be and how to help in a way that would not endanger either the veteran or his or her family.

In West Haven, Connecticut, I witnessed the work of one of the VA's thirteen Blind Rehabilitation Centers, which serve 157,000 veterans who are legally blind and hundreds of thousands more whose vision is sufficiently impaired that they have trouble navigating daily life.

In San Diego I talked to researchers doing pioneering work on the use of telehealth for delivering mental health care.

In Las Vegas I talked with nurses who monitor video screens, using telehealth to patrol the fluctuating blood pressures or blood sugars of the veterans whose chronic conditions they help manage. While in White River Junction, Vermont, I watched a veteran, again via telehealth, as a physical therapist in North Carolina coached him through exercises that would help him recover the use of a frozen shoulder.

At VHA clinics and hospitals across the country, I've observed veterans in salsa dancing classes that encourage them to socialize and relate more cooperatively, cooking classes to help them make healthy meals and read food labels, and mindfulness meditation and yoga classes to help them cope with their anger and frustration.

Over and over again, veterans told me—and you will hear their voices throughout this book—that they would be "dead without the VA," "in a ditch without the VA," or otherwise "lost without the VA." And very few, even those critical of VA failings or shortcomings, proved to be enthusiastic proponents of having private health insurance instead.

This is the hidden reality of veterans' health care that is rarely seen. In recent years the buzz about veterans' health care has not been good, inside or outside the Washington Beltway. Open any major newspaper, watch any TV news report, or listen to any radio talk show, and you'll find that "VA" is invariably preceded by adjectives like "stumbling," "beleaguered," "broken," or "scandal-ridden." Every year, our federal government spends about $70 billion on medical care for the nine million men and women who use hospitals and clinics run by the VHA. But according to the media and Congress, much of this goes to incompetent employees, bonuses for corrupt managers, indefensible expenditures on hospital art, failed suicide prevention programs, and doctors who dispense opioids like breath mints.

This steady stream of invective was unleashed in April 2014, when a doctor, Sam Foote, exposed serious misconduct by a few VHA hospital managers. The VA central office had imposed what some considered an unrealistic goal of wait times no longer than fourteen days for an appointment at the VHA. In Phoenix and several other cities, managers had falsified data that suggested that facilities were meeting this goal. The local administrators involved got undeserved performance bonuses.

Meanwhile, they papered over the need for more doctors and nurses to handle the high volume of veterans seeking VHA care in the Sun Belt. This wait-time cover-up triggered a political uproar on Capitol Hill and a journalistic feeding frenzy that has yet to subside.

Conservative Republican Jeff Miller of Florida, then chairman of the House Committee on Veterans' Affairs, kicked things off by insisting that forty patients died while waiting for an appointment at the VHA in Phoenix. Pressure from veterans' organizations like the American Legion led to the resignation in May 2014 of General Eric Shinseki, the first secretary of veterans affairs under Barack Obama. When the claim of forty deaths was later investigated by the VA inspector general, it was found that six, not forty, veterans died while they were on waiting lists to see a physician. The report noted, "We are unable to conclusively assert that the absence of timely quality care caused the deaths of these veterans." Many people die while waiting for a medical appointment. This does not mean, however, that they died because of the delay.[3]

Whatever the truth, the damage had been done. That July, President Obama replaced Shinseki with Robert A. McDonald, a West Point graduate and former CEO of Procter & Gamble. McDonald changed the reporting protocols of local VHA hospital administrators, fired or suspended those responsible for disguising appointment delays, and, most important, began recruiting more clinical staff to ensure faster patient access, particularly to primary care. Assisting McDonald's reform efforts was physician David Shulkin, a VA undersecretary for health appointed by Obama, who had private-sector experience as a hospital administrator in Pennsylvania.

None of the media reports on the Phoenix scandal highlighted the problems of chronic underfunding—and thus understaffing—of the VHA.[4] In February 2014, well before the much-needed whistle-blowing in Phoenix, Senator Bernie Sanders, then chairman of the Senate Committee on Veterans Affairs, had recognized the VHA's staffing shortage and proposed a budget allocation of $21 billion that would have fast-tracked the hiring of thousands of additional caregivers. Conservative Republicans opposed this expenditure. So after the problems in Phoenix erupted, Sanders was forced to negotiate with Senator John McCain on compromise legislation, eventually passed in the summer of 2014.

The Veterans Access, Choice, and Accountability Act of 2014 allocated $6 billion to care at the VHA, $18 billion less than Sanders initially sought. An additional $10 billion was earmarked for a three-year trial program known as Veterans Choice. Under Choice, patients who lived more than forty miles from the nearest VHA facility or faced appointment delays of more than thirty days could seek care from private hospitals and doctors at VA expense.

Despite this initiative, the drumbeat of conservative and media criticism continued. During his final two years in office, President Obama never vigorously defended publicly provisioned veterans' care. He didn't do what Senator Sanders did, which was point out the VHA's many strengths as an integrated national health care system (and personally encourage journalists like me to check it out more closely). Instead, the White House and Congress appointed a "bipartisan" Commission on Care to develop strategies for the future of the VHA over the next twenty years. This panel included some genuine experts, like Washington journalist Phillip Longman, author of the widely acclaimed book *Best Care Anywhere: Why VA Health Care Would Work Better for Everyone*, and Vietnam veteran Michael Blecker, executive director of the San Francisco–based veterans' group Swords to Plowshares.[5] But commission members like Longman and Blecker were far outnumbered by those from private-sector hospitals or representatives of the Koch brothers–funded Concerned Veterans for America, which favors further outsourcing of VHA services or total privatization of the agency.

The commission did conduct an independent assessment of the VHA's effectiveness. The resulting consultant report faulted the agency for various management shortcomings. But researchers from the RAND and Mitre Corporations also confirmed, in great detail, that the quality of the VHA's frontline care was equal or superior to that delivered in the private sector. And their study noted that wait times for appointments with primary care providers or medical specialists at the VHA were actually shorter than those experienced by patients using private doctors and hospitals.[6]

These findings were rarely reflected in any reporting or commentary in major media outlets. Instead, the VHA was indicted for failing to prevent veteran suicides (*New York Times*),[7] gaming internal ratings by keeping veterans out of small rural hospital (*New York Times* again),[8] and doing nothing to stem our national epidemic of opioid overuse, whose victims include many veterans (Fox News).[9] VHA wait times remained terrible, perhaps even lethal (according to CNN),[10] plus its operating rooms were filthy

(*Boston Globe*).[11] Women veterans got no services (*Philadelphia Inquirer*).[12] VHA services should be provided by private hospitals, its own facilities closed, and homeless veterans housed in them instead (*Boston Globe*).[13]

VHA staff—three hundred thousand employees in all, one-third of whom are veterans—were malingerers and a drain on the federal treasury (*USA Today*). Further displaying its profligacy, the VHA wasted US taxpayer money on artwork in its hospitals (*USA Today* again). And that was before Donald Trump targeted the VA in his campaign for the White House in 2015 and 2016. Trump declared that the treatment of veterans by their own government was "horrible, horrible and unfair." He pledged that, if elected, he would fire those responsible and greatly expand VHA patient access to private-sector care.

Trump's Electoral College victory unleashed what the *Times* called a "potent new effort" by "deep-pocketed conservative activists" to allow "private health care to compete with Veterans Affairs hospitals for the patronage of the nation's veterans." To advance its "campaign against government-provided medical care," the Kochs' Concerned Veterans for America "pledged millions of dollars for advertising and outreach and unleashed a small army of lobbyists and donors to pressure the Trump Administration and Republican lawmakers."[14] The Koch brothers and other conservative activists are determined to defund and dismantle the VHA, and use any hint of problems at the VHA to discredit the notion that government can serve the public good. They also use problems at the VHA to delegitimize efforts to create a more rational, national health care system in the United States.

Fearing the worst, many observers were thus surprised and relieved when Trump nominated Dr. David Shulkin to remain as head of the VA, becoming the only Obama administration holdover in Trump's cabinet. Shulkin was approved by unanimous consent of the Senate. Under Obama, Shulkin praised the VHA, pledged that he would never privatize it, and even helped compile a 440-page collection of VHA case studies titled *Best Care Everywhere* (published in June 2017) that hailed his agency's little-publicized role as an incubator for health care innovation.

Shulkin's collection is dedicated to veterans, their VHA caregivers, and Longman, the Commission on Care member who "showed us that VA provides some of the best healthcare anywhere, and who inspired us to disseminate our best practices and pursue the audacious goal of delivering the best care everywhere to our veterans." In his personal introduction to the collection, Shulkin noted that "it takes an average of 17 years for new medical evidence to reach patients in clinic or at the bedside. VA, the largest health system in the U.S., is not exempt from this problem. But VA is leading American health care in fixing it."[15]

Nevertheless, in his first "State of VA" address, delivered a month before *Best Care Everywhere* was published, Shulkin contradicted his own broader assessment of the VA, declaring that his agency was "still in critical condition and require[d] intensive care." Part of this assessment applied to the state of VA infrastructure and bureaucratic performance issues, like delays in handling claims for VA disability benefits, not directly related to health care delivery.

Among the VHA-related problems Shulkin cited were "absurd" delays of three to six months in hiring new nurses or nurse-practitioners, plus "low salaries for health care providers" at the VHA, which "make it difficult to recruit and retain critical positions." In fact, by mid-2017, the VHA had an estimated thirty-five thousand open positions.[16] Yet, instead of seeking money to fill these vacancies, Shulkin sought additional funds from Congress for more outsourced care through Choice, a program with $2 billion worth of cost overruns since it was created, including $90 million in overbilling by its two main contractors, TriWest Healthcare Alliance and Health Net Federal Services.[17]

In an approving profile of Shulkin, the *Times* reported that he wanted to focus the VHA on its "core mission of caring for the wounded," which required making "hard decisions" about outsourcing services like optometry and audiology. ("We make eyeglasses for our veterans. Last time I checked, every shopping mall in America has a place where you can get glasses in an hour," he told *Times* readers.)[18]

At the same time, Shulkin was floating an internal proposal to shut down VHA patient safety centers—a model program central to its core mission—to free up more money for reimbursement of private-sector providers. He has tried to shift a billion dollars in funding for—among other things—mental health programs, women's health, and social workers who help homeless veterans, to cover shortfalls in the revenue that finances the operating costs of VHA facilities. And he embraced a scheme to outsource the VHA's already state-of-the-art medical record-keeping system.[19] Instead of resolving the current problems in the groundbreaking

Veterans Information Systems and Technology Architecture (VistA) in house, Shulkin, with no competitive bidding, declared that the VHA would purchase the Cerner Millennium system, a move that would enrich the company with billions in federal money.[20] In February 2018, Shulkin would tell a House Veterans Affairs Committee hearing that he did not oppose a proposed hiring freeze for federal employees that would make recruiting to the VHA harder. He also supported limiting VHA services to labor-intensive chronic conditions and outsourcing the kind of expensive, episodic treatment that would further enrich private-sector providers.[21] As we will see, this kind of outsourcing—or stealth privatization—would constitute an additional wound from which veterans would suffer.

My Pathway to the VA

Although I am not a veteran myself, the campaign to dismantle the VHA and outsource veterans' care has been as dismaying and disturbing to me as it has been to longtime advocates in the field. I'm a seventy-two-year-old civilian whose family tree includes more health care providers than former military personnel. My father was a doctor, and my younger daughter is a nurse and former primary care provider at the VHA. Before I embarked on this project, my friends and acquaintances with military experience numbered just a few. Now they are legion and include scores of dedicated VHA caregivers around the country.

I do bring to this project more than forty-five years of journalism experience. That career includes three decades spent observing and writing about the work of doctors, nurses, and other health care providers and studying their interaction with patients and the health care systems that employ them, here and abroad. In addition to writing, editing, or coediting ten health care–related books, I have published the work of other journalists, academics, and health care practitioners as coeditor of the Cornell University Press series Culture and Politics of Health Care Work.

One focus of my own recent work is patient safety and how it can be improved through better workplace communication and information sharing among health care professionals. In the course of my health care industry consulting work, I first met VA hospital staff members, who were trying to reduce medical errors and accidents at a VHA facility in

Northern California. In many other clinical settings I have encountered, it was common for hospital administrators to pay lip service to patient safety and related training without actually institutionalizing the best practices of doctors, nurses, and other staff that can save patients' lives and spare them medical complications resulting in longer hospital stays or costly readmissions.

When I worked with the VHA, however, I was struck by its far more serious approach. Although many VHA managers displayed the same kind of bureaucratic mind-set and obsession with micro-management I had long observed in private-sector health care, frontline staff exhibited a distinctive ethic of service and a strong personal commitment to serving veterans. Unlike many other hospitals or health care systems, their employer was actually investing time and money in team training and often-neglected follow-up implementation measures. Several years after I did patient training at one veterans' hospital, my initial impression was confirmed when I met VHA leaders in this field, like Rajiv Jain, a physician who was the director of the VHA MRSA Prevention Initiative and later became head of Patient Care Services at the VHA in Washington, or Rebecca Shunk, an internist who is codirector of the Center for Excellence in Interprofessional Education at the San Francisco VA.

Jain and his colleagues had pioneered methods for reducing the spread of a terrible hospital-acquired infection, known as MRSA, throughout the VHA system. To accomplish this goal, they created high-functioning hospital teams—including bedside nurses, housekeepers, and transport workers—that took collective steps to reduce MRSA risk factors.[22] Meanwhile, Shunk introduced me to VHA teamwork training initiatives designed to improve the quality and delivery of primary care nationwide.[23]

I was also very impressed by how sensitive the VHA is to patient complaints. In any private-sector health care system, incidents involving substandard care tend to remain a far more private matter, even if they lead to litigation (often settled on a confidential basis) or result in reprimands from state or federal regulators like the Centers for Medicare and Medicaid Services. The VA is, without a doubt, a big government bureaucracy, more top-heavy than it should be. But the very fact that it is a public institution, with an exceedingly well-organized, vocal, and politically connected patient population represented by many veterans' service organizations, ensures a degree of transparency and responsiveness I had never encountered before.

VHA staff were very aware that if veterans didn't get services they expected—and on time—they or someone in their family would contact their representatives in Congress about it. In periods of major controversy—for example, during the aftermath of the Phoenix wait-time disclosures—patients of the VHA, through their national veterans' service organizations, have even demonstrated sufficient clout to secure the resignation of the VA's top national official, plus the disciplining of local hospital administrators.

In private industry, concerted action on this scale by health care consumers is very rare. It's likely to occur only in situations where hospital employees are unionized and their whistle-blowing (about short staffing or other unsafe conditions) generates sympathetic local media coverage and community pressure for change.[24]

More to the point, it's hard to recall the last time that the CEO of any major private-sector health care chain or hospital network even a fraction of the VHA's size was fired or forced to resign over administrative practices or clinical failings protested by patients. To cite only one example, the CEO of the Cleveland Clinic, Delos "Toby" Cosgrove, was rewarded with huge salary increases even though his hospital system was under threat of suspension from the Medicare program between 2010 and 2013,[25] faced $650,000 in fines by CMS (the Centers for Medicare and Medicaid Services) for lab violations at one of its hospitals in 2015,[26] and saw its Medicare payments reduced because of high hospital infection rates.[27] Nor was there any decrease in Cosgrove's pay or calls for his resignation when, in 2016, the Cleveland Clinic paid $1.6 million to the US Justice Department to settle "accusations that it implanted cardiac devices into patients too soon after a heart attack or surgery."[28]

The VHA's Multiple Missions

The VHA is held to a much higher standard as it performs its multiple missions. Although very few members of the public actually understand how the VHA works, what we'll see in this book is a genuine health care system in action. But first, a further word about where the VHA sits in what is known as the VA.

What is often referred to as VA health care is, in fact, the Veterans Health Administration, which is only one of three agencies within the

Department of Veterans Affairs. The VHA is the largest of the three. The others are the National Cemetery Administration (providing burial for eligible veterans) and the Veterans Benefits Administration (VBA), which determines and administers a host of veteran benefits, like the GI Bill, housing benefits, vocational rehabilitation and employment, pensions, home loans, life insurance, and access to VHA care.[29] It's critical to understand the difference between the three arms of the VA. When veterans complain about "the VA" and its hassles and wait times, they are almost never talking about the National Cemetery Administration. Their complaints, however, may not be about the VHA but about the VBA. In order to get access to the VHA, veterans have to provide documentation and file claims with the VBA. Because the claims process is unnecessarily complex (thanks to Congress) and the agency is chronically underfunded and understaffed (also thanks to Congress), there is a huge backlog of claims at the VBA, and veterans may be understandably frustrated because they have to wait for needed health care services.[30]

The VHA delivers care to almost nine million eligible veterans at over seventeen hundred sites, including acute care hospitals, outpatient clinics, rehabilitation facilities, nursing homes, inpatient residential programs, and campus- and community-based centers. With a salaried staff of nearly three hundred thousand, a third of whom are veterans, the VHA is the nation's largest and only integrated health care system that has full public funding.

The VHA is not a hospital chain competing with others for "market share." It is not a collection of physician practices or specialty services. Nor, like Medicare, is it only a "single payer" for care. It resembles the health care systems of almost all other industrialized nations: a full-service health care system that both pays for and delivers all types of care to those it serves. The VHA delivers more services more comprehensively to its patients than any other system in the United States. Not only can veterans who move from one part of the country to another get services at any VHA facility; the services they get are also fully integrated. Mental health care and primary care in the VHA are closely combined, and rehabilitation services are integrated with specialty services. What's more, much of this care is delivered in teams, often communicating face to face about their complex patients, rather than through truncated notes and "orders" entered into computerized medical records that may or may not be read or implemented. Plus, the VHA offers help with housing, employment, and even legal issues its patients might have, and, when necessary, it deals with family and community problems.

The VHA has four primary missions. First and foremost, it delivers clinical care in 153 hospitals, 900 clinics, 300 mental health centers, and other facilities that assist more than 230,000 people every day. At the VHA, health care professionals are not paid in a fee-for-service system but are all salaried. They do not have any incentive to engage in the kind of overtreatment of patients that is now epidemic in our health care system. Nor do they experience the kinds of insurance company denials and hassles that plague those in the private sector. In VHA primary care clinics, providers can actually spend more time with their patients, often two to three times as much as in the private sector, where you are lucky to get more than ten minutes with your doctor.

The VHA's second major mission—unappreciated by the general public—is research. Because it has more patients that it can track more consistently over a longer period of time than any other health care system in the country, the VHA is uniquely positioned to use this data for innovative research projects. One that is now under way involves a million veterans (the Million Veteran Program) and is exploring the impact of genetics on health and various medical treatments.[31]

As a research powerhouse, the VHA has made advances in medical care, medical equipment, and pharmaceuticals that now benefit all Americans, not just veterans.

Among such breakthroughs was the shingles vaccine, the product of a research partnership between the VHA and the National Institutes of Health. The VHA also pioneered the nicotine patch and the first implantable cardiac pacemaker.[32] VHA researchers also did pioneering work documenting that postoperative mortality rates among patients with known cardiac risks could be greatly reduced if they were given beta blockers before surgery, a practice now standard in US hospitals.

In 2016 alone, VA researchers published 9,480 papers. The VHA is currently researching the link between genes and suicide risk and the use of probiotics for veterans with traumatic brain injury.[33] In 2016 the VHA received a $50 million grant from the Prostate Cancer Foundation. Its CEO, physician Jonathan Simons, told me that the foundation was eager to work with the VHA because it is the largest health care system in America, with the most men suffering from prostate cancer of any health care system or institution. Because of this, he said, the VHA provides a unique opportunity to help solve some of the most vexing riddles about prostate cancer, democratize treatment through the VHA's superior telehealth capacity, and accelerate the pace at which new drugs and treatments are made available to the nation's veterans.[34]

The third VHA mission—also insufficiently publicized—is teaching. Since 1946, the VHA has been affiliated with major academic medical centers throughout the country. It now trains 70 percent of the nation's medical residents and 40 percent of all other health care professionals. Schools that educate nurses, physicians, psychologists, social workers, physical therapists, and many other health care professionals who rotate through hospitals and other facilities during their training depend on the VHA for clinical placements. At the VHA these future professionals learn how to perform concrete tasks like taking a patient's history, doing a physical exam, making the correct diagnosis, or delivering the proper treatment. They also learn lessons in teamwork and patient–staff communication, and they get to work in the VHA's unprecedented system of telehealth and one of the largest medical simulation centers in the country.

The fourth mission of the VHA, of which even fewer people are aware, is emergency preparedness. When I visited the VHA in Honolulu, the system had set up an incident command to deal with a volcano eruption on the big island of Hawaii. VHA staff were frantically calling veterans impacted by the disaster to make sure they were not hurt and had housing, medications, and medical services. In 2015 and 2017, during the disastrous California fires in Lake, Sonoma, and Napa Counties, the VHA set up similar incident commands and was calling thousands of veterans who had to flee their homes as a result of the fires. Two weeks after the fires were under control, staff were still making calls to veterans to help them recover from the trauma of lost or damaged homes or any health problems that occurred because of the terrible pollution that enveloped the area.

In this book I focus on how the VHA accomplishes its multiple missions and functions differently from its private-sector counterparts, whose care delivery is more costly, fragmented, and market-driven. As the largest health care system in the country, the VHA has its share of problems. But overall, as the studies and experiences I will cite convey, the VHA provides high-quality care to a very complicated patient population. In most health care systems, younger patients are usually the healthiest and least expensive to treat and are therefore the most sought after. That's not the case in the VHA. Because of a complex set of eligibility requirements imposed by Congress, not all twenty million veterans can be cared for in the VHA. Only those who have service-related health conditions or low incomes are eligible for VHA care. Apart from the low-income patients served by Medicaid, no other health care population in the United States includes as many poor, unemployed, or homeless people or ones suffering from mental illness, drug addiction, or alcohol addiction. With the exception of our national Medicare population, no other group of patients has so many seniors—in this case, surviving members of the World War II generation, plus those who served in Korea and Vietnam or were in the military during these conflicts.

As directed by Congress, the VHA has waived its standard eligibility requirements and is providing care to veterans of post-9/11 conflicts for five years after they leave the military. Veterans of our occupation of Iraq and ongoing military intervention in Afghanistan have returned with combat-related injuries, illnesses, and mental health problems that are no less challenging to treat than the myriad afflictions of Vietnam veterans. Because of the military's highly advanced methods of battlefield triage and fast transport to field hospitals, some of these young men and women have survived wounds that would have proven fatal in prior conflicts. One in six veterans who served in these conflicts also has a substance-abuse problem.[35]

The veterans the VHA serves have service-related disabilities. But as we will see, not all these conditions, of varying severity, were the result of combat. In fact, most are not. Those who serve our country by joining the military risk injury—and, in some cases, lasting mental or physical trauma—because their "working conditions" include a training regime that can be brutal and callous. Their later active duty exposes them to a variety of occupational hazards even if they never leave the continental United States. Most important, those who have, in the past, been conscripted or, in the era of the "professional military," volunteered to serve were promised later pensions and health care coverage, among other things, if their length of service made them eligible. Health care for low-income veterans and those with service-related conditions, regardless of how long they served, is one of those benefits. In this book, we will explore how the federal government delivers on this promise and how all Americans, not just veterans, benefit as a result. Far from being broken, the VHA serves as a model for how health care could be delivered, more effectively, for everyone in our country.

A Few Notes for the Reader

The VHA is a huge system. In the course of writing this book, I could not visit every one of its seventeen hundred sites of care. I did, however, visit many of them, and I observed many patient and caregiver interactions and talked with hundreds of veterans and their family members and VHA care-givers. No matter how harrowing their stories, these veterans and their families shared them with me because they felt it would help other veterans. Many of them wanted me to use their full names. Some asked me to change identifying details and give them a pseudonym, which we sometimes chose together. When an asterisk follows the name of a veteran, it indicates a pseudonym. And when a quote is not followed by a citation, it's because it came from a personal interview I conducted. I also refer to people in the military as service members rather than as soldiers, because, as I have learned, the term soldier refers to someone who served or serves in the Army (Marine is used for a Marine, sailor for someone in the Navy, airman for someone in the Air Force, and for the Coast Guard, it's Coast Guardsman).

Because the VHA is a comprehensive, full-service health care system delivering hundreds, if not thousands, of different services to veterans, I could not report on all that the VHA does. I chose instead to focus on areas of health care delivery that are particularly problematic in our larger, market-driven health care universe.[36] These include primary care, mental health care, rehabilitation, and outreach to the homeless, as well as help with legal issues, and geriatric, palliative, and end-of-life care. In the beginning of the book, I also describe our nation's often neglectful treatment of veterans in the past and the challenge of caring for VA patients today. Interspersed throughout are shorter profiles of specific VHA programs and employees. (Because this book took over four years to research and write, some of the people profiled here are no longer in their jobs—some have shifted positions or retired.)

Finally, I ask a question few reporters, media commentators, or legislators seem to address these days: How does the VHA's record of health care delivery compare to that of the private sector? I conclude by looking at the VHA's problems and consider how they might be addressed, and I argue that solving those problems and providing high-quality health care to veterans cannot possibly be accomplished by dismantling and privatizing the most successful—really the only—health care system in the country.

1

PROMISES BROKEN AND KEPT

A Short History of the VHA

The Department of Veterans Affairs is now the second-largest department of our federal government, comprising three separate agencies with a total workforce of about 370,000 and an annual budget allocation of nearly $186 billion (of which 36 percent goes to health care). How that bureaucracy developed over time from its underfunded, fragmented, state or federal predecessors is worthy of note. If the multiple reorganizations, consolidations, and political battles over veterans' benefits and services reflect any single historical thread, it's our persistent societal ambivalence about the burden of caring for former military personnel or offering them income support.

Since its inception, the United States has celebrated the patriotism and sacrifice of its soldiers—while they were on active duty. But after hostilities ceased and troops were mustered out, former combatants have been forced to struggle, repeatedly, for recognition of their pressing postwar needs. In *Wages of War: When American Soldiers Came Home—from Valley Forge to Vietnam*, Richard Severo and Lewis Milford trace this sad pattern back to the 1780s.[1]

Veterans of George Washington's Continental army were paid in paper currency that was nearly worthless and not accepted by banks, merchants, or local governments demanding overdue property tax payments. Many citizens who had volunteered to liberate the colonies from British rule ended up impoverished as a result. Some suffered humiliating eviction from their small farms or postwar incarceration in debtors' prisons.

Continental army officers fared better, of course. They received pensions and, under limited circumstances, so did their widows and orphans. But rank-and-file soldiers elicited little sympathy from the same business and political elites who had strongly encouraged them to enlist. When the financial desperation of some veterans led them to take up arms again—in Shays' Rebellion in western Massachusetts in 1787—that uprising was quickly suppressed.[2]

A Pledge by Lincoln

Between our War of Independence and Civil War, any postwar assistance for former enlisted men and officers came primarily from their individual states, which operated homes for disabled veterans. In 1862 the US Sanitary Commission conducted a study of what national governments in Europe did for their veterans. Its findings led to congressional authorization of a National Home for Disabled Volunteer Soldiers shortly after Abraham Lincoln's reelection as president. In his second inaugural address on March 4, 1865, with the Civil War nearing its end, Lincoln famously pledged "to care for him who shall have borne the battle and for his widow and his orphan."[3]

Unfortunately, even the able-bodied among the hundreds of thousands of demobilized Union army veterans faced multiple postwar difficulties. In August 1865 one former volunteer asked readers of the *New York Herald*, "What are the returned soldiers who were mustered out honorably from the service to do for employment? Are our wives and children to starve? All are willing to work, I am sure, if they can find employment. If a soldier asks for a situation, the response generally is, 'we are full' . . . or 'we engaged a clerk this morning.'"[4]

Such pleas for better treatment too often fell on deaf ears. Even a military publication like the *Army and Navy Journal* warned veterans not to "slump and become a dirty loafer" if they wanted to succeed in civilian life. Those who developed "new muscular habits," rather than succumbing to personal despair and reliance on charity, would find postwar housing and employment; those who sought special help would simply become dependent on it.[5]

Nevertheless, the post–Civil War need for national homes for disabled veterans was so great that they grew from one facility to six around the country by 1887. Their mission, carried on today by the VHA, was to assist veterans seriously injured during military service and then left jobless and impoverished. Both the Army and the Navy had their own facilities for professional soldiers in need of such care, but admission required twenty years of military service. The National Homes were a critical place of refuge for those who volunteered or were conscripted for shorter tours of duty during the Civil War.

Residents received medical care, social support, and even employment opportunities. As VA historian Darlene Richardson explains, "These homes were like little towns, with churches, theaters, and post offices. They were self-sustaining communities" filled with veterans who raised vegetables, tended to cows, and worked in manufacturing shops that produced products, like shoes, for use by residents themselves.

In the late nineteenth century, of course, formal hospital care of any type was very limited, so most wounded Civil War veterans, from North and South, were dependent on family caregivers. To support their role, the federal government provided some funding for relatives assisting Union Army veterans. But, as Richardson notes, recent immigrants to the United States often lacked the family connections or resources necessary for in-home care.

In addition, one large cohort of disabled veterans—those who served in the Confederate army—was excluded from the National Homes. (Exceptions were former rebels who were captured, took an oath of allegiance to the Union, and changed sides until honorably discharged.) As the twentieth century approached, the volume of newly disabled soldiers—mainly from the Spanish-American War—was just a tiny fraction of the patient population produced by conscription and enlistment between 1861 and 1865. The National Home network continued to serve Union veterans who were aging and no longer able to support themselves. But when these old soldiers began to die off, federal policy makers considered closing the homes because they were now underused.

Expanded Federal Role

US involvement in World War I canceled those plans. Prior to joining that murderous fray, the Wilson administration created a Bureau of War Risk Insurance (BWRI) within the Treasury Department to insure cargo ships bound for Europe and threatened with German attack. In 1917 the bureau also began offering life and personal injury policies for active-duty military personnel, veterans, and families of servicemen.

Of the 4.7 million Americans who served in World War I, 116,000 died, and 240,000 were wounded, creating a burden of care that could not be met by either existing military hospitals or the National Homes (now numbering just ten). So the BWRI created a new two-track system of veterans' health care. The National Homes continued to serve survivors of the Civil War, Spanish-American War, and other pre–World War I conflicts, and the newly wounded returning from Europe were moved into private and public facilities of their own.

In 1919 President Wilson transferred responsibility for all veterans' care to the US Public Health Service, also then housed in the Treasury Department. The Health Service began building its own facilities for veterans and acquired several former Army hospitals, including Fort Miley in San Francisco and two similar sites in Virginia. Because new hospital construction took several years to complete, many World War I veterans were assigned, in the meantime, to the old National Homes. Adding to this makeshift mix, the federal government leased some private hospital space for veterans' care.

In 1921 Congress merged all World War I veterans' programs—the BWRI, the Public Health Service, and the Federal Bureau of Vocational Education—into a single Veterans Bureau. The Bureau of Pensions under the Interior Department and the post–Civil War National Homes were not initially included in this consolidation. Eight years later, however, the bureau took over the New York Soldiers and Sailors Home, the last surviving National Home.

Overall, veterans' affairs were still handled by multiple federal bureaucracies throughout the 1920s. To access services, veterans had to fill out myriad forms and apply to different agencies. "If you wanted burial services, you had to go to the War Department, which administered the national cemeteries," says Richardson. "Where you were buried depended

not on where you lived, but what war you served in. If you needed prosthetics and had served before World War I, you went to the War Department. If you were a World War I veteran, then you went to the Bureau of
Insurance and the Veterans Bureau. Vocational and rehabilitation training and compensation depended on a different agency. And pensions—or
compensation, depending on the year a veteran was applying for funds—
were a function of the Bureau of Pensions under the Interior Department."

To make matters worse, the first director of the Veterans Bureau, Colonel Charles R. Forbes, was fired after just two years on the job, fined, and
jailed for defrauding the government on hospital contracts. This Harding
administration scandal in 1923 led to the appointment of Brigadier General Frank T. Hines in 1923. Hines began consolidating veterans' services,
establishing subdistrict offices of the bureau, and improving health care
delivery. In 1924, eligibility rules were even "liberalized to cover disabilities that were not service related."[6]

The Bonus Marchers Debacle

Nevertheless, six years later, veterans battered by the Depression were
still so frustrated by bureaucratic red tape that the American Legion
demanded further change from Congress and the Hoover administration.
In 1930 President Herbert Hoover signed Executive Order 5398, which
created a Veterans Administration to consolidate and coordinate all federal activities involving former military personnel, including pensions and
health care (but, for another forty-three years, still not their burial places).

The newly formed VA worked with the American College of Surgeons
on an overhaul of the hospital network created for World War I veterans. The facility mix that emerged included hospitals providing general
medical and surgical services, plus specialized facilities devoted to the
treatment of tuberculosis and mental health problems. Between 1931 and
1941, the number of VA hospitals increased from fifty-four to ninety-one,
with the number of beds rising from 33,669 to 61,849.[7]

Meanwhile, in 1924, Congress passed the World War Adjusted Compensation Act, setting the stage for a major confrontation with veterans.
This legislation provided veterans with service certificates guaranteeing them a bonus payment twenty years later. As the Great Depression

deepened, impoverished veterans demanded that their bonuses be paid immediately, rather than in 1945. President Hoover, a fiscal conservative, rejected these pleas. In desperation, forty thousand destitute vets—dubbed the Bonus Army—rode the rails or marched to Washington, DC, to lobby his administration. They camped out near the Anacostia River in a protest mode adopted by Occupy Wall Street eighty years later. Although Hoover found time to give visiting Boy Scouts a warm White House welcome, he staunchly refused to meet with any delegation of veterans.

Instead, the president and his political allies dismissed the marchers as radical troublemakers who threatened to overthrow the government. To quell their protest and drive them from the capital, Hoover dispatched federal troops led by Army chief of staff General Douglas MacArthur. Officers, including Dwight D. Eisenhower and George S. Patton, organized an infantry and cavalry assault that used tear gas, fixed bayonets, and six tanks. At least two marchers were killed, their makeshift camp was burned, and the bonus marchers dispersed. Of those subjected to this brutal treatment, 94 percent were in fact veterans, 67 percent had served overseas, and about 20 percent suffered some sort of disability.[8] But they left Washington empty-handed, for the time being.[9]

The federal government's responsiveness to veterans' needs did not initially improve under Hoover's successor in the White House. In 1933 the Roosevelt administration actually reduced veterans' allowances for service-related disabilities by 25 percent.[10] Despite a second veterans' march on Washington that year, it was not until 1936 that Congress finally authorized payment of veterans' bonuses before their stipulated due date—action that required overriding a presidential veto.[11]

Post–World War II Changes

During World War II, however, veterans' benefits increased dramatically. "After the attack on Pearl Harbor, Congress liberalized service-connected disability policies," Richardson notes. It also approved aid to families of servicemen who were killed or disabled before they had an opportunity to take out insurance. During the war, many of the VA's physicians, dentists, nurses, and administrative staff were called to active duty or volunteered for military service. To replace these employees, the VA reduced minimum age and physical requirements for many jobs. Women were hired for positions previously filled only by men to address the rapid increase in the volume of VA patients.

The Disabled Veterans' Rehabilitation Act of 1943 established a vocational rehabilitation program for disabled veterans who served after December 6, 1941. As a result of this law, the VA provided more than 620,000 of them with job training.[12] During World War II, Congress also authorized the provision of artificial limbs to amputees, paving the way for the VA to become a world leader in the development of prosthetic devices.

By 1946, when General Omar N. Bradley replaced Hines as VA administrator, the agency operated ninety-seven hospitals, capable of handling more than eighty thousand patients. Bradley recruited Major General Paul R. Hawley to lead the VA's Department of Medicine and Surgery (rebranded forty-five years later as the Veterans Health Administration). Hawley created a separate outpatient treatment program for veterans whose disabilities were not service related. With the nation still facing an enormous burden of care for patients who served in World War II, Bradley ordered the construction of twenty-five new hospitals and additions to eleven existing facilities. By 1950 the VA had 151 hospitals nationwide—and needed that additional capacity after three years of military conflict in Korea.

Hawley pioneered what is today one of the VHA's most important but lesser-known programs: providing medical resident and teaching fellowships at veterans' hospitals throughout the country. In addition to developing these medical school ties, Hawley persuaded Congress to endow the VA with a research capacity greater than that of any other hospital chain in the United States. "After the 1940s research programs took off, nuclear medicine takes off, collaborative research with the National Institute of Health, Academy of Science—all of it exploded," Richardson says. "The VA worked with [the Department of Defense] to do clinical trials to find out how to end [tuberculosis]."

The Vietnam Years

Changes in battlefield weaponry and resulting injuries, combined with the enhanced lifesaving ability of modern technology, have spawned different postwar challenges for veterans' health care in every era. For example, the use of mustard gas during World War I created a whole host of debilitating health problems for former soldiers who survived their initial exposure to it. Fifty years later, much faster, helicopter-assisted evacuation of the wounded to field hospitals and naval vessels saved the lives of many soldiers who would have succumbed to their injuries in earlier conflicts. But these same higher survival rates taxed the veterans' health care system in often unexpected ways, particularly after wars waged with many "citizen soldier" conscripts.

In Vietnam the United States suffered its first military casualty in 1959. Over the next sixteen years, 2.7 million draftees and enlisted personnel were deployed to Southeast Asia, 58,000 lost their lives, and 153,000 were wounded.[13] By 1972 more than 300,000 veterans had physical or mental disabilities they could prove were connected to their Vietnam-era military service. Hundreds of thousands more had yet to establish their eligibility for care based on PTSD symptoms or their exposure to Agent Orange, a toxic herbicide sprayed throughout Vietnam as a counterinsurgency measure.[14]

It is not surprising that the same US politicians who started or expanded the Vietnam War failed to anticipate the terrible burden of human suffering, disease, and disability it produced. During his second term in office, President Richard Nixon became particularly distracted by the Watergate scandal that eventually forced him from office in 1974. "Seemingly anxious to demonstrate his fiscal virtue, now that his political vulnerability had been exposed," Nixon actually "vetoed a VA healthcare bill that would have given the agency more doctors."[15] With characteristic duplicity the president cut the VA budget while publicly claiming that his administration was "doing more," rather than less, for veterans.

Congress—and the VA doing its bidding—also rejected benefit claims by former military personnel who developed multiple diseases after being exposed to some of the twelve million tons of chemical defoliants used in Vietnam. It took several decades of lobbying by veterans and their organizations, as well as the supportive research and advocacy of practitioners within the VHA, to win compensation for both Agent Orange–related illnesses and PTSD. In 1991 the VA finally stopped requiring victims to document their individual contact with the herbicide. Today any veteran who served in Vietnam is presumed to have such exposure and is now entitled to some kind of service-connected disability rating if he or she develops Agent Orange–related conditions.

Returning Vietnam vets with more recognizable battlefield injuries too often found themselves in hospital settings where VHA underfunding and understaffing produced hospital conditions shockingly exposed in Ron Kovic's famous memoir, *Born on the Fourth of July*, and much protested by veterans' organizations.[16]

The Vet Center Concept and VistA

Because of their distrust of the VA and alienation from a society seemingly uninterested in their wartime sacrifices, many Vietnam veterans avoided its acute care network. Ironically, this wariness of bureaucratic, institutional care produced a very positive and enduring legacy—the community-based Vet Center.

Authorized by Congress in 1979, Vet Centers were facilities funded and staffed by VA personnel but not located on hospital grounds. Although their mental health and social services were originally provided only to Vietnam-era veterans, Vet Center access was later expanded to include former combatants in Lebanon, Grenada, Panama, the Persian Gulf, Somalia, and Kosovo–Bosnia. In 2003 the VA further extended eligibility for Vet Center services to former participants in Operation Enduring Freedom, Operation Iraqi Freedom, and any military operations related to the "war on terror." Military family members also became eligible for help at three hundred off-site locations. Since 2003, Vet Centers have also provided bereavement counseling to surviving parents, spouses, children, and siblings of service members who die of any cause while on active duty.[17]

Like the Vet Center concept of decentralized, community-based support, the VA's cutting-edge system of electronic medical record keeping resulted from a grassroots initiative within its own nationwide information technology staff. Beginning in the late 1970s, a group of computer programmers and physicians known as the Hardhats, who formed what they called the Underground Railway within the VA, became frustrated by the VA's cumbersome handling of medical records in paper form. It's a story well told in Phillip Longman's *Best Care Anywhere*[18] and a shorter history by George Timson, one of the most influential VA developers of a new computerized record-keeping system (known as VistA), which micromanagers in the VA central office tried to thwart.[19]

The fact that the Hardhats all worked at the VA allowed them to contact and connect with one another and serve as a support group that provided knowledge and skill and served as an early social network for innovators, providing them with mutual support and constant contact. Like many other innovators within the system, the members of the Underground Railway cleverly leveraged resources to further their innovations and shared information. Because they worked in a not-for-profit, mission-driven system, they did not compete with one another for funding, sales, or markets (or, once the system was developed, for market hegemony), but rather collaborated to meld the innovations they each pioneered in their individual facilities to serve both local and national needs.

Although they were an almost textbook example of grassroots, front-line innovation, they managed to benefit from a top-down structure by going to the national media, making a case, and getting Congress to align with their goals. As we shall see, innovators in mental health, inter-professional teamwork, palliative and hospice care, pain management, suicide prevention, geriatrics, and the treatment of epilepsy, PTSD, Agent Orange, Gulf War syndrome, and more—in short, pioneers within a large system like the VHA—have definite advantages.

It is ironic that the work of the VHA's in-house computer system modernizers was finally producing results when President Bill Clinton took office and decided that VA services should be rolled into a larger system of market-driven managed care (also known as the Clinton Plan).[20] Veterans' groups vigorously protested this privatization threat. So the White House reform team, headed by first lady Hillary Clinton, backed off its original position and proposed instead that the VHA compete for patients with private health care organizations, an approach prefiguring today's Trump-expanded Choice program.

As the *Washington Post* reported, Senator John D. "Jay" Rockefeller IV (D-WV), chairman of the Senate Veterans' Affairs Committee and a key White House adviser, lauded this feature of the Clinton Plan as one of its principal attractions. Donald L. Custis, a health care consultant and former VA administrator, was less bullish. He warned that federally funded veterans' health care was "going to have a lot of trouble" under the Clinton Plan. At best, he predicted, the VHA network will "be a smaller system over the short term." It was clear to informed observers that the VA would need "a large infusion of cash and personnel" if its hospitals were "to successfully shift focus from in-patient care for an elderly male population to providing a broad range of preventive medical services to a more diverse population of veterans."[21]

The Kizer Revolution

The Clinton health care reform scheme crashed and burned because of Republican opposition in Congress. But Bill Clinton pursued a different approach when he named Kenneth W. Kizer to head the VHA in 1994. Kizer is a former US Navy medical officer who worked in emergency and occupational medicine and then served for seven years as California's director of health services. During his single five-year term as undersecretary, Kizer introduced a series of structural reforms designed to be more than just changing "boxes on organizational charts," as he put it.

Instead, Kizer has written, his team created change by "implementing a focused and meaningful performance management system, decentralizing day-to-day operational decision making, moving to a value-based resource allocation system, nurturing innovation, and modernizing information management, including deploying the most effective electronic health record in the world at the time."[22]

Under Kizer the VHA was reorganized into twenty-two Veterans Integrated Service Networks (VISNs) to bring administrative decision making closer to patients and frontline staff. In a document titled "Vision for Change," Kizer wrote: "Whenever feasible, implementation of policies and control of processes, operations and decision making will be vested with the field. The authority and responsibility to accomplish these functions will be similarly vested in the field leadership who will be held accountable for meeting defined levels of patient satisfaction, access, quality and efficiency."[23]

After assembling a leadership team that shared his vision, Kizer himself, as he described in a 1998 book titled *Straight from the CEO*, became deeply involved in leadership recruitment for the new VISNs, developed the questions that such job candidates would be asked, and personally interviewed "all ninety finalists for the 22 positions. In the end, eight of these positions were filled by outsiders, some from private industry—a big break with VHA tradition."[24]

In addition to promoting decentralization, Kizer helped steer the VHA away from its past emphasis on acute care delivery and toward the integration of inpatient and outpatient services that makes it such a unique health care provider today. The VHA did not reduce the number of its acute care facilities. In 1994 it set up the first of what would become, over two decades, a network of more than eight hundred Community-Based Outpatient Clinics (CBOCs).

By 1995 primary care physician and expert in the field Barbara Starfield and her colleagues were so impressed by the transformation beginning at the VHA that they wrote the following in a report published in collaboration with VA researchers and the Foundation for Health Services Research: "Although the VA was initially slow in responding to the changing U.S. health care environment, it is now engaged in far-reaching and innovative changes in American health care. In fact, the veterans health care system is poised for one of the most profound transformations of any organization in American history. The VHA has assured that 'each and every patient has a designated generalist physician or physician-led team of caregivers that is responsible for providing readily accessible, continuous, comprehensive and coordinated care.'"[25]

Kizer also helped the VHA pioneer patient-safety initiatives like full disclosure of medical errors. Building on the advanced health information technology of VistA, the VHA set up a Patient Safety Event Registry. Its top managers encouraged lower-level staff members to report safety problems by assuring them that they would not be blamed for errors. The good news was that more clinicians began reporting errors; the bad news was that there were still too many of them.

In response, the VHA began to implement critical components of the safety culture in commercial aviation that has dramatically reduced crashes in that industry over the last several decades. Air carriers employ a system known as crew resource management (CRM). Pilots, flight engineers, flight attendants, ground crew workers, and many others are all trained and encouraged to work in teams, communicate and share crucial information, solicit the input from those lower in the hierarchy, cross-monitor one another, and engage in a variety of team activities. To incorporate CRM-type training and safety protocols more systematically into the VHA, Kizer created a new, Michigan-based Center for Patient Safety, with former astronaut, flight surgeon, and NASA investigator James P. Bagian as its first director.

Patient safety initiatives like this put the VHA way ahead of most private hospitals. In 2005 two of the country's most prominent patient safety advocates, Lucian Leape and Donald Berwick, assessed patient safety progress in the United States in light of the Institute of Medicine's 1999 report *To Err Is Human*. This report estimated that ninety-eight thousand patients a year died from preventable medical errors.[26] According to Leape and Berwick, hospital practices were not improving fast enough in the private sector to reduce this annual toll of preventable deaths and injuries. However, they deemed the VHA to be "a bright star in the constellation of safety practice, with system-wide implementation of safe practices, training programs, and the establishment of 4 patient-safety research centers."[27]

Kizer also began the process of rigorous scrutiny and purchasing controls governing medication prescription practices. This approach helped protect patients from potentially harmful drugs, ones not fully tested, and, in some cases, drugs overpriced in comparison to equally effective alternative remedies. This drew the ire of major drug manufacturers. As Phillip Longman reports, "Kizer set up an elaborate drug review process to establish what is known as a 'formulary of recommended drug therapies.' Field investigations by VA physicians and pharmacists compared the effectiveness of new drugs with current therapies, considered safety concerns, and decided whether the VA should include these news drugs in its formularies."[28]

In the five years that Kizer served as undersecretary for health, he and his team challenged the prevailing philosophy that divided a veteran into service- and non-service-related problems. The notion that the system should focus exclusively on service-related medical and mental health conditions in isolation from the other problems veterans had with their health or lives, he argued, was not only medically but ethically indefensible.

As Kizer told me recently, what he feels he brought to the VHA was the kind of understanding of the intersection between public and population health that was needed to deal with the complex problems of a very particular group of patients. "If you're a paraplegic and you have a headache, is it the same as when I have a headache?" Kizer asked. "In health care most people don't understand that people's lives are messy. Overall, the patient population the VHA takes care of has messier lives than those taken care of in the private health care system. Thirty-five percent of patients the VA serves have psychiatric or behavioral health diagnoses. In the private sector, the mental health system, such as it isn't, is a disgrace by many people's accounts."

To serve these messy lives and complex needs, Kizer and his team focused on far more than how to book episodic medical appointments with primary care providers or specialists, diagnose a particular medical condition, or prescribe the latest drugs or procedures. "American medicine," he commented acerbically, "is so enamored with dramatic saves and rescues and technological breakthroughs that we too often don't recognize the day-to-day mundane stuff that you have to get right." He wanted to do more than expand an integrated health care system that delivered services to veterans all across the country. His goal, he told me, was the creation of an integrated care system, which integrated all the care veterans received at the local or national level in the ways we will see throughout this book.

To create what was a radical culture change in the agency, Kizer said he and his team depended not on leaders delivering harangues about what people were doing wrong (and punishing them for lapses) and exhorting them to do right. The change required top-level support for frontline action. "When I first came to the VHA," Kizer recounted, "I had, like many people, stereotypes of the VA and the people who worked in the VA. When I was actually at the VA, one of the things that struck me was the degree of dedication, commitment, and sense of mission that staff had. This was much higher than I had ever seen in all my experience in the civilian sector. I was also impressed with how good the care was despite all the rules and interference from VA headquarters. RNs and MDs were, and so many others were, trying to do the right thing in spite of the rules."

Kizer proceeded to, as he put it, "take down the barriers that keep people from doing the right thing and help them do it. We created a lot of awards, and recognition, certificates for things, call-outs for things trying to change culture." He also was very careful to support them if they make mistakes. "We allowed people to use their brains. We made them feel it was safe to do things and experiment because headquarters had their backs. They could do things, like transform healthcare IT, that needed to be done."

Kizer left the VHA in 1999, but over the two decades since his departure, the VHA has become a leader in providing high-quality care to veterans in many different areas. By the turn of the twenty-first century, the VHA was applauded by some of the most prominent business publications. *Fortune* ran a story on the VA with the banner headline "How the VA Healed Itself."[29] *Businessweek* trumpeted that the VA had "the best medical care in the U.S.,"[30] and the *Harvard Business Review* called the VA transformation the largest and most successful "turnaround" in US history.[31]

Although all this good press in the early twenty-first century validated the "turnaround" efforts at the VA, Kizer told me recently that they may have provoked a conservative backlash. As Kizer explained, when the nation's preeminent business publications lavished such positive attention on a government program that is essentially a successful example of socialized medicine, albeit for veterans only, this was not what the George W. Bush administration wanted to hear. It also contradicted the idea that only the private sector and the market can solve problems like health care. Congress and the Bush administration began to reverse what Kizer and his team had begun to build. "Congress, in its wisdom," Kizer said, "pulled information technology out of the VA." VA leadership began a slow but steady recentralization of leadership; rather than supporting frontline staff, leadership began to micromanage. VA central leadership also introduced the kind of poorly thought-out performance measures that led to the Phoenix crisis.

"In part why the American health care system is so screwed up is that it is so influenced by health care economists who tend to think money is the only thing that drives behavior," Kizer commented. "These views reflect how out of touch some people are with the reality of patient care and what needs to be done to achieve high quality and reliability. While money can drive behavior in the short term or improve production processes, there are many other kinds of incentives that drive people to perform well—things like autonomy, mastery, and commitment to a higher purpose."

These performance measures were antithetical, said Kizer, to everything he and his colleagues had done at the VHA to motivate staff. The kind of supportive environment that Kizer and his team created has been largely replaced by a punitive one. "When your boss (i.e., Congress) is talking about how many hundreds of thousands of people are going to be fired, that tends to dampen the spirit of those who work for you. In fact, what you want to do is the exact opposite—you want to encourage and support the workforce by the kind of messages you send out."

During the early 2000s, the Bush administration and Congress also began to tighten up restrictions on VA eligibility, an issue that is crucial to our understanding of how the current system works and how it should be organized in the future.

Eligibility

Ever since the United States began to provide health care services to disabled veterans during the War of 1812, there have been stipulations and qualifications on—and a tremendous amount of haggling about—what kind of benefits veterans would receive and who was eligible to receive them. As the system has grown and become more complex, the rollercoaster ride of requirements has also become more confusing. You know there is a complexity crisis when someone writes a book titled *VA Benefits for Dummies* and a lot of people who work at the VHA can't necessarily explain who is and is not eligible for services and why. Here is a short version of a very, very complex and contentious problem.

Among the factors that determine eligibility for VA services are minimum duty requirements. In most instances veterans have to have served for twenty-four continuous months or the "full period for which they were called to service." These requirements may be adjusted if someone was hurt in the line of duty, or for hardships incurred.[32] The discharge status of the service member determines eligibility for VA benefits. These assigned categories range from "honorable" to the punitive "dishonorable," which can encompass severe crimes as well as bad conduct that is serious but not enough to require a court-martial. In the middle spectrum are "other than honorable" discharges—administrative, nonpunitive sanctioning of people with performance or disciplinary problems also not considered serious enough to warrant a court-martial.

This group of some five hundred thousand veterans is excluded from VHA services and the broader array of VA benefits. Many of these vets suffer from mental or physical illnesses arising from their military service; their allegedly dishonorable behavior while on active duty may even have been triggered by a job-related health condition. Some may have been drunk on duty, tested positive for drug use, or engaged in fights. Some were simply mustered out unfairly—during the era of Don't Ask, Don't Tell or before it—because of their sexual orientation.

Yet all are ineligible for any VA benefits, from the GI Bill to health care to homeless services and more, because of the discharge characterization the DoD assigned them when they separated from military service, which the VA has accepted.

Veterans' advocacy groups and attorneys who work on veterans' benefits have identified significant problems with this classification system, which, in the case of dishonorable and other than honorable discharges, leads to denial of VHA benefits. Swords to Plowshares, a San Francisco–based advocacy group, notes that the exact same workplace conduct can result in a different type of discharge in different branches of the service. An airman testing positive for drugs might get sent to rehab, complete the program, and get an honorable discharge. A Marine Corps commander with a zero-tolerance policy may just boot a Marine with the same problem right out of the service.

Commanders often fail to consider the full circumstances of an individual's discipline problem. Did the veteran have service-related PTSD or another mental health problem? Was he or she in combat? Where? For how long? Was the female veteran a victim of military sexual trauma who drank because of the abuse? Did a woman report harassment or rape by a senior officer and get kicked out of the service on trumped-up charges?

Although the VA functions essentially like a workers' compensation system, it is unlike the one that operates in the civilian world. In civilian life a worker who gets fired, with or without just cause, doesn't automatically lose current or future access to state workers' compensation systems. Eligibility for partial compensation for lost income caused by job-related injuries or illnesses and related medical insurance coverage for those conditions is not contingent on someone having a good work record, although employers can contest claims on the grounds that they are not job related. For example, a coal miner applying for state or federal black lung benefits just has to prove that he or she worked in the industry and supply sufficient medical documentation of resulting lung damage. Disabled miners with a proven diagnosis of pneumoconiosis can't be denied benefits because they were fired from their last job (or fired in other circumstances before that).

Because of their discharge characterization, more than eight thousand veterans a year are denied services that many desperately need. Although they can apply for a discharge upgrade from the DoD, these appeals are rarely granted. The process of establishing initial eligibility at the VA is also too cumbersome. And veteran advocates argue that the VA could challenge discharge characterizations far more effectively and frequently than it does. Although both the DoD and the VA are aware of the problem and trying to address it, Congress is ultimately responsible for the complex set of eligibility requirements and discharge characterizations that unfairly limit veteran access to health care and other benefits. Congress could begin to remedy this injustice by at least directing the VA to deny eligibility only to veterans with punitive discharges. This would automatically expand access to VA benefits to those with other than honorable discharges. If Congress chose to give these veterans the care and service they deserve, it would, of course, also have to allocate the additional funding to pay for these services. Under the Trump administration, VA secretary David Shulkin has ordered the VHA to deliver emergency mental health services for up to ninety days to veterans with other than honorable discharges. In January 2018, the president also issued an executive order giving all those who separate from the military a year of mental health care services. There was, however, no funding or additional staff allocated to serve the tens of thousands of veterans with acute mental health needs who could be brought into the system.

Another thing that determines eligibility today is a service-connected disability. Not all eligible veterans have seen combat, but all of them—if they served after 1980—must provide evidence of a "service-connected disability."

The level of service connection can range from zero to 100 percent. A partial disability finding might result from back or knee injuries incurred while carrying sixty- to one-hundred-pound packs during basic training or combat—a problem few civilians connect to military service. Other, more serious, conditions warranting VHA coverage include amyotrophic lateral sclerosis (or Lou Gehrig's disease) or other diseases that were a side effect of Agent Orange exposure during the Vietnam War and the traumatic brain injuries (TBIs) and amputations suffered by targets of improvised explosive devices in Iraq or Afghanistan. VHA and DoD researchers are also discovering that many service members, like football players who experience repeated concussions, are suffering from mild TBI because of the exposure to blast pressure from firing heavy weaponry.[33]

Most members of the military, as we shall see, are not counseled about VHA or even VA eligibility when they enter the service. They don't know that veterans have to provide documentation to the VBA to prove that any physical or emotional condition they have was acquired during military service. In other words, they may not know that there has to be a paper trail that verifies that a Marine hurt his knee, or an airman or sailor or soldier had an emotional problem like PTSD, while in the service. Maintaining a paper trail is further complicated by the fact that, as we shall see in later chapters, many service members are discouraged from going to the doctor or medic to report even physical problems. Most are terrified that admitting to an emotional one will lead to an immediate discharge or the end of a career in the military. Even service members about to be discharged from the service may not reveal physical or emotional problems because that will delay their discharge.

Veterans are also eligible for VHA services if they have low incomes or are indigent. Over the objections of many veterans' organizations, in 1986 Congress mandated means testing for eligibility for health benefits. Up until 1996 the only people eligible to go to the VHA were service-connected and economically indigent. In 1996 Congress enacted eligibility reform to allow more veterans to enroll in a system that was moving its focus from inpatient care toward outpatient and prevention care. Its goal was to provide timely access to quality health care—the right care, at the right time, in the right medical setting. Under this reform the VHA initially established seven priority groups to make sure that the most severely disabled veterans had the timeliest access to care. People who suffer from 50 percent or higher service-connected disabilities are in Priority Group 1. (Service-connected veterans unable to work because of their medical condition are rated at 100 percent.) If you were a prisoner of war or awarded a Purple Heart, you're in Group 3, and then, going on down the list, come other priority groups with a lower service-connected rating. Indigent veterans do not have the highest priority, although they are eligible to enroll (they are in Priority Group 5). Means testing today applies only to Priority Groups 5, 7, and 8 (Group 8 was added in 2003 and includes higher-income veterans).[34]

Reserve components (this includes Reserves and the National Guard) who are not considered to be on active duty add another complexity. Members of the National Guard are not eligible to enroll in the VA health care system until they obtain "veterans' status" by having served on active duty.

If you are eligible for VHA services, you receive all the benefits that are available under the veteran's medical benefit package, not just care for your particular service-connected problem. (If you have PTSD and get an unrelated lymphoma, for example, you are treated for both). Although, just to make matters more confusing, if you are treated for a service-connected problem and get better, your service-connected rating may be reduced. If you have a service-connected problem and are affluent (say, an attorney who served in Vietnam), you are covered for that service-connected problem but may have a co-pay for the treatment of non-service-connected medical conditions. Again, all this depends on the degree of your disability rating.

Recently Congress has made VHA benefits available to all veterans returning from Operation Enduring Freedom, Operation Iraqi Freedom, and Operation New Dawn (as the military refers to these wars), for five years, no questions asked. Also, you don't have to prove military sexual trauma (even for a member of the National Guard who was in training) to receive services. The VHA has engaged in a big push to enhance care to female veterans.

With multiple exceptions (Purple Hearts and veterans of current wars, for example), very high-income veterans with no service connection are not eligible for VHA care. The Veterans Affairs Health Care System also serves as a backup to the DoD, and active-duty service members can utilize VHA health care under specific circumstances, usually when it is part of their rehabilitation or recovery.

Veterans must prove that they are eligible for VHA care. This requires assembling an impressive dossier and may also involve undergoing what are known as compensation and pension ("comp and pen") examinations, usually conducted by a doctor at a VA hospital or clinic. (At the time of this writing, many of these comp-and-pen hearings are being outsourced to private contractors.) These exams are designed to verify that a veteran has a disability for which he or she can receive compensation. If a veteran claims more than one disability, there can be more than one comp-and-pen exam. Whatever the complexity of the veteran's condition, the first step in the process of obtaining benefits from the VA involves passing through the doors of the VBA, which has been, for decades, chronically underfunded and understaffed. When a veteran complains about wait times at the VA, it's important to ascertain whether those waits are at the VHA or the VBA. It's even more important to understand who the veterans are who are waiting, what their problems really are, and what they are waiting for.

Those Who Have Borne the Battle

The VHA's Patient Population

Fred Fuller*

Fred Fuller's house seems as remote as you can get if you live in the middle of the city. The last on the road, it hugs the edge of the mountain. This way, he tells me, he can patrol the perimeter and prevent any stealth attacks. Fuller, a burly forty-year-old with curly black hair and several days' worth of black stubble flecked with gray, apologizes for the fact that we can't park in a driveway cluttered with tools, sawhorses, and other construction equipment. "I'm building myself a shop. It's driving my wife crazy," he offers by way of explanation.

When we go inside and sit down at the kitchen table, he gives me his military history. The son of a Vietnam veteran, Fred joined the Army when he was eighteen because, he says, "I just wanted to fight." He ended up defusing mines in the DMZ. "Korea," he acknowledges now, "was not a great place to be when you were a nineteen-year-old kid prone to drinking, partying, and running after girls—from South Korea, Russia, New Zealand, you name it. Korea had all of them."

When he left the Army, he had knee, foot, and shoulder trouble from carrying around a hundred-pound pack day in and day out. Fuller tells me that, like other soldiers, he was discouraged from going to the medic or doctor for any "owie," as he dubs injuries. Complain about something— even something serious—and they had a name for you, in addition to "wuss" or "pussy." It was "sick-call ranger," or just plain malingerer.

When he came back to Hawaii, he signed up for the GI Bill and went to a community college, finished an associate's degree, and then went on to get a bachelor's degree in diplomacy and military studies. While in school he met a National Guard recruiter who, as he puts it, waved a magic wand. He told Fuller that if he signed up for the Hawaii Army National Guard, he wouldn't have to spend his GI Bill money on education but could use it for getting a mortgage and taking care of his family.

This was too good a deal to pass up. "So," he continues, "for the eight years I owed them, I went to doing part-time one weekend a month, two weeks a year, what I was paid to do in the Army." He finished college and had fun on the weekend, almost finished grad school, got married, and received $129 a month. In 2004 he thought he was "out the door." Then he got a phone call informing him about orders for Iraq. He couldn't believe it and hung up. They called back. "Dude, you need to come down to the unit. We're going to Iraq."

Fuller spent the next twenty-two months working in force protection in Iraq. "We were the guys who prevent bad stuff from happening. Barriers, counterblast barriers, stopping suicide bombers from getting in."

When he left the military and returned to his family, he got a job in the county sheriff's department. He had all the aches and pains he had acquired during his first stint in the military, plus some new problems. He was having nightmares, drinking himself to sleep, and constantly irritable. "I was a total cockhead," Fuller admits. "I was angry, bitter, violent. Being in the sheriff's department, well, you know . . . ," he says, trailing off, inviting me to fill in the blank. Finally, his wife had had enough and kicked him out of the house.

Fuller had lost enough over the years. He did not want to lose his family. So he checked himself in to Dr. Kenneth Hirsch's Post Traumatic Stress Recovery Rehabilitation Program at the Honolulu VA. When Fuller entered the six-week residential program, Hirsch asked him what his goals were.

"That was simple," Fuller says. "I told him I just wanted to save my family. He said, 'Okay, we can help you do that. But you, in turn, have to do two things.'"

One, Fuller says, was come to Jesus. By that he did not mean get religion, but rather admit there was something wrong. For Fuller, that would not be easy. "Honestly," he says now, "I thought I was perfectly sane and the rest of them were crazy. Iraq just totally cemented in me my ideals of what the world should be versus what it is. That ended up being my issue with my wife and kids."

The second thing Hirsch wanted the veteran to do, Fuller reports, was "use the tools we give you. If you use the tools properly, we can't guarantee that your wife won't leave you, but we can guarantee it will be a little bit better."

He agreed, and the results were dramatic. The VHA "helped me save my wife and kids," he says. "They gave me the one thing I needed more than anything else: that four seconds to think before I act. This guy just cut me off in traffic because he's a dumbass. This person is just some idiot in a lowrider who's just blasting his music seventy-five decibels too loud." Instead of taking them on, Fuller says, he fought the impulse—successfully.

But twelve months later, Fuller explains, "My wife had again gotten tired of my ass, and drove me back up to VA and said, 'Throw him back into PRP [the post-traumatic stress rehab program].' Dr. Hirsch said, 'Yeah, we got a bed for him.'"

When he left the program the second time, Fuller realized that he could not move forward if he remained in law enforcement. "I don't like gray areas," he confesses. "If I'm in for a penny, I'm in for a pound. What that means is I can play cop, or I can play family man. If I'm going to be a cop, I'm going to be the best damn cop this place has ever seen." That involved, he says, fighting and being angry and irritable—all the behaviors he was trying to overcome.

The VA provided him with $25,000 worth of vocational rehabilitation services, and he has gone into construction work. He continues to get treatment for his ongoing emotional problems and for his knees, feet, neck, and shoulders. He volunteers in his children's schools every day, he tells me. "That way, I have a reason to go in there and make sure they are safe." After his stint in the military, safety is not something Fuller will ever take for granted again.

Fuller is one of millions of veterans who have significant problems acquired or exacerbated by military service. You cannot understand how the VHA functions without understanding the conditions from which these men and women suffer. To grasp the challenges the VHA confronts, it's also essential to explore the process of socialization most service members undergo while in the military. This shapes veterans' ability to ask for and get needed help, as well as their responses to those who try, with the best of intentions, to offer them help. Finally, it shapes their responses to the obstacles they may encounter coping with complex health conditions and navigating a large health care system.

Service-Related Physical Problems

Military veterans suffer from the usual chronic and acute problems that beset so many Americans today: obesity, type 2 diabetes, and asthma, for example. They break their bones in accidents, have strokes, fall off ladders, or experience bouts of back pain or other musculoskeletal issues. They also cope with mental illness and stress-related health conditions. On top of this, military veterans also suffer from problems (both emotional and physical) created or exacerbated by military service.

The first time I met him in the lobby of a hotel near San Francisco International Airport, Rick Weidman, executive director of government affairs for the Vietnam Veterans of America, gave me a crash course on the facts with which too many politicians and even health care professionals are unfamiliar. "The military," the burly, balding, then sixty-six-year-old Vietnam veteran explained with a combination of palpable frustration and patient effort, "is a collection of very dangerous occupations." Whereas the average elderly private-sector patient may have three to five presenting problems, the average Vietnam veteran has nine to fourteen. Almost every military activity, in basic training or after, carries with it health care consequences. And, Weidman added, one doesn't ever have to go near a field of combat to experience many of them.

Learning about the complexity and specificity of military-related health problems has been one of the most fascinating aspects of researching and observing VHA care. When I began writing this book, I assumed, like so many civilians, that what prompted most veterans to sign on with the

VHA were service-connected conditions like PTSD, amputations, or TBIs. It never would have occurred to me that the most common ailment that brings people to VHA care is hearing loss and tinnitus.[1] This is because almost every branch of the military exposes personnel to high levels of noise. In the Air Force and Navy, there's the rumble of airplane engines. In the Navy there's the metallic clanking that rebounds through the echo chamber of a submarine or other vessel. You don't have to go to the Middle East to be at risk for the ear-popping effect of explosions—just go through basic training. Nor do you have to be in a shootout with the enemy to do irreparable damage to your ears. One well-heeled lawyer from Marin County that I met at a VHA cooking class at Fort Miley signed up with the VHA because he served as an honor guard at Arlington National Cemetery during the Vietnam War. Day after day, month after month, he fired his rifle at military funerals without wearing any protective sound gear. The result was both predictable and preventable.

At our first meeting, Weidman presented me with a VHA Pocket Guide that outlines how clinicians should take a military health history. They should ask, it instructs, the following general questions of their patients at the very first visit: When and where did you serve? What do you / did you do while in the service? How has military service affected you?

It then advises following up with five other queries: Did you see combat, enemy fire, or casualties? Were you or a buddy wounded, injured, or hospitalized? Did you have a head injury with loss of consciousness, loss of memory, "seeing stars," or being temporarily disoriented? Did you ever become ill while you were in the service? Were you a prisoner of war?

There are questions about sexual harassment, sexual assault, or other trauma. And there are questions about the veteran's living situation: Are you in safe housing? Did you lose your home? Do you need assistance caring for dependents?

It then catalogs the various exposures—chemical, biological, or physical— to which service members are subject. These include pollution, solvents, radiation, noise, heat, car crashes, shell fragments, and explosions, to name only a few. No matter what the war or era, military personnel are exposed to pit smoke, contaminated water, nerve agents, mustard gas, pesticides, and an array of other chemicals, pollutants, and environmental hazards. As if this were not enough, each war in which the United States has participated recently—World War II, Vietnam, Korea (and the later patrolling of the DMZ), and the various wars in the Middle East and Afghanistan—has its own particular set of contaminants, signature injuries, and infectious disease risks. There was Agent Orange for Vietnam and chemical warfare agent experiments and nuclear weapons testing and cleanup during the cold war. There are Gulf War syndrome and the chemicals and contaminants military personnel inhale because of the burn pits in Iraq and Afghanistan. Added to these are exotic infectious diseases like visceral leishmaniasis, West Nile virus, and mycobacterium tuberculosis, to name only a few. There is also the problem of chronic pain and resulting opioid use. When I have shown this guide to my friends who are private-sector primary care providers (the informal survey included nurse-practitioners, physician assistants, and primary care physicians), they were surprised to learn about the complex problems from which service members and veterans suffered. They also told me they would be hard-pressed to ask even a fraction of the questions listed. When she scanned the list, one physician assistant in a busy rural clinic that has some veteran patients laughed. "You must be kidding. I have ten to fifteen minutes with a patient. I have no time for this."

Chronic Pain, Musculoskeletal Injuries, and Other Exposures

The news has been filled with angry denunciations of the VHA's failure to deal with veteran pain and the epidemic of opioid use that plagues the veteran community. What we don't often learn about is why so many veterans are in so much pain in the first place. It's because military service produces serious problems with musculoskeletal diseases and injuries. In every branch of the service, basic training involves hauling around sixty- to one-hundred-pound packs that place an excessive burden on the bodies of service members.[2] Many of the veterans I interviewed, like Fuller, talked about back, knee, ankle, foot, and shoulder problems they acquired during their military service. A 2014 report on the burden of musculoskeletal diseases in the United States documented that these injuries impacted three hundred thousand active-duty Army soldiers annually, leading to one million medical encounters.[3]

In 2014, *JAMA Internal Medicine* published research that surveyed an Army infantry brigade made up of soldiers between the ages of eighteen and twenty-four three months after its return from Afghanistan. It found that 44 percent were in chronic pain. More than 48 percent reported that their pain lasted over a year, "55.6% reported nearly daily or constant frequency, and 51.2% reported severity of moderate to severe; 23.2% reported past-month opioid use, and 57.9% of those reported few or several days use." This burden of chronic pain was almost twice as high as in the civilian population.[4] Chronic pain also increases the risk of suicide.

The high rates of injury and pain have surprised many researchers. "We expected pain after a long war and many injuries, but we didn't expect it to be nearly one out of two, given that these are otherwise young, healthy soldiers," Annette Boyle wrote.[5]

Then there are the toxic exposures from which veterans suffer. Agent Orange exposure can lead to the following:

- AL amyloidosis
- Chronic B-cell leukemia
- Chloracne (or similar acneiform skin conditions)
- Diabetes mellitus type 2
- Hodgkin's disease
- Ischemic heart disease
- Multiple myeloma
- Non-Hodgkin's lymphoma
- Prostate cancer
- Respiratory cancers and soft-tissue sarcomas[6]

Gulf War syndrome consists of "a cluster of medically unexplained chronic symptoms that can include fatigue, headaches, joint pain, indigestion, insomnia, dizziness, respiratory disorders, and memory problems."[7] In the current wars in Iraq and Afghanistan, veterans are suffering from asthma and other respiratory problems; skin and eye conditions; heart, stomach, and intestinal problems; cancers of the brain, lungs, and other organs; memory problems; chronic fatigue; and other health issues.

One of the most famous casualties of burn pit exposure was thought to be Vice President Joseph Biden's son Beau, who served in Iraq and died of a brain tumor in 2015. The toxic brew to which service members have been exposed on bases and other military facilities include the burned residue of animal carcasses, asbestos insulation, biohazard materials, cleaning supplies, dangerous chemicals, hydraulic fluids, pesticides, paint and paint strippers, lithium batteries, and human waste.[8]

Mental Health Problems

Veterans also suffer from complex mental and behavioral health problems that were either acquired in or exacerbated by military service. When the RAND Corporation conducted a four-year study of VHA mental health care, it reported: "Veterans with mental illness and substance use disorders represent a large and growing population with severe and complex disorders. Despite representing only 15 percent of the U.S. Department of Veterans Affairs' (VA's) patient population in 2007, veterans with these problems accounted for one-third of all VA medical costs."[9] In 2015 the VA reported that more than "1.6 million veterans received specialized mental health treatment from VA; this number has risen each year from over 900,000 in FY 2006. VA believes this increase is partly attributable to proactive screening to identify Veterans who may have symptoms of depression, Posttraumatic Stress Disorder (PTSD), problem use of alcohol or who have experienced military sexual trauma."[10]

Over 30 percent of male Vietnam veterans are estimated to suffer from PTSD, compared to 6.8 percent for all American adults. Between 18.5 and 42.5 percent of service members and veterans returning from the conflicts in Iraq and Afghanistan have some sort of mental health problem, with over 18 percent suffering from PTSD.[11] The problems from which these veterans suffer were eloquently chronicled in David Finkel's book *Thank You for Your Service*.[12]

Because of the coverage of PTSD, the public may erroneously believe that this is the major mental or behavioral health problem from which veterans suffer. In fact, not all veterans with mental health problems have PTSD, and for those who do, as Harold Kudler, chief VHA mental health consultant, puts it, PTSD "rarely travels alone." Many veterans may suffer from schizophrenia, bipolar disorder, major depressive disorder, personality disorders, or substance abuse disorders, among other problems. Veterans with PTSD can have any—or even many—of these problems. Thus, patients may have what is known as a dual diagnosis: PTSD and substance use disorders, or major depression and alcoholism.

Many veterans of the conflicts in Iraq and Afghanistan have also suffered from traumatic brain injuries, which add yet another dimension to their treatment.

Since the 1990s, clinicians and researchers have identified another kind of trauma-related mental health problem: military sexual trauma, the result of sexual assaults or harassment experienced while in the military.[13] Military sexual trauma is a risk factor for developing PTSD, as well as anxiety, depressive disorders, and alcohol and drug abuse. More female service members and veterans report military sexual trauma, but men are also victims of unwanted sexual attention or assault.

A 2008 study reported that "annual prevalence of sexual assault for women was 6.8 percent, and 1.8 percent for men. When it came to sexual coercion—promises of jobs, benefits [in exchange for sex] or threats of job loss . . . the prevalence was 9 percent for women and 3 percent of men, while unwanted sexual attention was experienced by 31 percent of women and 7 percent of men. Former reservists reported even higher numbers."[14] According to other studies, more than half of women who served in the military have experienced "offensive sexual behaviors such as repeatedly being told offensive sexual stories or jokes or unwelcome attempts to be drawn into a discussion of sexual matters." More than half of women in the military have experienced some form of sexual harassment. Because sexual assault, harassment, or offensive behaviors occur in settings in which people are taught to depend on others for their very lives, women who experience such trauma have special difficulty. They may feel "isolated," develop issues with trust, and have even greater difficulty adjusting to civilian life than their male counterparts.[15]

Anyone who suffers from severe trauma (whether physical, emotional, or sexual) or mental illness is also at a higher risk for committing suicide. Studies have documented that, whether because of trauma, mental illness, or other factors, compared to the rest of the American population, veterans have a higher suicide rate. This is particularly true for service members deployed in the recent conflicts in Iraq or Afghanistan. For those deployed in Operation Enduring Freedom or Operation Iraqi Freedom between 2001 and 2007, the rate of suicide was greatest during the first three years after leaving military service, according to a recent study.[16]

Suicide is increasing for white males over fifty years old, a fact that is also reflected in the veteran population, which, as we have said before, is older, sicker, and poorer than the average patient in private-sector health care. In the United States, suicide in general is on the increase. Suicide was the tenth leading cause of death in the United States in 2014. According to 2016 data from the Centers for Disease Control, after declining between 1986 and 1999, suicide rates began a steady increase between 1999 and 2014. Suicide rates jumped for both males and females of all ages in the general population. Although rates increased overall, they are higher for men over seventy-five.[17] In an article in the *New York Times*, experts speculated that divorce and economic downturns may contribute to suicides in the over-fifty age group.[18] Studies also note that more than half (55.4 percent) of men who kill themselves use some sort of firearm.[19]

Veteran suicide is part of this escalating trend. Mental health issues and social isolation, as well as economic deprivation, play a big part in the problem of veteran suicide. According to a major report released in 2016 by the VA, on average twenty (not twenty-two, the figure commonly cited) veterans kill themselves each day. Only six of the twenty are users of the VHA. The rest are not. Veterans account for 18 percent of all deaths by suicide among US adults, down from 20 percent in 2010. The risk of suicide is 21 percent higher among veterans than other Americans, 18 percent higher among male veterans, and 2.4 percent higher among female veterans. Middle-aged and older veterans are more likely to kill themselves—in 2014, 65 percent of vets who committed suicide were fifty or older—but there has been an increase in the rate of suicide among veterans between eighteen and twenty-nine. In 2014, 67 percent of all veteran suicides involved firearms.[20]

The Problem of Adjustment to Civilian Life

No matter what their motives for joining up, what branch they were in, or whether they saw combat, service members all went through military training, which could have made a significant impact on their developing brains. And military socialization could have made an equally serious impact on their adjustment to civilian life.

"We now understand that the brain is not fully developed until you are about twenty-five or twenty-six," Edgardo Padin-Rivera, former chief of psychological services at the Louise Stokes Cleveland VA Medical Center, explains. "The prefrontal cortex is the last thing to develop. Yet it is what controls many of our most important reactions and interactions with the outside world. It impacts empathy and impulse control and helps us develop a more nuanced view of the world.

"Kids who go to college don't only learn how to think about academic subjects," Padin-Rivera points out. "Higher education, as well as vocational training and civilian work, hopefully produces adults who interact in more nuanced ways with other people. When, on the other hand, we take young people and send them into military training and then perhaps to war, they learn more than how to use a weapon and defeat an enemy; they learn to cultivate very particular ideas about trust, intimacy, and vulnerability, as well as how to enter into and negotiate relationships."

All this is complicated by the fact that some recruits may come from families that face serious economic, social, or psychological challenges. "Many of today's volunteers may have histories of juvenile deprivation," says Karen Parko, a neurologist and epileptologist who directs the National VA Epilepsy Centers for Excellence. "Recruits often come from backgrounds in which there were family problems and few emotional or economic resources. Their families are in need themselves and have little or no ability to take on the additional problems that being in the military brings to their loved one. So when they develop problems as veterans, they don't have the support systems that give them the ability to deal with what we have thrust them into. If this kid went into the military because he had problems in the past, he needs help now from his family or community, and he may not get it."

Several years ago, I attended a lecture at San Francisco's Commonwealth Club, where three veterans described the process of trying to turn suffering into art. One of them was Ari Sonnenberg, an artist and then thirty-one-year-old Iraq and Afghanistan veteran who spent fourteen years in the service. Slight, still wearing his military-style buzz cut, his face etched with pain and his words a rapid-fire staccato blast, Sonnenberg expressed the dilemmas that Padin-Rivera says produce an existential crisis for so many veterans.

"I joined the military at seventeen and was raised by wolves, basically," he said. "I learned all my values, all my morals, all my skills—everything I needed to stay alive, I learned in fourteen years. And it kept me alive in all these combat tours. And it's funny because all those skills are now being told to me, they're all wrong. Here, in the civilian world, if you communicate loudly, you're being called aggressive. If you're always watchful and you're always making sure you're not sitting with your back to the door, you're being hypervigilant. Basically, my whole life now is being turned upside down, and I'm being told that you can't be in this world, it's all wrong."[21]

Padin-Rivera not only treats these problems, but, as a Vietnam veteran, he has grappled with them himself. He warns that private-sector providers "may misdiagnose the veteran's sense of doom, loss of meaning, and alienation from society with PTSD, or depression, or anxiety, or some other psychiatric disorder. We at the VHA, where dealing with veterans is our specialty, understand that, for many veterans, there may be five different things going on all at once."

What VHA caregivers recognize is that military socialization is life-changing in many different ways. "The whole military experience is sold as an opportunity for a life-changing transformation," says Joshua Jackson, a psychology professor at Washington University in Saint Louis and the lead investigator of a study of the impact of military training published in *Psychological Science*. "Recruiting materials of military forces around the world bolster the idea of military experience as being a catalyst for change. For example, recent slogans in the United States, such as 'Be all you can be,' 'Accelerate your life,' and 'Aim high,' all imply that military experiences affect life trajectories."[22]

In his study on military training and personality traits, Jackson found that military training did indeed have an impact on those who entered the service. Compared with those in his study of German military personnel, "military service was associated with lower levels of agreeableness than civilian community service.[23] It's one of the few situations in life where an individual's daily actions and expectations are completely controlled by someone else. Where, from the moment you wake up in the morning until you go to bed at night, someone is actively working to break down anything that's individual about you and to build up something else in its place."[24]

In more colorful language, Anthony Swofford, in his book *Jarhead: A Marine's Chronicle of the Gulf War and Other Battles*, described a lecture by his Marine drill instructor when he was at boot camp. "He yelled, addressing us all, 'I am your mommy and your daddy! I am your nightmare and your wet dream! I am your morning and your night! I will tell you when to piss and when to shit and how much food to eat and when! I will teach you how to kill and how to stay alive! I will forge you into part of the iron fist with which our great United States fights oppression and injustice! Do you understand me, recruits?"[25]

Jerome Serdinsky joined the Army at nineteen in 1999. He candidly explained that he volunteered because he was a troubled teenager from South Milwaukee who needed to get his life together. In the Army, Serdinsky did maintenance work, served in the Reserves, and in 2005 was deployed to Iraq.

"I wanted to serve," he says. "It was a privilege to go. That's why I joined the Army, to serve my country. This was the only way to make sense of all the training I had." It was also, he added, a way to help other people. "I genuinely thought I was in Iraq to help the people there."

As a young man, he learned many skills in the military but didn't master many others. "The food was put in front of me," he says. "I always wore the same clothes." And most important, he emphasizes, "I didn't need to think about me. When you're in the military, you don't have to think about me. People have your back. Your buddies are thinking about you. You don't have to think about yourself."

Members of the military are trained to repress their sense of individuality and adopt the kind of group identity that fosters the sense of mission and unit cohesion that Serdinsky and so many others describe.

A PowerPoint presentation on Military Culture 101, created by a program called Veterans Integration into Academic Leadership (VITAL) that is designed to help veterans succeed in higher education, notes: "Every enlisted service member goes through some sort of Basic Training, while officers go through ROTC (Reserve Officers' Training Corps) or Officer Basic Course. This is a stressful environment designed to tear a person down and then build them back up with values of camaraderie, team work, leadership, Loyalty, Duty, Respect, Selfless Service, Honor, Integrity, and Personal Courage."

Military training not only teaches self-sacrifice; it also trains service members to accept, as part of their normal duties, taking the lives of other human beings. In all the talk about service and sacrifice, it may be easy to forget that when you join the armed forces, "you are being trained to kill other people," says Padin-Rivera, who vividly remembers his initial indoctrination. "This goes against everything people have been taught in the civilian world. We've all heard the terms krauts, gooks, japs—these are terms you learn because the first thing you need to do to kill someone is dehumanize them."

Military training also encourages service members to deny their own needs, vulnerability, pain, and suffering. The US Army's Infantryman's Creed, which so many soldiers recite every day, is quite explicit about the connection between being a man, being a soldier, being hurt, and being weak.

I am the Infantry.
I am my country's strength in war,
her deterrent in peace.
I am the heart of the fight.
I am what my country expects me to be.
I yield not to weakness,
to hunger,
to cowardice,
to fatigue,
to superior odds,
for I am mentally tough, physically strong,
and morally straight.[26]

Asking for Help, and Moral Injury

In our highly individualistic society, one that values independence and self-help and has long viewed mental illness as shameful, it is difficult for many people to admit that they need help. The military magnifies broader cultural ideals, often creating a pernicious dichotomy: you are either a victim or a victor. This message, anthropologist Erin Finley, who works at the San Antonio VA Medical Center, writes in her book on PTSD *Fields of Combat*, "can run into direct conflict with the need to reach out for help when injured or unwell. . . . Men may find it difficult to identify with the idea of being traumatized (which can carry the implication of being a victim) or may, when they experience uncontrollable emotion, see it as a threat to their sense of themselves as invulnerable and tough."[27]

"In the military," Padin-Rivera elaborates, "you become hardened and learn to repress or deny vulnerability." With so little emotional flexibility, the only choice for many service members is to "push away feelings of pain, anxiety, depression, or questions about the morality of what you are doing and why you are fighting."

I have observed this pattern in my interviews with veterans over the last four years. Many veterans I talked with had, for years, even decades, tolerated sleeplessness, nightmares, and terror. They had lost jobs and marriages and had become alienated from their children, all because they could not, or would not, admit their problems and seek help. Way too many of them ended up going to the VHA after they were found with a gun in their mouths, or after, as they describe it, they had "hit rock bottom." As Finley documented, in spite of all the societal attention to PTSD and other mental illnesses, these men and women and their loved ones still viewed the very overt manifestations of their problems as symptoms not of mental illness but of bad behavior or a bad character.

The Anger Problem

If vulnerability is to be shunned at all cost, military culture promotes anger and aggression. Service members, Padin-River explains, "learn what we call a behavioral—not a negotiated—reaction." Whether they are in combat or not, service members learn to live in a state of high arousal. "Many of these men and women become very reactive, with hair-trigger responses, and may roll right from pain to anger." This is, of course, functional in warfare, where assuming the worst—that a garbage bag at the side of the road is an improvised explosive device, or a person walking on a highway overpass or looking out the window of a building near you is a sniper—can save your life.

Anger and aggression are also, Padin-Rivera continues, byproducts of "the constant beating soldiers take, getting shot at, losing friends. The tension and anger may stay with people when they leave the military. In high-stress situations, it may become hard to distinguish who is and who is not your true enemy, whom one is angry at."

As one Iraq veteran who worked in supply told me, "Eventually, you just get permanently pissed off. They're lobbing mortars at you all the time. You can't get a full night's sleep. You go to eat, and you can't eat because they've shot off a mortar round. You just get irritated. Can't I just fucking eat my dinner, please? Really?" And then, of course, your friends are getting killed, and you may be narrowly escaping death on a routine, daily basis. As VA psychiatrist Jonathan Shay noted in his 1994 book, *Achilles in Vietnam,* "For many veterans in our treatment program for combat post-traumatic stress disorder, replacement of grief by rage has lasted for years and become an entrenched way of being."[28]

All of this may be exacerbated if service members have experienced the kind of hazing that has made the news in a variety of military training programs. At the Marine Corps East Coast Training Depot at Parris Island, South Carolina, recruits were treated so brutally that one of them killed himself and others have suffered from PTSD and other chronic mental problems. Because of this, several staff sergeants have faced court-martial for, among other things, cruelty and maltreatment.[29]

The problem of anger and aggressiveness among both active-duty service members and veterans is a serious one that is receiving more systematic attention. One study, titled "Prevalence of Mental Health Problems and Functional Impairment among Active Component and National Guard Soldiers 3 and 12 Months following Combat in Iraq," published in 2010, surveyed 18,305 members of active component and National Guard soldiers.[30] The 13,226 surveys the investigators received back revealed that serious impairment from PTSD ranged from 8.5 to 14 percent, whereas milder impairment was between 23.2 and 31 percent. Of these soldiers who had returned from combat in Iraq and Afghanistan, half had problems with alcohol use and aggression. Sadly, problems with functioning in daily life and aggression increased over time.

Another study of service-related anger, conducted by researchers at the VA Puget Sound Health Care System in Seattle, Washington, found that, among Iraq and Afghanistan veterans, anger was "independent from, albeit related to, PTSD." Veterans who had been diagnosed with PTSD or had what is known as "subthreshold PTSD" reported increased levels of anger, hostility, and physical aggression, particularly in their intimate relationships. As evidenced by Vietnam War veterans, these problems may go on for decades.[31]

"You can turn off the stress response," Serdinsky told me in a recent conversation. "I can't. I am stuck there every minute of every day."

Living in this heightened state of aggression, anger, and arousal without an enemy on the battlefield may mean that one's target can quickly become friends, family, the civilian world in general, government, or anyone else in positions of authority. This response is part of what Shay termed "moral injury" in his two books, *Achilles in Vietnam* and *Odysseus in America*. As he studied veterans of the Vietnam War, Shay began to understand that members of the military were experiencing moral injury.[32] As he defines it, "Moral injury is present when (1) there has been a betrayal of what is morally correct; (2) by someone who holds legitimate authority; and (3) in a high-stakes situation." Shay also describes another critical byproduct of military culture and combat: "the persistence in civilian life of adaptations necessary to survive battle," which in turn leads to the "destruction of the capacity for social trust."[33] This applies particularly to trust in those in authority who have put soldiers in harm's way, but also to other civilians in positions of authority.[34] "The boss who hires and fires him, writes recommendations for him, raises or lowers his pay, and otherwise disposes of his destiny is nothing but a soft civilian. . . . While the veteran was risking his life for his country, the boss and the foreman were having an easy time of it."[35]

For a small subset of veterans, particularly those who suffer from mental illness or have problems with substance abuse, angry, aggressive behavior poses a danger not only to family and friends but to the caregivers who try to help them. Angry patients are, of course, a problem in the private sector as well, which is why nurses and other health care workers have often asked the institutions in which they work to implement programs to deal more effectively with violence in the workplace. In fact, many nursing organizations have fought for and won legislation to force health care institutions to act more vigorously to protect them from such danger.

The problem of violence in the veteran patient population can be more acute if the brew of anger and alienation that veterans experience—coupled with mental health or substance abuse problems—becomes toxic. Then veterans who have been trained to physically assault or even kill those they perceive to be enemies can become a serious threat to the people who care for them.

Anger and Alienation from the Civilian World and Even Other Veterans

In responding to their caregivers in the VHA and to the VA itself, veterans may be fueled by the sense that they now find the civilian world to be unfamiliar, if not alien or even hostile. Vietnam veterans did, in fact, come home to antiwar protesters who seemed to hold them in contempt. Today's veterans have instead come home to parades and "thank you for your service." Yet they may feel equally isolated, detached, and dismayed by a civilian world whose values they fought to uphold but whose behavior and ethics they may decry.

This kind of alienation may be a byproduct of the kind of military socialization that teaches service members to view themselves as more noble, self-sacrificing, loyal, and accountable than those whom they are defending. "Many people know what the words Loyalty, Duty, Respect, Selfless Service, Honor, Integrity, and Personal Courage mean," an Army recruitment campaign asserts. "But how often do you see someone actually live up to them? Soldiers learn these values in detail during Basic Combat Training (BCT), from then on they live them every day in everything they do—whether they're on the job or off. In short, the Seven Core Army Values listed below are what being a Soldier is all about."[36]

It is no wonder that so many veterans I have spoken with view the civilian world in black-and-white terms, attributing nobility and self-sacrifice to active-duty service members and veterans while condemning many civilians as selfish, rampant individualists. "Here, people only think about themselves. In the military there is always accountability. Where is the accountability here?" Where in the civilian world to which he has returned, this Iraq veteran asked me, are people willing to sacrifice for one another?

Disaffection with the VHA may result from veterans' feelings that those who care for them should somehow be members of the same culture, or at least familiar with the culture from which they just separated. One Vietnam War veteran I talked with said he despised the VA. Why? Because when he returned from the service and went to the VA, the clinician he saw didn't even know what a DD214 was. He may have relevant medical or psychological knowledge that could have served the soldier well, but he didn't know the relevant military jargon. When I probed further, the veteran said that, almost fifty years later, he doesn't like to tell people he was in Vietnam because he worries about their reaction. Without skipping a beat, he then told me that whenever he meets VA personnel today, he can't stand hearing "Thank you for your service." He said, "How phony is that?"

Alienation from the civilian world may also be fostered by veterans' conviction that civilians are hopelessly out of touch with the realities of human evil—with what, as they often say, life is really like. When he came back from Iraq, Serdinsky told me, it was with the knowledge that the world is a scary place. "You come home, and people don't understand that the world is dangerous and dark. I saw how horrible the world is, and I am alone in this knowledge." To make matters worse, "People are bitching about all this trivial shit, and you want to tell them, 'Hey, don't you realize it's a privilege to have a toilet or running water?'"

"This is a symptom of feeling different from other people," Padin-Rivera says. "You feel alienated and alone, so you find a reason for this sense of alienation. You look at the civilian world, and it starts with 'They don't understand what the world is really like.' And then it escalates to 'They're all for themselves, never for the team.' You've been taught to work for the team, not an individual. You are mission driven, and then you look at society, which is very individualistic, and you can't connect. When you hear veterans put down the civilian world, it all stems from the fact that the traumas they have experienced make them feel so apart from it all."

Sasha Best, a psychologist at the CBOC in Martinez, California, who works in cognitive rehabilitation with veterans who have PTSD as well as traumatic brain injury, is very familiar with this dilemma. As service members develop an intense sense of camaraderie, an almost tribal trust in one another, the byproduct is sometimes an intense distrust of the rules, etiquette, and even concerns of people living in the peacetime world they set out to defend. "One of the wonderful things about military service," she points out, "is the deep and powerful connections that are developed between members of the team. These are very powerful connections that many veterans find hard to replicate in the civilian world."

This complex dynamic of anger and alienation may not only result in a schism between the veteran and the civilian population. It can also create divisions between veterans—as well as active-duty service members. Many veterans who could successfully navigate the VBA's eligibility maze don't even try because they think that the VHA is for combat veterans only. And some don't want to be treated at the VHA because they are combat veterans and don't want to associate with vets who are not. After Vietnam, civilians have largely been socialized to consider that all those who served in the military have, in some way, sacrificed for their country, to view them as heroes and warriors. We have also come to recognize that veterans who have not actually been in combat may still have serious health problems.

The civilian population, ironically, may have more sympathy for these noncombat wounded warriors than many other veterans do. One Vietnam vet told me quite bluntly that he resisted seeking help for his mental and physical problems for decades because he didn't want to sit in a VHA waiting room next to a bunch of guys who had been to Nam but never fought there. "You go to the VA for an appointment, and there's a guy in the waiting room who has never been in combat, and he's telling war stories. Was this guy really in the shit? In a combat zone, only 15 percent of the guys may have really been in combat. The rest are in supply or logistics. The number of wannabes is incredible. These are the guys who were in the rear with the gear, and forty years later, they want to tell war stories, and that's a big turnoff to those of us who were actually in combat. I have friends who went into the VA for benefits and sat next to someone like that and got disgusted and won't go back to the VA. It's a big source of upset."

Younger veterans who have fought in Iraq and Afghanistan have echoed these comments. At the inpatient PTSD / mild TBI program in Martinez, California, I sat in on a session with seven young veterans. All were in their late twenties and early thirties and had served and suffered in either Iraq or Afghanistan or both. They were complaining about the civilian world and then turned their anger on another patient who was also suffering from severe PTSD. He had not left his room since he entered the program and had barely interacted with the other patients. Yet he had become an object of their scorn because he had not served in a direct combat role in the military.

How could he have PTSD or a brain injury or any other problem that would make him worthy of their sympathy? He had not gone through what they had gone through. Upon hearing this, their therapist, Jeff Kixmiller, who helped to found their program, immediately moved to action. Deeply empathetic to the plight of his patients, he told them in no uncertain terms that they could not rag on a fellow patient. This is a safe place for everyone, he told them, emphasizing that whether veterans or civilians, other human beings who have experienced terrible trauma—as had this other patient—are equally deserving of empathy and care.

"When veterans are in groups," Padin-Rivera explains, "they can really start nitpicking other people's experience. 'I had it worse than you did. You didn't really experience what I experienced. I was in the shit, you weren't. Or the shit I was in was worse than the shit you were in."

Veterans are, of course, not the only ones to engage in competitive martyrdom. As those who study the mysterious workings of the human brain have explained, we all tend to overestimate our own suffering while underestimating, or sometimes even denying, the suffering of others. In the process we create the kind of hierarchies of suffering that may exclude anyone—even those within our own particular band of brothers or sisters—who has not gone through precisely what we have.

"A very common symptom of traumatic stress disorder is that people who go through traumatic events feel both disassociated from themselves and other human beings," says Padin-Rivera. "You find this across the spectrum of traumatic events. People who have been raped or in airplane accidents or earthquakes are searching for someone who's been through similar traumatic events because they believe only people who have experienced the same thing can understand them."

One of the advantages of group therapy, VHA clinicians say, is flexibility. A group can be made up only of combat veterans. Or it can include patients who have had different military experiences but ended up with similar problems. "The job of the therapist," says Padin-Rivera, "is to really get in there and put a stop to people ragging on each other and help them have greater sympathy for other human beings."

Therapists also help veterans adjust to the more muted tones of the civilian world. "You've experienced an incredible level of connection and sense of purpose in the military, and then you come back to interactions in the civilian world that seem to pale in comparison," says Best. How, veterans ask, do you return to what seem to be workaday, banal, and sometimes even silly relationships with a wife or husband, with kids, other family, friends, or coworkers? "It's as though you've lived in color, and now you're coming back to black and white. It's our job to help them do that."

"They need to learn to stop," Padin-Rivera explains. "We have to help them to turn the thermostat from hot to cooler. People also have to learn to stop pushing people away. It is very difficult to teach people how to react when people push their buttons, how not to react like they did when they were soldiers but to have a more modulated approach."

What It Means to Be a VA Volunteer

It is seven forty-five on a morning in late October 2014, and Bill Avants stands at attention for two hours—maybe more—in the entryway to Building 200 at the VA's Fort Miley hospital complex in San Francisco. Avants, who is seventy-five, wears neat khaki slacks and a San Francisco Giants leather jacket and baseball cap. To everyone who walks through the double doors and into the facility, he offers a greeting and a smile. He does this day in and day out. Not because he has to or is paid to—Bill Avants is a volunteer at the VA.

When we talk in the quiet, glassed-in Emergency Department waiting room, adjacent to Avants's post at the building's entryway, the veteran volunteer tells me that he joined the military in 1957 and served until 1959. It was between the wars, so he never saw combat. When he left the military, he found it hard to get a job but eventually worked as an airline mechanic, got married, had three kids, and became an alcoholic. "It didn't come from the service, my alcoholism," he tells me. "I can't even explain why that came to be." Avants started going to AA meetings and sobered up.

Like so many veterans I have met, Avants came to the VA late in his life. He had medical coverage when he worked as an airline mechanic. When he turned sixty-five, he discovered he could get coverage at the VA. His belated decision to utilize the VA also enabled him to support other veterans. First he was in the escort service, and then he served coffee (which, he reminds me, is an AA symbol of sobriety). While volunteering, he noticed a lady who was greeting people as they came in the lobby. "I thought she was doing a marvelous job," he smiles broadly as he talks, "like she was doing something mystical or magical, making people smile and feel welcome. I wasn't sure if I could do that."

When she was no longer available as greeter, Avants decided to take a chance and apply to replace her. He got the job. He was given a short orientation, consisting, he says, mostly of what not to do. Don't give people medical advice. Don't feed people. Don't give people medications. There were, of course, a few dos, apart from smiling and greeting people, such as supplying a wheelchair for someone who needs it.

Avants says that both AA and his work as a volunteer help him to maintain a spiritual attitude toward life. Not religious, he adds, with emphasis. "I was never raised in religion," he says. "A lot of people were trying to get you to go to religion, but I never went for that."

Although he may not have a religious perspective on his work, he definitely sees its spiritual side, as he explains: "I stand here and say hello to you. And you say hello to me. We both get something out of that. You go on your way, and I stand here and say hello to someone else. When I say hello to two people, each one of them has one hello, but I have two. And at the end of the day, each person has one hello, but I have two hundred or three hundred. I don't know if it's selfish, but it sure helps my spirituality."

Avants recognizes how important the greetings are to his health. "If I stopped doing this, I know that the old self would come back again, and that's not pleasant," he says. "It's a twelve-step cliché that you must give it away to keep it. I'm seventy-five years old, and I've come to the realization that the old Bill was locked in for years. When I started looking at things and getting rid of things, Bill was there all along, like the sculpture of David by Michelangelo. David was in that big rock, and he just released it. I'm not an icon or a movie star, just Bill. The new Bill is out; if I stop, the old one will come back. The Bill I'm liking now was there all along. Hopefully, I won't lose my position."

Primary Care
the Way It Should Be

At twelve forty-five one afternoon in October 2016, Rebecca Shunk, a tall, blond primary care physician from South Carolina who speaks with a pronounced drawl, arrives at the medical practice clinic at Fort Miley in San Francisco. She takes off her Birkenstocks and changes into low-slung heels. Then she meets with some of the members of her Patient Aligned Care Team: Marilyn Oblanca, a petite nurse with long dark hair, and Bing Pablico, a short, stocky licensed vocational nurse (LVN) with long straight hair. All three spend the next fifteen minutes planning the rhythm of their day.

Oblanca informs Shunk about patients who have recently been discharged from the hospital and gives her suggestions for their home care needs. Pablico has already consulted with the clerks, who are stationed at a panel of desks in the large waiting room. She has information about which patients may show up on time and who will be late, as well as why some are coming to see their doctor today. One of Shunk's longtime patients called only a half hour earlier, complaining about a sore hand. Fortunately, a last-minute cancellation opened up the one-thirty slot.

The question is can he make it from Sebastopol, fifty-five miles across the Golden Gate Bridge to the north of San Francisco, on time?

"I can't tell him to go home if he's late and has rushed in. I want to see him," Shunk tells her colleagues, and they strategize about how staff and patients will be affected if Shunk is running late. Shunk wonders if she should call another patient whose appointment is at three. Because of the complicated problems of so many of her patients, Shunk knows she'll probably be running a half hour late. They all agree that the three o'clock appointment should be saved the wait, and Shunk picks up the phone to notify him of the delay.

Pablico then updates Shunk about their other patients. One veteran has asked to come in but refuses to say why. Another, who served on the ground in Vietnam, needs a comprehensive Agent Orange workup. Shunk wants to make sure he is on the Agent Orange registry. They discuss how this will impact not only his health but also the level of his VA compensation. After the meeting, Shunk is ready to begin seeing patients.

Shunk, who is now fifty, has worked at the VHA since 2001. She graduated from the Medical University of South Carolina, did two years of internal medicine training at the University of Chicago, and then finished up at Johns Hopkins Bayview, where she occupied the prestigious post of chief resident. She stayed at Johns Hopkins for four years, both practicing and teaching internal medicine. Her husband, who is an interventional cardiologist, was recruited by the University of California at San Francisco (UCSF). Rick Shunk was offered the choice of being cath lab director at USCF or at the VA. Rebecca could have worked in other academic institutions in San Francisco. Both Rebecca and Rick chose the VA.

"Other providers at the SFVA had nothing but good things to say about the system and the patients," she recalls. "I didn't know much about veterans, but I decided to take a risk."

From her very first week on the job, she says, she felt she had found her own medical home. "I never knew I had a mission or a calling until I spent one week with veterans. Then I found this was it." Shunk continues practicing internal medicine in the primary care clinic and, along with nurse-practitioner Anna Strewler, is codirector of one of the seven VHA Centers of Excellence in Primary Care Education.

What she loves about the VHA, Shunk says, is the model of team-based care she has been encouraged to practice, as well as the time she is given to really get to know her patients. Unlike private-sector care providers, whose patient load can exceed twenty-four hundred, the average patient load for full-time providers at the VA is twelve hundred. As a result, she doesn't have to rush through her appointments. Shunk's routine visits are at least thirty minutes long.

Which is how long she spends with her first patient of the day, Alfred Marsden.* A small African American veteran in his mid-seventies, Marsden has raced to make it on time and is a few minutes late. He wears a bright red US Marine Corps baseball cap. As he sits down and catches his breath, he apologizes for being late. Shunk tells him not to worry, that she's just happy to see him.

He says that he has been having pain radiating from his neck that has been keeping him up at night. He has also been having some trouble with one of his hearing aids. Shunk immediately calls down to audiology to make sure they can see him after he is finished with their appointment.

One of many patients who combine VHA with other health plans, Marsden says that he has gone to Kaiser to get acupuncture treatments, which have helped his neck, and has used some capsaicin for the pain. Shunk suggests over-the-counter Tylenol and the prescription medication Gabapentin, which, she explains, can change the way the body senses pain. Would he be willing to try those? she asks, simultaneously warning him away from ibuprofen, which can harm his kidneys. She also wants to make sure the VHA pays for all these meds, even the over-the-counter ones. She then demonstrates some neck stretches he should do three or four times a day and suggests physical therapy. She asks if he would prefer to see a physical therapist at the VHA or Kaiser.

He doesn't hesitate. "Frankly," he confides, "I would rather do it here. I have more confidence in people here. The doctors don't seem the same to me at Kaiser. They don't really care there. It's not like you get the same individual attention."

Shunk beams and thanks him. "We really appreciate it that you like the VA," she says.

As has been recommended by the Institute of Medicine's report on enhancing patient safety, Shunk then inquires about his inhalers, carefully going over the function and proper use of the three she has prescribed.[1] Again following best patient-safety practices, she asks him to explain to her how he will take them so she can be sure he has actually heard and understood what she has said. They conclude with a plan for a phone follow-up visit, and she reminds him that he needs to go down to audiology while he is at the facility to check out his hearing aids and then to the pharmacy to get the medicine she is entering into the computer.

Shunk's next patient is the veteran from Sebastopol, Mr. Silver,* who made the fifty-five-mile trip on Highway 101 by, he admits, some creative driving. As with so many of her patients, Shunk has a long history with Silver. Ten years ago, when he first came to see her, he was wracked by PTSD—not from combat but from horrendous childhood abuse. He spent most days drinking himself into a stupor. Now he is clean and sober, has full-time work in construction, and shares the care of a daughter he had abandoned for years. He goes to AA meetings every day and is the sponsor for four AA members, whom he shepherds through the kind of one-day-at-a-time journey he has made.

He and Shunk begin their visit by catching up on their respective children. And then Silver offers her his hand. She palpates the palm and looks at the area he describes as red, throbbing, and sometimes warm. She turns his hand over and scrutinizes his knuckles, which are gnarled by overuse.

"What makes the pain worse?" she asks.

"Work." Particularly, Silver says, when he's scrubbing his tools.

"What makes it better?"

"Rest."

Shunk points out that her patient definitely has osteoarthritis. What she worries about is the onset of rheumatoid arthritis. She orders X-rays and blood work to ferret out any signs of an inflammatory process. She also looks at the patient's chart in the electronic medical record, which has tracked his aches and pains, PTSD, and substance abuse history, among many other things, ever since he came to the VHA so many years ago. She wants to review previous X-rays and other relevant information.

After Shunk and Silver consider how to proceed, Shunk leaves the room to consult with the pharmacist, who has an office in the primary care clinic. I ask Silver about his experiences with the VHA.

"From my point of view, the VA is awesome," he says. "These guys are awesome," he repeats. He compares his treatment at the VA with what he received in the private sector. "I've gone to Petaluma Valley Hospital when I had a broken rib," he says. "I was lying on the table, and this doctor came in and saw me trying to get up and just stood there. He didn't even try to help. I was there waiting four and a half hours, and the doctor came in, and I saw him for, what, maybe fifteen minutes, and it was fifteen hundred bucks. I called today at 12:36, and they said 'Come right in,' and here I am."

The Crisis of Primary Care in the United States

It is by now a commonplace that primary care should be the centerpiece of any efficient, affordable, and productive health care system. If a health care system has an effective primary care system, costs are lower, quality indicators are higher, and there are fewer unnecessary treatments, tests, and procedures and far fewer visits to the emergency room and even hospitalizations. According to primary care guru Barbara Starfield, the four pillars of a good primary care practice are "first contact care, continuity of care over time, comprehensiveness, or concern for the entire patient rather than one organ system, and coordination with other parts of the health care system."[2] These pillars are embedded in the current concept of the patient-centered medical home, which has been promoted by organizations like the American Academy of Physicians.

The patient-centered medical home is "accountable for meeting the large majority of each patient's physical and mental health care needs, including prevention and wellness, acute care, and chronic care," according to the Agency for Health Care Research and Quality. "Providing comprehensive care requires a team of care providers. This team might include physicians, advanced practice nurses, physician assistants, nurses, pharmacists, nutritionists, social workers, educators, and care coordinators."[3]

Although there is a lot of discussion on the need for patient-centered medical homes and an efficient primary care system, America has, for decades, been plagued by a primary care provider shortage that has made this more of a dream than a reality. Between 1997 and 2005, the number of US medical school graduates choosing primary care dropped by 50 percent.[4] (The growth of physician assistants and nurse-practitioners as primary care providers is a direct result of this crisis, with both promoted as potential solutions to the primary care crisis.)

Some estimates suggest that today, only 15 percent of medical students are choosing primary care. In an article titled "First Teach No Harm,"

Phillip Longman dissects the alarming facts. America's teaching hospitals receive over $13 billion in federal subsidies, but "of the 759 institutions sponsoring residency programs, 158 produced no primary graduates at all. Overall, only a quarter of all residents go into primary care, and far fewer than that go to work where they are needed." What is worse is the fact that institutions that receive the most federal largesse—Massachusetts General Hospital, with $85 million in taxpayer subsidies, or the Johns Hopkins University School of Medicine—produce the fewest primary care physicians.[5]

Studies are also documenting that more and more nurse-practitioners and physician assistants are choosing to work in specialist practices rather than in primary care because the pay is better and the demands fewer. The result of this is that there are simply not enough primary care physicians—or physician assistants and nurse-practitioners—to accommodate the number of Americans who need a primary care provider. In 2016 the American Association of Medical Colleges reported that "under every combination of scenarios modeled, the United States will face a shortage of physicians over the next decade. The projections show a shortage ranging between 61,700 and 94,700, with a significant shortage showing among many surgical specialties. . . . By 2025, the study estimates a shortfall of between 14,900 and 35,600 primary care physicians. Non-primary care specialties are expected to experience a shortfall of between 37,400 and 60,300 physicians."[6] One of the reasons the VHA has so much trouble finding primary care physicians is that it depends on the larger American medical educational system. That system is simply not doing its job.

Experts like Thomas Bodenheimer and Kevin Grumbach suggest that there are numerous solutions to the problems that plague primary care. These include congressional efforts to not only allot more residency slots but to assure that they are adequately redistributed between primary and specialty care and penalize medical programs that do not produce enough primary care physicians.[7] Other solutions include paying primary doctors more and specialists less; relieving school debt for doctors, nurses, and physician assistants; lightening the burden of paperwork and data entry that primary care providers carry; and reducing the number of patients that primary care providers have from their current load to a more manageable load of eleven or twelve hundred. Critical also is the model of team-based care, which would include a registered nurse, social worker, pharmacist, and behaviorist, as well as nonclinical staff who "agree on ground rules that establish a respectful culture, perform daily huddles, and write standing orders empowering non-clinician staff to share the care."[8]

Experts also suggest health coaching, particularly of chronically ill patients, as well as what they call complex care management, where social workers or registered nurses lead teams of other clinicians and staff. Others have also recommended using telehealth to deal with shortages in rural areas.

The VHA has been implementing each of these recommendations throughout the entire system and has produced a primary health care system that is extremely attractive to many of the clinicians who work in it and those who are exposed to the model during their years as students, interns, or residents. The VHA employs about ninety-three thousand nursing personnel, which includes registered nurses and licensed vocational nurses. At the VHA, nurse-practitioners can practice without physician supervision. Because the VHA is a federal health care system, its rules supersede those of any state in which a facility is located.

Primary care providers at the VHA are not subject to what Bodenheimer and Grumbach term the "tyranny of the 15-minute visit."[9] This is a result of the fact that VHA primary care providers have the recommended twelve to thirteen hundred patients—not twice or three times as many. This allows a routine primary care visit of thirty—not ten or fifteen—minutes.

VHA primary care providers are thus able to manage the many acute and chronic health care conditions of their population, which are far more complex than those in most private-sector primary care practices. As one young nurse-practitioner told me, "One of my veterans is the equivalent of four patients in private-sector health care."

Those who practice primary care in the VHA are able to implement what is known as "population management"—managing not only individual patients but a population of patients with specific problems. They learn how to diagnose and treat the problems not just of individual patients but of the specific veteran population they serve.

Perhaps most important, the VHA has implemented the precise model of team-based care that experts like Starfield, Bodenheimer, and Grumbach recommend.

Teamwork and the Huddle

Mr. Silver told me that he had benefited from the VA's—and Shunk's—dedication to a model of primary care different from the one practiced in the private sector. As we saw when Shunk started her day, before seeing patients, physicians at the VA meet with nurses, unit clerks, and nurse-practitioners, as well as residents and other professional trainees, so they can all plan their day together. This daily routine is known as the huddle.

A huddle is a "structured brief (five to fifteen minutes) routine (i.e., daily or multiple times a day) face-to-face communication of a team's full members." Content covered during huddles typically includes pre-visit planning for scheduled patients, strategizing care plans for patients with special or complex needs, addressing work-flow and communication issues through collective problem solving, and ensuring awareness of what team members do and what actions are happening among the team and in practice.[10]

"The huddle is a commonly used tool in patient-centered medical homes," says Shunk. "However, huddles may not realize their full potential because they are not given enough time and intellectual attention. At the San Francisco VA, we realized that to fully utilize what the huddle has to offer, we would need to rigorously and systematically train learners and staff to participate in the huddle, study its value, and research its effectiveness. We set up structural interventions, which include designated space and scheduled time for huddles. We instituted process interventions, like making sure there are expert coaches for the huddles, as well as a checklist to make sure all tasks are accomplished, and that all participants participate. The final thing we did was develop relational interventions. Twice a year, we have team retreats to support relationship building and communication."

Shunk tells a story that illustrates how the huddle has improved the medical practice at the San Francisco VA. A Filipina clerk had worked in the clinic for a long time. Before the huddle, Shunk now says shamefacedly, she did not even know the woman's name—Maria Famy-Abadilla. One morning during a huddle, Shunk suggested canceling the appointment of a patient who was scheduled to come in that day. Famy-Abadilla, who would never have thought of challenging a physician prior to her training in the huddle, interrupted Shunk and told her that this was not a good idea.

"She told me," Shunk says, "that she had to make three different phone calls to arrange for a visit and that scheduling the appointment I was about to cancel required extensive cajoling. She added, 'Do you remember he has trust issues? I am not sure he will ever come back if we cancel this appointment.'" Shunk immediately acquiesced and saw the patient.

"I've never been all that hierarchical," Shunk says, "but I was never trained to appreciate the value of all the team members and the critical nature of their role. I didn't purposefully ignore people or dismiss them because I thought I was better than they were. I was oblivious to their critical role in patient care. Now I recognize that they are an integral part of safe care delivery."

As Shunk's anecdote about Famy-Abadilla demonstrates, one of the most important functions of the huddle is to encourage nonphysician staff to speak up to doctors and help them learn to listen. To make sure this happens, huddles are routinely led by nonphysician team members like clerks or LVNs. And the checklist ensures that everyone attends the huddle, that it is appropriately led, and that everyone has a seat at the table rather than the periphery.

Another critical aspect of the huddle is the fact that it incorporates intensive coaching. Huddle coaches who may be nonphysicians make sure that everyone in the room speaks up and that those higher up on the health care ladder do not dominate or intimidate.

As Rina Shah, deputy chief of staff at the San Francisco VA, candidly acknowledges, "Physicians aren't trained to do huddles." The huddle, she says, teaches physicians what a registered nurse or LVN or clerk can bring to the table. Learning how to work on teams through vehicles like huddles, she says, has transformed her practice.

"If you ask me what my life was like five years ago," she pauses, reflecting on the stress she put herself through, "I think I thought I had to do all of it and constantly make sure I didn't miss anything. But here, I realize there's something the nurse brings, the LVN, the clerk. It's a place where everyone works together."

LVN Donna Soriano told me she was initially reluctant to participate in huddles. "When I heard about this, I thought, this is not going to work. It's going to take too much time and won't change anything. I'm sure not going to do it," Soriana recalls. "Now," she says, laughing at her former resistance, "I do it every day." She says it has entirely changed her relationship to her work and those she works with. "Oh my God, when I first started here," she says, "I wouldn't even talk, and then I started talking one day, and I haven't stopped."[11]

Oblanca feels that the huddle has increased not only her ability to better care for her patients and establish trust with them but to get to know her team on a personal level as well. "We feel like, 'I belong to them, and they belong to us,'" she says.

Lead medical support assistant Antonio Spann, an African American veteran who was in the Army from 1988 to 1995, where he participated in Desert Storm, echoes these sentiments: "I feel great about huddles. It gives everybody a voice, everyone the opportunity to voice a complaint or concern—no matter how big or small. The group considers it and then acts on it or doesn't."

For medical residents like Thomas Cascino, the huddle training "breaks down the traditional medical hierarchies" and teaches doctors "to listen to other members of the team."

Patient-Aligned Care Teams

The huddle did not come out of nowhere. It is part of a comprehensive approach to teamwork that the VHA has implemented nationwide as part of its Patient-Aligned Care Team (PACT) model, which was established in 2010. Gordon Schectman, the chief consultant for primary care at the national VA central office, who has worked at the VHA since 1984, says the PACT model has revolutionized the way the VHA delivers care.

"When I first began working at the VHA, veterans didn't expect much from VA health care," he says. "Yes, they expected their doctors to be knowledgeable and have expertise in their field. But as for timely care, coordination of care, having enough nurses who were also helpful—that was not an expectation. In 1984, when I began working in the ER, we had a huge sign, like maybe four by eight feet, saying, 'If you have not been called or seen in more than six hours, please see the nurse at the nurses' station.'"

Back then, veterans would come for an appointment with a book because they knew they would have to wait a very long time to be seen. All of this, he says, has changed, beginning with the profound improvements that former VHA undersecretary for health Kenneth Kizer instituted in the 1990s and continuing today.

The integration of teamwork into the primary care setting has been one of the most significant improvements over the last decade. In 2010, Schectman explains, it was becoming clearer and clearer that veterans—especially aging ones—had increasingly complex problems that, if they could be managed at all, could not be managed with a single provider. Veterans needed more comprehensive care and greater continuity of care, which meant that staff needed to work together more effectively. "We needed larger, better-informed, and better-equipped teams who were able to more effectively coordinate resources," says Schectman.

The model of what is called a "patient-centered medical home" was being implemented in a number of private-sector systems, and a group of VHA providers and leaders explored how the model functioned and adapted it to the VHA.

In April 2010 the VHA's PACT model was rolled out nationally at a meeting in Las Vegas, attended by more than four thousand health care workers. "These included national leaders, regional and local leaders from every facility, and," Schectman pauses for emphasis, "we made a point to also include frontline providers, not just physicians or [nurse-practitioners], but everyone who would work on a PACT team, from the pharmacist to the unit clerk."

Once the idea was introduced, the challenge was to initiate the kind of culture change that would help staff work together, even though they had been trained in the silo system of health care, where different professions and occupations function in their own little fortresses. In typical VHA fashion, a national training program was launched to accomplish this mission.

This effort was supported with adequate funding by then undersecretary for health Robert Petzel. The VHA then developed a curriculum to teach PACT and launched a national training program to educate staff at every level about how to function as a team.

"We trained twenty-five to thirty trainers and took the show on the road from site to site," Schectman recounts. "Training was mandatory for all staff. For the first two years, every facility had training teams, and staff attended three-day trainings for the first two years. We also created learning Centers of Excellence around PACT." Because one of the VHA's fundamental missions is teaching, these Centers of Excellence would teach the team-based model.

There are now seven Centers of Excellence in primary care education, and they are located in Boise, Cleveland, Houston, San Francisco, Seattle, West Los Angeles, and West Haven, Connecticut. At these Centers of Excellence, rather than having residents who would come to a random half-day primary care clinic now and again, the new requirement was that residents spend 30 percent of their total training time in a medical home. Another requirement was that these Centers of Excellence use a practice partnership model in which doctors and nurse-practitioners work side by side—not in a superior–subordinate relationship but as equal colleagues.

Within these and other guidelines, the centers are given flexibility to shape their own curriculum. Rebecca Brienza, an internist at the West Haven VA, and Shunk at Fort Miley became leaders in the effort to integrate team-based training into graduate medical and nursing education. As Brienza recounts it, when the VA rolled out its PACTs in the patient-centered medical home, she and other faculty wondered just how they could incorporate medical trainees into the model. "Trainees were outside of the PACT. How could we integrate them into the PACT in a meaningful way? This involved turning the traditional training model upside down."

In West Haven, Brienza paired medical residents with nurse-practitioner residents, a model that did not exist outside the VA at the time it was introduced. West Haven was also the first setting to start a nurse-practitioner residency program within the VA where recent graduates would train for an extra year in the ambulatory setting alongside medical residents. This pairing of nurse-practitioner and doctor trainees, Brienza argues, is one of the most successful parts of the model.

More Than TeamSTEPPS

The VHA has a much more serious commitment to teaching teamwork at every level in the health care hierarchy than medical facilities in the private sector. Although it is now recognized that failures in teamwork and communication result in the majority of preventable patient deaths and injuries, only about one-sixth of America's six-thousand-plus hospitals have staff trained in a program called Strategies and Tools to Enhance

Performance and Patient Safety (TeamSTEPPS), which was developed by the Department of Defense and the Agency for Healthcare Research and Quality to enhance patient safety and workplace communication. Even those hospitals that teach TeamSTEPPS tend to do so in a perfunctory manner. The two-and-a-half-day training may be reduced to two hours, with no plan for follow-up or team coaching. Most TeamSTEPPS training, moreover, focuses on emergency or crisis situations rather than on routine communication.

One nurse whose hospital sent her to TeamSTEPPS told me that even two hours was considered to be too much for her hospital's executives, who asked her to try to teach complex teamwork skills to her nursing colleagues at the bedside when they were caring for patients. This was called "just-in-time teaching."

At another major California hospital, a patient safety physician told me the hospital had done a two-hour TeamSTEPPS training. It never repeated the training because (surprise, surprise) a year later, no patient outcomes had changed as a result. By contrast, as Shunk explains, in her primary care clinic alone, twenty people, including key nursing staff, a chief resident, psychologists, nurse-practitioners, and physicians, were sent to their first TeamSTEPPS training, which was followed by a two-and-a-half-day, hands-on, nuts-and-bolts team training delivered by the VHA.

The Boston VA Medical Center has also initiated a program that encourages better teamwork and helps lay the groundwork for working on health care teams. Although this program is not centered in the ambulatory environment, Cecelia McVey, the chief of nursing and patient care services in the Boston VA, created the program with chief of medicine Michael Charness to counter the traditional training of physicians and nurses and other health care professionals, which usually occurs in their own professional silos. They created a program called "The Other Side of the Bed," in which Boston University School of Medicine students are paid twenty dollars an hour to participate in a seven-week course in which they do eight-hour shifts with nurses.

Students choose a nurse who will serve as their mentor in a variety of nursing settings, from a medical surgical ward to the intensive care unit. After four days of intensive orientation, they learn nursing skills, and they learn to understand the nurses themselves, about whom they learn little in their training. A clean-cut, fast-talking med student said he had a much better sense right now of what nurses do than what doctors do. Twenty-six-year-old Brenna Hogue said that she knew in theory that nurses were skilled and knowledgeable, but she didn't know to what extent. She said it was "awesome" to be learning best practices from nurses. She also said she was "shocked" that doctors don't do much hands-on patient care. "My perspective has changed about what doctors do."

Another critical initiative that is impacting primary care at the VHA is the effort to implement a nationwide model of what is known as "whole health care," which links poor health and quality of life (and chronic conditions like cancer, diabetes, chronic pain, obesity, and heart disease) to mental and behavioral health conditions and to environmental issues, social and economic issues, and changes in lifestyle and self-care. The VHA has created a new office of Patient Centered Care and Cultural Transformation, directed by physician Tracy W. Gaudet. At medical centers like Fort Miley it comprises, among many other things, health coaching with peers, health planning in primary care, teaching mind-body skills like yoga, meditation, and tai chi, and researching the impact of mind-body wellness interventions on both patients and staff.[12]

The Warm Handoff

A central part of the VHA's teamwork model is something that one rarely finds outside the system—the warm handoff. When a primary care provider has a patient who has to see a specialist or a social worker or a psychologist or a dietitian, for instance, the provider doesn't simply enter a referral for such an appointment into a computerized medical record and tell the patient to be sure to follow up. Instead, the provider walks these patients down the hall or around the corner to introduce them to the appropriate colleague. This is very doable in the VHA because everybody practices together in the same facility.

A research study by VA internist Karen Seal and her colleagues examined the effectiveness of different modes of transferring information about, and responsibility for, a patient from one clinician to another. The most frequent handoff is through notes in a chart. In an electronic handoff, one provider enters an order on the computer for a referral to another clinician, and information about the patient is transferred via the electronic record. The electronic handoff, like an e-mail or text, is often truncated and lacking in any human interaction, and it does not permit on-the-spot collaborative communication, clarification, or problem solving.

Another way information and responsibility are exchanged is through a provider-to-provider handoff through telephone conversation, or what is known as curbside consultation. I have watched many of these so-called conversations, and they tend to be characterized by their brevity, impatience, and lack of rigor. These handoffs often involve one provider talking brusquely to another as they pass in a corridor. After spending decades watching these curbsides in various hospitals, I have come to think of them as one person talking to the fleeing back of another. Needless to say, neither of these handoff mechanisms ever includes the patient, and they don't serve to reinforce team communication or tighter team relationships.

What Seal and her colleagues refer to as "collaborative handoffs," or warm handoffs, occur when a provider notes a problem that requires consulting and input with another clinician. The provider then asks the patient if he or she would agree to talk with another clinician, and if the patient consents, the provider walks the patient to meet this clinician, and the three discuss what is to be the next step. There are, of course, limitations to this kind of exchange—providers aren't always available to meet with patients, clinicians may be wary of sharing concerns in front of the patient—but this method is far and away the most patient centered.

"The patient is an active participant in the care transfer," Seal and her coauthors write. "She or he has the opportunity to help shape what clinical and social information is discussed." And it helps create what they call "a multidisciplinary therapeutic alliance."[13]

The warm handoff doesn't just encourage a new kind of communication among providers. It is also central to making sure that patients get the care they need. It helps patients overcome the stigma of getting help for mental health issues, for instance. And it eases the reluctance of some patients to talk to a pharmacist about problems with medication or a nutritionist about losing weight or doing more exercise. And the warm handoff helps solve the vexing problem of patients who won't follow through on making an appointment with another clinician or showing up for an appointment they have already made.

Getting to Wellness

When I watched patients interact with pharmacist Shirley Chao after a warm handoff from a psychiatric nurse-practitioner, I saw the teamwork model in action. Chao has worked at the VHA for ten years and is embedded in the Fort Miley medical practice. Her office is a sixty-second walk from the primary care providers with whom she partners. Chao's patients may be referred by a primary care physician but can also call about questions or ask to see the pharmacist themselves. Because her patients are so complex, she says, they need a lot more attention than the patients she dealt with as a resident at California Pacific Medical Center, a large private-sector hospital in San Francisco.

"What we do is help patients understand how to take their medicine correctly," Chao says as we sit in her small office near the clinic entrance. "They can come out of the primary care physician's office thinking they should take their meds all at once with food, when in fact some need to be taken in the morning or without food."

Chao also does what she calls "brown-bag" teaching. "Patients come in with a brown bag full of medicines," Chao explains. "They may be seeing a doctor from Kaiser or someone else in the private sector because they have Medicare. As a result, they have confusing medication lists and don't understand what to take, or the medication side effects or potential interactions, or even what medications may have been discontinued. We need to go over all this very carefully and make sure all this is being well coordinated. We also help them organize their medi-sets so they can remember to take their medications."

This attention helps not only the patients, but the doctors and nurses, too. "We get a list of all the patient's allergies," Chao says, "a list of all prescription medication, all over-the-counter medication, even vitamins or supplements the patient is taking. Then we compare this to the list on our formulary. All of this is very time-consuming and takes a burden off the provider—which is why we get such positive feedback from providers about our work."

Each appointment I observed with Chao and her patients took about forty-five minutes to an hour. Two of her patients were diabetics with whom she has worked for years. She knows their history, when their blood sugars zoom up and when they dip down, when they take their meds, when they forget, how often they stick their fingers to check their blood sugar, what they understand about their conditions and medication regimens, and what they don't.

One of her patients is Mr. Kennedy,* a fifty-seven-year-old veteran who works two menial jobs to make ends meet. Chao knows he is the primary caregiver for his sick wife, and she recognizes that when Kennedy's wife takes a turn for the worse, he can't sleep well and is perpetually agitated. As he relates the story of his wife's latest hospitalization, Chao nods sympathetically, and the two strategize about how he can better control his illness and food intake. Kennedy confesses to eating too many meals from KFC, whose mashed potatoes, gravy, and biscuits he loves but which send his sugars off the charts. With Chao's help his weight has gone down in the past, so she gently encourages him to try to avoid these sugar-bending episodes and do more exercise than walking up two flights of stairs at work twice a day, which she explains patiently is not a substitute for the more vigorous walking he has done in the past.

Outside the VA, diabetics like Kennedy are not generally cared for by teams, but rather by different specialists who rarely coordinate their care. Because of this, a diabetic patient may not be effectively coached to take his insulin correctly, monitor blood sugar levels, get necessary foot or eye exams, or make sure he adjusts his diet and gets enough exercise. It is no wonder studies show that the diabetics treated by the VA do far better on many critical measures than those using private insurance or Medicare.[14]

Chao spends hours with patients like this every day and often works in conjunction with Gary Yee, the PACT dietitian whose office is just outside the entrance to the medical practice clinic. Yee, a Chinese American who just turned forty, has worked for the VHA for seventeen years. He is a trim man in a blue plaid shirt, his cropped black hair fashionably swept up into a miniature Mohawk at his forehead. Yee tells me he learned—or learned to be oblivious—about food while working in his family's Chinese restaurant as a teenager. "I would watch the cooks ladle in at least a quarter cup of oil into the wok for every dish," he says. "I never realized that that was four hundred calories or more. Now I advise people that if they get Chinese takeout, they should eat from the top and leave the oil at the bottom."

Yee greatly values the warm handoff model. He says it is critical to getting patients into his office and the series of programs available to help veterans adjust their diet and exercise. Not only in the VHA but nationally, getting people to come to appointments with dietitians and nutritionists is notoriously difficult. "There's about a 20 percent no-show rate for appointments everywhere," says Yee. So if you can bring the patient to the dietitian, that at least yields better results. Once Yee and his colleagues have veterans in their offices, they identify what the patients want to work on, what is problematic about their current diet, and what reasonable changes can be made.

What he tries to do is get people to understand the concept of calories and think more judiciously about their eating habits. The patients who come to him because they are overweight or have type 2 diabetes or hypertension or high cholesterol are often unaware that even healthy oils like olive oil have one hundred calories per tablespoon. Some who focus on weight loss try to get patients to fill out food logs. Yee does not consider that to be an effective weight-loss strategy.

What he does is ask his patients to take pictures of their food. "I had a patient who lived in a very small apartment, and he came in with fifteen pictures of food that he took in just one day," Yee says. "That was very revealing. It showed the patient how often he mindlessly went into the kitchen and just grabbed something to eat, even though he wasn't particularly hungry. So we strategized about how he could get out of the house more, and he decided that rather than read the paper in his house, he would go to the library to read."

Because many people have a cell phone that takes pictures, it's easy for patients to take pictures of what they're eating, and this provides a vivid record—and a concrete way for them to chart their progress. "If they go from fifteen to ten pictures a day, that's real progress," Yee says. "What we want is for people to make little changes. Eating in a more healthy manner doesn't require people to turn their diets upside down."

Yee and his colleagues also encourage patients to join the national VHA MOVE! strength and wellness program, where veterans work with a dietitian, recreation therapist, and behavioral psychologist in group classes that meet weekly at the VHA. In these classes they learn about healthy exercise and eating habits. Then they spend several more hours a week working with a recreational therapist at the YMCA, which partners with the VHA to help veterans exercise.

Another resource available to clinicians and patients is a program the VHA has created with a private not-for-profit, Cooking Matters.

This award-winning program helps veterans learn not only how to cook but how to shop and prepare healthy food. In partnership with the organization called 18 Reasons: Empowering Your Discovery of Good Food,[15] the VHA provides a chef for cooking classes, offers space in its auditorium for weekly cooking demonstrations and education in healthy eating, and encourages referrals of veterans to the program.

At each class that I attended at Fort Miley, veterans who had never cooked a healthy meal or even read a food label were taught how to make two or three healthy dishes. They were guided through the process of food safety and food preparation skills and then given a bag of groceries so they could replicate the process in their own kitchens. In the fifth week of the six-week course, veterans don't cook. Instead, they are taken on a shopping expedition to the local grocery store. They are given $10 to buy three main meal components—meat or protein, grain, and fruits and vegetables. They are also given help reading labels on food so they can figure out what is really healthy, regardless of whether the food is hyped as natural or healthy.

Watching patients talking to a dietitian embedded in their facility about how to adjust their diet or exercise reminded me of a close friend who was morbidly obese. She was seeing a primary care provider who was very worried about her weight and wanted her to see a nutritionist, but none worked in her primary care practice (the very idea of having a nutritionist, pharmacist, social worker, or mental health provider in this large, stand-alone primary care office was unheard of). To find a nutritionist, the primary care provider had to search the Web to ferret out someone who would accept my friend's insurance. Although seeing a nutritionist could have helped save my friend's life, her insurance company would pay only for part of the fee (although it would pay a great deal more if my friend had to amputate her foot because of out-of-control type 2 diabetes). As it turned out, insurance didn't have to pay for any resulting hospitalization because, several years later, my friend dropped dead of a heart attack while she was unpacking a grocery bag stuffed with processed food and pastries.

Motivational Interviewing

Meetings with primary care providers, nutritionists, and other clinicians don't guarantee that veterans like the ones Chao counsels lose weight or take their medications as prescribed. To try to help both clinicians and patients attain their goals, the VHA has launched a national effort to teach clinicians what is known as motivational interviewing (MI).

William R. Miller and Stephen Rollnick, clinical psychologists who originally worked with people who had problems with alcohol, developed the motivational interviewing model.[16] Miller and Rollnick realized that traditional approaches to behavioral change were not working. Clinicians were often very judgmental with their patients. Adopting a confrontational and adversarial stance, they would flood patients with information about the negative consequences of their behavior and then tell them to stop drinking. The patient was then expected to comply with this advice or be viewed as either "difficult," "in denial," or "noncompliant."

To counter this traditional definition of clinical expertise, Miller and Rollnick developed a model to engage their patients' "intrinsic motivations." Rather than talking at the patients, they tried to listen to them and find out why they were drinking, why they might consider making a change, and what that change might look like.

Jennifer Manuel is a clinical psychologist at the San Francisco VA Medical Center who trained with Miller and has played an integral role in the VA's motivational interview initiative. "Ambivalence about one's behavior is normal," she says. "People both like and dislike things about their habits or behaviors."

Motivational interviewing assumes that patients and their caregivers may not share the same concerns. "I might be concerned that a heavy smoker will develop cancer," Manuel continues, "while, to the patient, cancer isn't their biggest worry. Their biggest worry may be how much they're spending on cigarettes. So in MI we structure the conversation so that it's about why the patient wants to change—not about why we want the patient to change."

Manuel gives me another example. "In the traditional model, someone would ask a patient a series of closed questions. 'How long have you been smoking? How many cigarettes do you have a day?' Then they would explain why smoking is so bad for them, tell them to quit, and outline what would happen if they don't."

Manuel begins the conversation very differently, listening for what is known as "sustain talk" and "change talk." "I would ask the patient what their thoughts are about smoking," she elaborates. "Then I would listen very hard to their answer. They might regale me with sustain talk: 'I love to smoke. I've smoked for thirty years, and I really like the fact that it allows me to get out of the house or office and take a break.'"

"If I let them talk," she continues, "they will also give me these little gems of change talk: 'Smoking is such a huge part of my life. I can't imagine quitting.' But then comes the change talk. They will say, 'It's getting so hard to smoke. It's really a lot of work.' And I will try to pursue that, asking 'Why is it so hard?' And helping, over time, to direct them to attend more to the intrinsic motivation to change."

This approach has been proven to be far more effective, and so a technique that was once used only in psychology and therapy settings has migrated into primary care and other medical settings. I attended a three-day motivational interviewing course at Fort Miley for about thirty different health care professionals: primary care physicians, nurse-practitioners, psychologists, social workers, occupational therapists, and psychiatrists. These included Alison Ludwig, physician chief of medical practice, and addiction psychiatrist Tauheed Zaman, who directs a number of addiction programs at Fort Miley. Both not only function as administrators but also see patients in their own clinical practices.

Manuel and clinical psychologists Brian Borsari and Joni Utley taught the group how to help motivate their patients to stop smoking, eat less, do more exercise, take their prescribed medications, or otherwise change the habits that were compromising their health. The group listened to material about the theory and practice of motivational interviewing, watched videos that illustrated its techniques, and engaged in role-plays that put them into practice.

Throughout the course of the three-day workshop, it became clear that motivational interviewing involves more than addressing the ambivalence of patients. Clinicians who were studying the technique had their own ambivalence—not so much about its utility but about abandoning an expert command-and-control approach in which they had been socialized for years or, depending on their age, even decades.

"Providers went to school, studied incredibly hard, and have all this information they feel they have to impart," Manuel explains. "They've also been trained to elicit information from the patient by asking a series of closed questions. Then they give their advice or information. They have not been trained in a nonconfrontational but nonetheless directive model that teaches them to gather information about what motivates the patient, which may have nothing to do with medical concerns at all."

To help clinicians learn this new model, the VA's workshops involve a pre-workshop assessment, the workshop itself, and then six months of ongoing supervision with an expert on staff. Before they attend the workshop, they record an encounter with a patient. Trainers then code the session to establish a baseline.

Then clinicians do the workshop. Over the course of the six months following the workshops, participants continue to record sessions in which they use motivational interviewing with patients, and then they meet weekly with a trainer. In these sessions they review the recordings and consult on what's working and what isn't.

"This part is absolutely critical," Manuel says. "When we review the tapes of clinicians after they have just done the workshop, we see a big jump in skills. There have been several studies looking at the best way to train providers in using MI, and they have documented that if they don't do the consultation process, we see an erosion of skills. We know that if we just send them off and don't do the six months of consultation, MI skills will fade, and they will go back to where they were before the training. So the whole thing will have been a huge waste of both time and money."

Ludwig was one of the primary care physicians attending the motivational interviewing sessions I observed. When I caught up with her in a small office in the medical practices clinic at Fort Miley several months after she had completed the training and supervision, I asked her if it had helped her deal better with her patients.

"It was super helpful," Ludwig says. Typically, she explains, "bread-and-butter communication skills isn't what's rewarded in medicine." When she was a resident, she recalls, "not much was focused on how you motivated your patients." Instead, everything was geared toward "your ability to give this incredible clinical diagnosis."

Lacking these communication skills, Ludwig says, makes it easy to get frustrated and even burn out because patients don't change. "In the VA's patient population, which has such an overwhelming burden of mental illness and substance abuse, you can feel like you weren't successful," she says, adding that it's like rolling boulders up hills, only to see them roll right down again. "They come back and back and back, and you think, 'What are we doing here? We're not getting anywhere.'"

To make any headway in terms of wellness or behavior change, Ludwig says, the provider needs to get at the patient's motivations. "It helps you understand that the patient is responsible for their own health," she says. If they're not ready to change, it's not the provider's fault. "MI doesn't blame the patient," Ludwig says, "but it doesn't blame the provider."

Ludwig is determined to teach this approach to trainees. Even today, she says, when there is supposed to be more of a focus on doctor–patient communication, residents are still coming to the VA with the same attitudes and preconceptions she had when she left medical school.

"They come into the preceptor room and tell me that their patients are coming back with the same problems over and over again," Ludwig says. "They tell me they offered the patient this or that, and that the patient isn't interested. I want to help them reorient the conversation so they can understand why the patient likes drinking or smoking and learn about how the patient got to that place."

Zaman echoes Ludwig's view. The workshop "has helped me motivate patients—particularly patients with addiction—to go from one stage of change to another," he says, adding that it's also been useful in "helping patients to take medications regularly and even come to appointments on time."

Zaman says he used to barrage his patients with a bunch of closed questions. Now, he says, he begins by asking open-ended questions about, for instance, patients' heroin use and how it affects their life.

"I try to be more curious about it," he explains. "I might say, 'Okay, gosh, it sounds like heroin has been a part of your life for some time. Tell me about what you've heard about how heroin impacts your health.' Then I listen to them tell me about their own experience. They might tell me that when they started using heroin it felt good, but they've also noticed X, Y, and Z that is not so good. So I will say something like, 'So it sounds like when you first started using, it felt good, but now there are adverse effects?' Then, rather than telling the patient what to do, I would ask, 'What would you like to do about it?'"

This approach, Zaman adds, strikes a balance between the role of medical expert and that of collaborator. "Obviously," he adds, "if someone is doing something life threatening or it's a medical emergency, I'm not going to say, 'How would you feel about going to the emergency room?'

I'm going to walk them right over there myself. Outside of this kind of situation, I can have more engaging and collaborative relationships with patients."

Zaman credits the VA for stressing motivational interviewing. "It has taken a tremendous amount of unlearning on my part to do MI, but MI has changed pretty much every conversation I have with a patient," Zaman says. "It has improved outcomes as well as my job satisfaction. It takes a lot of work and good supervision and practice to learn a new skill. It's worth it because it serves our veterans better."

As many veterans told me in the course of my research for this book, they really appreciate the patient-centered primary care they receive at the VHA. For instance, one week after my visit with Shunk and her team at Fort Miley, I was sitting in the primary care clinic at the Baltimore VA Medical Center with another primary care physician, Cathy Staropoli. One of her patients, Mr. Gill, is a buff sixty-two-year-old who looks ten years younger. His long dreadlocks cascade almost to his waist, and he is dressed in stylish black jeans, black T-shirt, and shiny cowboy boots. When he served in the Army between 1974 and 1998, he was a medical technologist, and he now works as a lab scientist. He's been seeing Staropoli for seventeen years. They go, he says, "way, way back."

For the first fifteen minutes of the visit, the topic is Gill's blood pressure. He has missed some doses of his medication, and the two consider what he might do to take his medication more regularly. Gill then complains of some chest pain, and Staropoli checks it out. She discovers that he's recently moved house and spent a lot of time lifting heavy boxes and furniture. After more conversation and a physical exam, she determines that he is not suffering from heart pain but rather a pulled muscle. Staropoli suggests stretches and maybe some physical therapy, puts in the order, and makes the therapy appointment for three days hence.

Staropoli goes over Gill's medicine list, orders lab work that, again, will be done on the same day, and, before the visit is over, asks him if he has any other concerns. There are none.

After Staropoli has left the room, I ask Gill what he thinks of the VA. "It never seems just like a visit here," he responds. "You know, fifteen minutes and you're out, which is what I've experienced in the private sector. They do what they need to here, and if they can't do it here, then they send me to Johns Hopkins or University of Maryland."

He does, however, have a complaint with the bureaucracy at the VBA. He has PTSD, he says. His claim was finally accepted, but it was a long and painful process. He couldn't prove it was from the military, but, on the other hand, he remarks bitterly, "I didn't get it from Disneyland."

4

Healing Minds and Bodies

Integrated Mental Health Care and Primary Care

Psychiatric nurse-practitioner James Caldwell immediately recognized that he had found his dream job when he arrived at the San Francisco VA Medical Center in 2007. Rather than working on his own or in a clinic where he would have to wait for a patient to be referred by a physician and then wait for a patient to call and show up—or not—he is part of an unusual and expanded primary care team, along with clinical psychologist Charles Filanowsky, at the Medical Practice Clinic at Fort Miley. When patients come to an appointment with a primary care provider, Caldwell and Filanowsky are available to talk with them and assess their problems as well as administer tests and provide on-the-spot treatment. They also manage patients on long-term medication and advise nurses, social workers, pharmacists, and dietitians on mental health issues, as well as teach students who train in the clinic.

Caldwell usually sports a two-day stubble and neatly trimmed hair, wears round, black-rimmed glasses, plaid shirts, and jeans, and displays the kind of quirky warmth that puts the veterans he treats at ease. He tells me that he is very comfortable with even the most "difficult" patients. To him it is no mystery why a veteran with PTSD or mental illness would avoid getting help. After his parents died when he was only nine, his sister and brother-in-law, who had PTSD after serving in the Korean War, raised him.

"For these guys from World War II and the Korean War," Caldwell observes, "this was all just part of the package. They thought of it, if they thought of it at all, as 'shell shock.' It was just part of what you dealt with. They didn't know how to ask for help. In my house we never talked about it."

Now helping veterans "talk about it" is what Caldwell does every day. To facilitate such conversations, he has transformed his small office into a cozy and inviting space furnished with two comfortable brown leather chairs, soothing photos on the walls, and a touch of whimsy: a male nurse action figure, a plastic dinosaur, a Car Jar, and other amusing oddities.

With the veterans' permission, I sit in on several sessions with Caldwell and his patients. One of them is a Vietnam vet dressed in cowboy boots, neatly pressed black jeans, and a black cowboy shirt with bright red trim. I'll call him Hank (he didn't want me to use his real name). Hank is a seventy-something gay man who lives alone; as he sits across from Caldwell, his legs seem to have a life of their own, rattling against the leather chair as he describes his inability to sleep, his PTSD, and an abusive father who sometimes appears in his nightmares swinging his fists. Instead of probing the man's early childhood, however, Caldwell zeroes in on his patient's current sleeping habits and how his insomnia might be fueled by his caffeine consumption.

How many cups of coffee or Coke does he drink, and when? Does he notice any correlation between caffeine use and his nightmares and insomnia? Hank admits that when he kicked caffeine for eight months, he slept better and had fewer nightmares. Since he went back to his old regimen of Cokes and coffee, nightmares about his parents are worse than ever.

But, he hastily interjects, "I am seventy-three. One of the pleasures of my life is drinking soda pop, and eating candy, and my cup of coffee."

Caldwell patiently explains that soda pop right before bed will not increase his long-term pleasure in life. "I don't want to do battle with you on caffeine," Caldwell tells Hank. "I'm just trying to troubleshoot with you about the problem of vivid dreams."

During the conversation Hank also reports waking up in the morning in severe pain. Caldwell asks Hank if he has made an appointment with the orthopedic service. Hank says he gets frustrated waiting on the phone. Knowing that patients with PTSD or other mental illnesses may experience even a very short wait on the phone as way too long, Caldwell offers to call and make the appointment before Hank leaves. Caldwell reaches the clerk in the orthopedic department and learns that Hank had an appointment, but it was canceled. Did Hank cancel it? he asks. Hank can't recall, so he and Caldwell walk over to the orthopedic department and sort it out. Hank leaves with a new appointment—and a promise to reduce his soda intake.

Caldwell's session with Hank illustrates the way that mental health care is integrated into primary care. This integration, which took decades to accomplish, is one of the national VHA's proudest organizational achievements, and it's one that many other health systems wish they could implement. It became possible because the VHA has intentionally fostered a community of caregivers both locally and nationally. Clinicians may pioneer programs and develop new models of care at the local level. These models are often connected with emerging trends and research in a clinician's particular field, and when they are proven effective, they eventually receive support from the national VA, which implements them across the entire system.

The clinician who helped develop the model of integrated mental health and primary care was family practice physician Andrew Pomerantz, who began practicing as a primary care physician (before that term was commonplace) in rural Vermont in 1972. Pomerantz went into medicine hoping to become a psychiatrist. In medical school, however, he became disillusioned with the traditional psychiatric model. Patients were seen as a kind of archaeological dig in which the psychiatrist sifted through the detritus of the patient's experience in an attempt to uncover a series of problems that were perhaps more relevant or interesting to the psychiatrist than the patient.

Instead of going into psychiatry, Pomerantz chose general practice (family medicine was just at the cusp of development), where he became convinced that mental and behavioral health issues could not be segregated from so-called medical issues. As later research has found, "70 to 80 percent of all primary care visits are related to psychological distress," and almost half of patients will eventually have a mental or behavioral problem at some point in their lives.[1] As a general practitioner, Pomerantz wanted to deal with these problems but felt that general practitioners had a "hole in their knowledge base about behavioral and mental health issues." It was a hole he was determined to fill.

After twelve years of general practice, Pomerantz began a psychiatric residency at Dartmouth Hitchcock Medical Center, where he spent much of his time training at the White River Junction VA. When he finished his psychiatric training, he went into full-time practice at the VA.

Pomerantz's first job at White River was serving as a consultation liaison psychiatrist who supervised medical students and residents as well as provided inpatient consultation services. Even though the word "consult" was constantly in use, the model used in primary care was not really consultative. Instead, physicians worked under a referral model in which primary care physicians passed along their patients to mental health or psychiatry with basically a "Here, you take care of it" attitude.

Pomerantz had a very different idea, what he considered to be a collaborative model in which the mental health provider worked on the primary care unit alongside the primary care physicians. He wanted mental health care providers to do more than share the same space; he wanted them to work together to manage their common patients over the long term. Pomerantz got an opportunity to make this kind of integrated care a reality when he was given office space in what was then the ambulatory care clinic at White River Junction. When he arrived at the clinic, he enthusiastically approached his colleagues with his ideas. "What are you talking about?" Pomerantz recalls their astonished, are-you-kidding reaction. "You're here to be part of our team? Really?"

Without others sharing his vision, Pomerantz found himself cloistered in an office, seeing patients—co-locating, not collaborating, with primary care physicians. Many of them viewed him simply as a referral source who was easier to access and who helped them to marginally reduce the no-show rate. About a year later, when primary care needed more office space, Pomerantz was out, back in the mental health clinic.

Things did not look promising until a young resident in psychiatry named Steve Spalding, who was about to leave his training to work for a psychiatric practice in Tennessee, came to him and expressed interest in his efforts to integrate mental health into primary care. Pomerantz sent him over to ambulatory care with the hope that he could both learn and help out.

He did that and more. Without an office, Spalding inhabited communal spaces—the lunchroom, the break room—with primary care physicians. Because he was ever present, he became a sought-after adviser, answering questions about what might help, guiding referrals, and triaging patients. The physicians in the clinic, Pomerantz says, came to value him and were distressed when his residency ended. Their distress did not, however, translate into a call for others to join them. Finally, after several more trials and errors, Pomerantz tried a "collaborative care clinic" that was housed in primary care.

"A psychologist, psychiatrist, or social worker had an office in primary care," he explains. "If a primary care provider felt that a patient needed mental health services, that mental health provider would meet briefly with patients to determine whom they should be referred to. He would make arrangements for an appropriate referral and might do some therapy himself if it was appropriate. We called it a collaborative care clinic. We at least wanted to keep the name 'collaborate.' We needed to demonstrate that we were useful in delivering a service, since the main service the physicians wanted was an appropriate and timely referral."

The primary care physicians and Pomerantz worked this way for five or six years. During this period Pomerantz joined a research project called Primary Care Research in Substance Abuse and Mental Health for the Elderly. From 2000 to 2002, this research was conducted at community health centers, VA facilities, and other community primary care clinics, and it tested two models of care for depression, anxiety, and at-risk drinking. One was an "enhanced" referral model, and the other was integrated care. Its initial findings reported that of the 23,828 patients in the study, those who received integrated care for depression were more "engaged" with mental health care. Providers also liked the integrated model better because there was "better communication between mental health and primary care providers, normalization of mental health services, and better care coordination." Other studies on this model reported similar positive results.[2]

Ironically, Pomerantz explains, what allowed his model to advance even further were the serious cutbacks in mental health services at the VHA both nationally and locally that occurred in the late nineties and persisted into the middle of the next decade. Because of cuts Congress imposed, medical center directors often failed to fill mental health positions left vacant because of attrition. The situation was so dire that a substance abuse counselor working for Pomerantz who was dying urged him not to tell anyone in charge about his illness—and not to mention it when he died—because they wouldn't let Pomerantz fill the position if they knew.

Because of these cutbacks, mental health professionals were overworked and exhausted, and an increasing number of veterans were subjected to unacceptable delays in getting services. "At White River," Pomerantz recalls, "our waits for a first appointment grew to six weeks or more. We needed to turn the collaborative care clinic into something more efficient and effective."

Pomerantz felt he could do this because of his approach in treating many mental health patients. The typical approach at the time was to view every problem a veteran had as a complex one that required one- to two-hour comprehensive evaluations. In those sessions clinicians were supposed to "probe every nook and cranny of people's lives looking for things that may or may not be relevant to the problem at hand," he recalls. "We wasted a lot of time by not focusing on the patient's presenting problem. I felt most mental health problems could be dealt with simply and straightforwardly."

Research studies, Pomerantz adds, were also confirming that things like depression could be effectively managed without an extensive psychiatric diagnostic evaluation. Addressing depression could begin if a primary care physician identified the problem, started treatment, and worked with a nurse to call the patient and ask about depressive symptoms and any side effects of medication. The nurse would also encourage the patient to do basic things like get up in the morning, get dressed, and get out of the house. The nurse served as a crucial link between patient and primary care provider.

After assembling a working group of interested clinicians, Pomerantz and his team held meetings and scoured data, with everyone looking for ways to eliminate waste, increase access and effectiveness, and thus find the best method to truly integrate mental health care into primary care. Each member of the group presented his or her own suggestions for an ideal process of integration, and then others would critique it. The group also hired a non-VA, Web-based system analyst to assess patients' needs and suggest how best to address them without inefficiencies. They discovered that questionnaires given to patients who then reported on targeted areas of concern were more effective than face-to-face evaluations that asked a lot of open-ended questions.

The group then designed four questionnaires to be given to patients before an appointment. Patients would report on their feelings of depression, anxiety, symptoms of PTSD, and overall functioning. Mental health providers would be in the clinic to assess patients immediately and initiate therapy with those who had less serious problems and refer on to specialists those whose problem was more complex.

"Warm handoffs," in which one clinician brought the patient to another, rather than computerized referrals, became the norm. The group actually disabled the computer function through which primary care physicians (PCPs) entered a consult/referral request. "We wanted the PCPs to bring the patient to us and introduce them. Our aim was same-day service, open access. Rather than taking the time to enter a referral request, the PCP could use that time to bring the patient to us."

When Pomerantz and his colleagues disabled the referral function on the White River Junction computers, they enabled people to talk to one another. In a world where technology has increasingly replaced and disabled human contact, this is a critical advance.

After a year of planning and also consultation with primary care staff, on July 5, 2004, the group launched its integrated care model. "We didn't want to phase the program in," Pomerantz explains. "We wanted to start overnight."

"The PCPs loved it," Pomerantz says. "They had immediate access for any mental health problem. Patients filled out questionnaires. Then they would see a therapist, all on the same day. That therapist would decide whether the patient could be followed in the clinic or by phone and whether they could see us more regularly or when they came back to the VA. They could determine whether the person needed to see a specialist or even a hospitalization."

The success was dramatic. "It worked for everyone," Pomerantz says. "The no-show rate for mental health specialists' appointments dropped by 75 percent. The number of new referrals coming to specialty mental health services was reduced by about 75 percent. Over 90 percent of those patients who were referred showed up. The waiting time for seeing us in primary care averaged out around twenty minutes. Waiting time for specialist mental health care dropped from six weeks to less than a week because the patient would leave with an appointment in hand."

Why did the program produce such impressive results? It is not surprising that when patients have more information about mental health care, they are more apt to embrace treatment recommendations. "Veterans had their first appointment with a mental health provider in the clinic and could see what it was like," Pomerantz says. "The patient would realize that, 'Oh wow, he's not going to delve into all these deep, dark family secrets. He's just going to talk to me.'"

Patients who were going to be referred were told what to expect and could decline or accept an appointment rather than saying yes to please the doctor and then not showing up at the scheduled time.

"We have to recognize," Pomerantz points out, "that many veterans coming back from Iraq and Afghanistan don't want to sign on to the kind of intense PTSD treatment that might be recommended. They don't want to go to appointments for eight to twelve weeks, do a lot of homework, and engage in that kind of therapy."

As is typical in the VA, many other clinicians had exchanged information with Pomerantz about the program and were interested in the same model. Meanwhile, word got out about the success of the program, and Pomerantz won two awards for his work: the American Psychiatric Association's Gold Achievement Award for innovative programs and an award offered by the secretary of the Department of Veterans Affairs called the Advanced Clinical Access Champions Award.

Because the VHA was under fire for its access problems, news about the program prompted Gerald Cross, then head of patient care services at the VA central office, to get in touch with Pomerantz. A few months later, the VA central office issued a request for proposals within the VHA seeking sites interested in replicating the same kind of model Pomerantz had developed. At the same time, Congress was fortuitously restoring VHA funding for mental health, so this helped expedite the expansion.

In a project known as Translating Initiatives in Depression into Effective Solutions (TIDES), some VA facilities around the country were given two-year research grants to use a model that eventually became known as the collaborative care model to test the effectiveness of a nurse care manager who would contact and follow by telephone a veteran who had depression. That model again proved to be effective. Another model that was also useful was the Behavioral Health Laboratory.

"What VA did at that time," Pomerantz explains, "was combine the nurse care manager model and the White River Junction Model to form the VA's Primary Care Mental Health Integration program, which was launched nationwide in 2007."

Rina Shah, who is now deputy chief of staff at the San Francisco VA Medical Center, told me more about how this model of care was disseminated throughout the VA. Shah, a primary care physician who has worked for the VA for sixteen years, is a slim woman with straight, dark hair and deep black eyes. She often dresses in a gray flannel suit, businesslike attire that belies the compassion she exudes in conversation. In 2007 she was asked to represent the San Francisco VA Medical Center on the national rollout of the primary care–mental health integration. At Fort Miley this meant starting with the Medical Practice Clinic, which cared for some ten thousand veterans.

Shah immediately partnered with psychiatrist Kew Chang Lee, the physician who did psychiatric consults and oversaw outpatient care. They hired Caldwell and Filanowsky and proceeded to get buy-in from the different disciplines, which, Shah tells me, was not a hard sell.

"From a primary care perspective, integrating mental health into primary care made a lot of sense," she says. "A lot of veterans felt stigmatized if you suggested they go to Building Eight to get mental health services. Patients didn't want to be labeled as having a mental health disorder. When you suggested a consultation for treatment, they would say, 'Oh no, I'll deal with it on my own. I don't want to go there.' So this was a great thing for us."

Shah searches for the right phrasing. "It's great when I talk to a patient and I say, 'I'm just going to walk you down the hall, introduce you to this person, and then let's see what comes out of it. Either they'll treat you, or we'll treat you, or you'll move on to more specialized care.' That's something we would have wished for. As practitioners we wanted to do it, but no one ever came to us with a model. And here it was, this great opportunity."

Shah remembers the first primary care patient she "integrated" into mental health in the clinic. Although she had worked with this older veteran for five years, she could not persuade him to get mental health care.

With this new model, she approached him and said, "You know, we have this great new thing here. I'd like to walk down the hall with you to talk to this person. If you don't like it, I am not going to force you to do this. It's totally fine if you don't like it."

He looked at Shah skeptically, and she told him: "Up to now we've worked together well in primary care. You've done well. Just do this one thing for me." He agreed but was surprised that the mental health professional was so close by.

"You mean that doctor will be in this clinic?"

Shah responded: "Yes sir, middle hallway. I'll walk you over there. You'll have a chair there."

"You mean, just like a chair in your office?"

"That's right."

After Shah walked him down to the middle corridor and introduced him to Caldwell, he talked to the nurse-practitioner. Because he had a good experience, he continued talking to Caldwell five or six times and then eventually accepted care in Building Eight. As Shah recounts, "He was very appreciative. To him, seeing was believing."

Seeing was also believing for primary care providers in the Medical Practice Clinic, Shah says. These practitioners had already become accustomed to walking down the hall to introduce a patient to dietitians and social workers. They walked down the hall to pick up their patients and get labs and patient appointment slips. Now they discovered that walking down the hall to mental health also saved time.

"We loved having someone in the clinic from whom we could get advice about a patient," Shah says. "Maybe we have an elderly gentleman with pathological reasons for severe back pain who is not a surgical candidate. He's on opioids, has neuropathy and also difficulty sleeping. The basic medications that we are most comfortable with haven't worked. I'll go to James and go over the chart with him and look at medications. We have a discussion. He will suggest a medication. After the patient starts the medication, we both call the patient to see how he is doing."

Over the last decade, the VA used this model to treat millions of veterans. In 2015 the VHA provided over 1.9 million primary care visits to veterans (up 28 percent from 2014). In that time period, more than 490,000 veterans whose illnesses would otherwise have gone unaddressed were diagnosed with depression during a primary care visit. Mental health providers embedded in primary care clinics treated nearly one-third of these patients. Other veterans were diagnosed with other mental and behavioral health conditions.[3]

Mental health providers like Caldwell and Filanowsky also emphasize how much they appreciate working with primary care physicians. "You know who to send people to, and they know me," Filanowsky says.

Embedding mental health clinicians into the primary care clinic creates an intricate web of connections, communication, understanding, and support. As Caldwell puts it, "They feel we have their backs, and they respect and support what we're doing, and they have our backs."

Caldwell gives the example of a veteran who worked in construction but had PTSD from combat trauma, as well as a brain injury. He could talk for hours on end, wandering from subject to subject. "I thought Chuck needed to do some testing on him, and so I asked him whether his inability to stick to one subject and follow through was a problem for him. 'Oh my God, yes,' he said."

Caldwell asked Filanowsky to come in and talk to the veteran. After meeting the psychologist, the veteran almost broke down. "No one had ever asked him about any of this or suggested there was a way to deal with it," Caldwell said. "They just listened, rolled their eyes, and gave him a pill. He's a lovely guy who was hurting in a way that I couldn't put my finger on. I just love being available, meeting people where they are at."

In the primary care clinics at the VHA, integration of primary care and mental health is a two-way street. Shira Maguen, a PhD psychologist at Fort Miley, is the director of the Integrated Care Clinic as well as a researcher and staff psychologist on the PTSD team. Maguen and her colleagues are also embedded in the Medical Practice Clinic. "A lot of veterans," she explains, "are hooked up to mental health but have never seen—or even considered seeing—a primary care provider. They're men or women who started using the GI Bill to go to a local college, say, City College of San Francisco. They go to the mental health clinic there and are diagnosed with PTSD or depression. A veteran may begin treatment for his PTSD or depression, but he also has an injury or other health needs. So rather than coming to the VHA via primary care, he or she comes in via mental health care."

Maguen and her mental health colleagues don't view their job as just treating the veterans' mental health problems. "We talk to the veteran and explain that our job is also to make sure any other health care needs are met," she says. "We ask if there is anything else we can help with. Are there any injuries, or are there social work needs that the veteran has—with housing, finances."

In a highly integrated system like the VHA, integration of mental health into primary care is also dependent on tight coordination and collaboration with mental health providers in Behavioral Health Services, which is housed in Building Eight. John McQuaid's office is located on the third floor, where I meet with him often to discuss the VHA's integrated care model as well as his teaching of psychology students and other mental health care workers. McQuaid, a PhD clinical psychologist, is associate chief of the Mental Health Service and has, like so many of the VA staff I have met, a long tenure at the VA—over twenty years. Early access to mental and behavioral health services, he knows, has been documented to lead to more effective treatment. But the issue of access is directly connected to the issue of stigma.

"In order to provide veterans with quick access to mental health care, it's important to begin in a setting that's perceived by the veterans as less stigmatizing," he says. "That may mean locating services outside what is formally labeled as a mental health building and decreasing the number of steps that can be an obstacle to care."

He cites the example of a real patient to whom he attaches the fictitious name of Jim Smith. Smith comes in to see his primary care physician and reports he's having panic attacks. Caldwell or Filanowsky gets him started on treatment. Then he is taken to the Access Center and begins prolonged exposure therapy, which helps him cope with the physical sensations that keep surfacing.

"The most rewarding thing about this model," McQuaid says, "is that we see people who would never find their way to mental health care any other way."

Dealing with a World of Hurt

VHA Treatment of Chronic Pain

Joshua Wilder Oakley joined the Army in 1995, when he was eighteen. "I wanted structure. I knew that if I stayed where I grew up, I would have ended up in a dead-end job or as a drug addict," the tall, thin thirty-nine-year-old recalls. "Who knew," he says with a wry smile, "that joining the Army would put me on a journey through inexorable physical and emotional pain and that I would, indeed, become a drug addict?"

I met Oakley in 2013, when I attended a special veterans' orientation at City College in San Francisco. The two-year community college, in conjunction with the San Francisco VA Health Care System, has made a vigorous effort to support its veteran students. In the roomful of mostly younger veterans returning to school on the GI Bill, Oakley stood out not only because of the mala beads strung around his wrist and the thick, wavy hair that contrasted with the usual buzz cut and standard-issue baseball cap. What I couldn't help noticing was the look of tightly controlled intensity, the sense that this guy was working really, really hard to keep it all together.

Which, he later told me, is just what he has succeeded in doing. It has only taken him seventeen years.

Oakley was stationed at Schofield Barracks in Honolulu, where his military occupation specialty was infantry medic. Medics, he tells me, go through the same training as every other soldier. In training, medics carry the aid bag they would use in battle, which adds an extra forty or so pounds to their load. This means even more foot, back, knee, and shoulder problems than are usual for infantry.

For Oakley there was an even weightier problem: in the era of Clinton's Don't Ask, Don't Tell policy, he was gay. "When I filled out all the forms," he told me, "they still had questions about being gay. They were all crossed out with Magic Marker, but there they were. So I knew when I signed on that I was committing myself to four years of living a lie."

Oakley loved the military. "Enlisting was a desperate move for me, but it was the best thing I ever did," he says. "I was really, really good at what I did, being a medic and a soldier. I got my expert field medic badge when I was still a private, and it's the hardest badge to get in the Army. I loved it, but then, when I was twenty-one, overnight everything changed."

While in Hawaii, he collapsed with a lung aneurysm and was immediately rushed into surgery. He woke up after the operation in Tripler Army Hospital in Honolulu to what he describes as a year of total hell. "For the surgery to rectify the problem, they went in through my femoral artery to cauterize my lung, and my nervous system didn't like that. I was in excruciating pain, and all the Army's docs did was give me drugs—heavy, heavy narcotics. By the time I was medically discharged, I was taking six OxyContin every eight hours, four to six Vicodins, or morphine, every four hours. And the doctor told me, 'Oh, you're fine, you won't become an addict.'"

During the eighteen months it took for the Army to figure out whether he could return to active duty, Oakley said the military tried hard to heal his body. "The military is pretty good at dealing with people with serious, visible injuries," he says. "For guys who got blown up or had a clear, noticeable injury—a leg or arm amputated—then there was all the sympathy in the world. They clearly had something wrong with them. But if you couldn't see it, if it was mental anguish, PTSD, the kind of chronic pain or vulnerability I was experiencing, that was a different story entirely."

Oakley did briefly see a psychiatrist. "But," he says, "I couldn't really talk about my problems because I was gay. I had to formulate very carefully what I could say because I was afraid. I'm only just beginning to understand the ramifications of that."

Finally, after a year and a half, Oakley was medically discharged and sent home. "When I was discharged, no one told me anything about the VA or the benefits to which I was entitled," he says. "When I went to the VA in Hawaii in 2000 for the first time because I was sick with postsurgical nerve damage, I was terrified that I would be stuck with a hospital bill. Nothing was explained on exit. I had a 70 percent service-related disability, and I thought I would have to pay for everything."

In retrospect Oakley has come to realize that his choice to use his GI Bill to go to culinary school didn't help. "The high-stress, macho environment of the restaurant kitchen attracted me because it was kind of like the military," he says. "It was really regimented, really high intensity, and there was a lot of drugs and alcohol. If I went to the VA for a physical problem, I didn't reveal my drinking, nightmares, or emotional problems. Why should I? I was a high-functioning, successful chef, working in some of San Francisco's best restaurants. So I got really good at using meds to suppress the symptoms of both my mental and physical pain."

Then, in 2012, Oakley injured his foot. "One day I was fine, and then the next day I felt like I had stepped on a needle," he says. "My foot ballooned up like a watermelon. I was reliving the trauma I had experienced after surgery in the Army. I lost my job and went into a deep depression and became suicidal. I was referred to a VA pain clinic for my chest and my foot. I met with a physical therapist twice week and had a nerve block, which allowed me to walk again. With the help of the therapist, we got the pain down, and I got through the depression. I went back to work. Trouble was, while I'd dealt with the pain in my foot and chest, I hadn't dealt with the psychological problems with which I'd been plagued for years."

Those problems got worse until he finally hit bottom, losing his job, his relationships, and even becoming homeless. That was when he finally went to the VA for help with his emotional issues. "The VA sent me to detox to dry out," he says. "I was enrolled in outpatient care as well as in outpatient rehab for substance abuse. We met three times a week. Anything I needed, they were there. I lived in a clean-and-sober house and connected with the veterans' advocacy group Swords to Plowshares. I was able to get a service rating for PTSD that went from 30 to 80 percent, and I also received monetary compensation."

Oakley received intensive cognitive behavioral therapy for his PTSD and went to the pain clinic. He also has learned meditation practice to deal with his issues. "All of this has given me a way to cope without using drugs or alcohol," he says. "I still have pain, but the pain doesn't control my life."

Oakley also learned that he could not maintain his recovery while working in the cutthroat kitchens of San Francisco. "With the help of the VA," he says, "I have been able to find the courage to do with my life what I had always wanted to do, formalize my education and become a professional artist. Thanks to the VA's vocational rehab program, I was able to afford tuition at City College of San Francisco, where I am earning a degree in graphic design. The VA pays for books, supplies, and even for a computer. "

At City College the VHA has established a Veterans Resource Center and lounge that Oakley says has been very helpful. "Dealing with community college counselors outside the Veterans Resource Center, you're just a number," he says. "At the Vet Center I see the same counselor, and she remembers me and gives me a hug. There's a real sense of community. For me, it's come full circle. I have the camaraderie of being in the Army with people with whom I share common experiences. I have found that people I never knew have all been through some of the same stuff. We get it."

Oakley maintained a 4.0 grade point average and was on the dean's list. He was accepted at the University of San Francisco, where he is now pursuing his bachelor's degree. "I tried private-sector health care, and it didn't work," he says. "Without the VA I don't know where I'd be. Well, on second thought, I guess I do. I'd be dead."

The Origins of the Problem

The epidemic of opioid overdoses is a particularly vexing and ironic problem throughout the American health care system. As one report outlined, "Drug overdose is the leading cause of accidental death in the U.S., with 47,055 lethal drug overdoses in 2014. Opioid misuse, abuse, addiction, and overdose accounts for over 60 percent of this epidemic, with four in five new heroin users starting out misusing prescription painkillers. In 2014, there were 18,893 overdose deaths related to prescription pain relievers, and 10,574 overdose deaths related to heroin."[1]

Veterans have been hard hit by this epidemic because, like Oakley, they suffer from pain from operations and amputations, pain from headaches created by TBIs and other concussive shocks, chronic pain from musculoskeletal injuries, and auditory pain from tinnitus, which is the number-one reason why veterans seek care at the VHA. Approximately 50 percent of veterans treated in primary care report one or more chronic pain complaints, disproportionately higher than American nonveterans. Pain is the most commonly identified risk factor when people examine the histories of veterans who have died from suicide.

In the VHA, and across the American health care system, the foundation of the problem of opioid overprescription was laid in the 1990s when the undertreatment of pain in American medicine became a major concern. Because most physicians had been trained not to prescribe opioids except in extreme cases of severe pain, they often paid little attention to a patient's acute or chronic pain. Researchers began to denounce what appeared to be the callous undertreatment of pain in both adults and children. The American Pain Society also worked diligently to make pain what is known as the "fifth vital sign."

Clinicians and patients alike were warned about failing to aggressively treat pain—and were tutored in the message that poorly managed pain can retard healing and significantly compromise a patient's quality of life. Patients who have recently complained about chronic pain or had surgery are shown a chart of scowling or smiley faces when they are asked to rate their pain. This is the result of a decades-long and highly successful effort to encourage clinicians to pay greater attention to pain management.

The pharmaceutical industry quickly exploited the new attention being paid to pain and encouraged the use of opioids to treat both the chronic and acute varieties. According to the Johns Hopkins Bloomberg School of Public Health, "Advocates for enhanced pain treatment successfully lobbied state medical boards and state legislatures to change statutes and regulations. One particular goal was to lift any prohibition of opioid use for non-cancer pain. In Washington State, for example, state law was modified to stipulate that 'no disciplinary action will be taken against a practitioner based solely on the quantity or frequency of opioids prescribed.'" In at least twenty states, these new guidelines, statutes, regulations, and laws dramatically liberalized the long-term use of opioids for chronic non-cancer pain, reflecting the prevailing thought at the time that there is no clinically appropriate ceiling on maximum opioid dosing.[2]

With the best of intentions, the VHA and the DoD took this message to heart. In 2000 the VHA published a "Pain as the Fifth Vital Sign Toolkit" that was designed to encourage clinicians to pay far more attention to pain and, among other things,

- provide a system-wide VHA standard of care for pain management that will reduce suffering from preventable pain;
- assure that pain assessment is performed in a consistent manner;
- assure that pain treatment is prompt and appropriate;
- include patients and families as active participants in pain management; and
- provide for continual monitoring and improvement in outcomes of pain treatment.[3]

Internist Karen Seal, who has been involved in the VHA's national response to the opioid epidemic, describes the ethos of the era. "I had never used long-acting opioids like OxyContin in my practice," Seal told me. "But suddenly drug companies began a huge campaign to push prescription opioids. There was this huge push to convince us that we were not only undertreating pain but failing to use long-acting, higher-dose opioids to treat it. Suddenly, throughout the broader health care system and inside the VHA, all of us were required to go to eight to ten hours of mandatory training on pain. The message was, 'You physicians are undertreating your patient's pain and have to stop making them suffer.'

"We took on the fifth vital sign," Seal continued, "routinely asking patients about their pain to rate its severity and do something about it. The public and our patients began to expect that doctors would be prescribing long-acting, high-dose opioids, which created the epidemic of fatal opioid overdose."

Within the military, overuse of opioids became a particularly critical problem for VHA providers like Seal. Like basketball or football players who are sometimes doped up so they can continue playing and ignore an injury, many service members who suffered from even worse injuries were given opioids to treat them. A *JAMA Internal Medicine* study found high rates both of chronic pain (44.0 percent) and opioid use (15.1 percent) in US military personnel after combat deployment. These rates were much higher than estimated rates in the general public (26 and 4 percent, respectively).[4]

"Military medicine is entirely different from medicine at the VA," says Rick Weidman of Vietnam Veterans of America. "In the military you get injured, and they pump you up with narcotics because the whole point is to get you back out to fight."

Although the DoD and the VHA, like the rest of the health care system, are now rethinking the wisdom of opioid use for chronic pain, neither managing chronic pain nor getting people off opioids is so easy. "You can't just tell patients who've been taking opioids for years, maybe even decades, to just cease and desist," Seal says. "If doctors abruptly cut off pain medication, this may lead veterans to seek out street drugs like heroin to deal with their pain, which then leads to increases in HIV, hepatitis C, and other health problems."

In 2009, to deal in a more comprehensive, nuanced, and effective way with the kind of chronic pain problems that plague so many veterans, the VHA introduced a stepped-care model. Following guidelines put out by the Centers for Disease Control and Prevention, VHA clinicians now "specifically recommend avoiding the use of opioids in favor of cognitive behavioral psychotherapy, exercise therapy, and non-opioid medications as *first-line* treatments for chronic pain." Using an interdisciplinary approach, the VA involves everyone from primary care doctors, psychologists, pharmacists, and physical therapists. Preliminary results show decreased disability from self-reported pain, opioid risk, and daily opioid use.[5]

VA hospitals and clinics across the country offer different levels of pain management and opioid safety programs to veterans. Payal Mapara, a pain psychologist, explained the menu of pain management options at Fort Miley: "There is no one approach that can address all the facets of chronic pain management, which is why we have so many pain services. Chronic pain is complex, and you need to use lots of different things to manage it best. But once you get into the mode of it, it just becomes a part of patients' lives in a way that they didn't realize it could be before. And they are living their lives and doing things that are pretty amazing."

At Fort Miley, for example, the first level of pain management begins with a primary care provider who evaluates the patient and comes up with an initial pain management treatment plan. For additional support, veterans can contact the pain pharmacy telephone clinic, which helps with medication safety and tapering off any medications. Clinicians who have questions or need extra information can consult with the pain pharmacy e-consult to discuss the risks and benefits of a patient's regimen. Primary Care Mental Health Integration Services provides extra support for primary care physicians working with veterans on pain issues. A veteran who has been in pain for years and has become dependent on opioids may become very frightened at the thought of getting off—even when the drugs are ineffective—and trying other alternatives. That is why pain psychologists, who may mobilize motivational interviewing techniques, are available to work with veterans on their anxieties or concerns. The VA also offers acupuncture, chiropractic services, nutrition counseling, and the MOVE! program, which helps veterans learn pain-relieving exercises. "The VHA," Karen Seal adds, "offers occupational, physical therapy and recreational therapy, which are free of charge and include complimentary and integrative modalities like Tai Chi and yoga."

The second level of pain-management programs offers even more support to both patients and busy primary care providers. The Integrated Pain Team at the San Francisco VA is a relatively new model of pain care that is being rolled out at a number of VHA facilities around the country. The team, directed by Seal, is embedded in the main primary care clinic and is also available via telehealth to community-based clinics in Ukiah, Eureka, and Clear Lake, California.

"Our emphasis," Seal says, "is on nonopioid, nonpharmacological management of chronic pain. We received a grant from the National Center for Complementary and Integrative Health to test structured primary care visits, plus motivational coaching, to help patients adhere to a pain care plan that they develop in collaboration with their doctor. We also discuss weight loss, yoga, meditation, walking, hobbies they love, like woodworking, and various other ways to distract patients from chronic pain and get them moving, since we know exercise is one of the best ways to alleviate chronic pain."

Patients who have been referred to the Integrated Pain Team by their primary care providers meet together with a pain psychologist, pharmacist, and primary care provider who is trained in pain management to create a plan of care that increases pain management and decreases reliance on opioids. The pain psychologist may recommend individual or group psychotherapy for cognitive behavioral therapy for pain. A registered nurse experienced in mind-body medicine leads a mind-body skills group, and some veterans who are using opioids to manage pain are gradually tapered off this medication and use other ways to manage their pain.

The pain service also offers a two-hour monthly Pain and the Brain Education class available to veterans. This is led by a specialized pain physical therapist and focuses on the neuroscience of chronic pain, which helps veterans understand how pain becomes chronic and what they can do on their own to alleviate it.

Because chronic pain may still be a serious problem for some patients, there are a number of other, more intensive, treatment options. The Intensive Pain Rehabilitation Program (IPRP) includes psychologists, pharmacists, occupational and physical therapists, a dietitian, and chaplains, all of whom specialize in chronic pain. For a period of twelve weeks, veterans attend the IPRP three days a week, four hours a day. To make the program accessible to people who live far from San Francisco, the VA has a contract with a local hotel and pays for their stay—plus three meals a day—for the duration of the program.

The Outpatient Chronic Pain Management Clinic provides diagnostic and therapeutic procedures, like spinal cord stimulation. Anesthesiologists also provide inpatient pain consultations.

Opioid Safety Initiative

The VHA has also launched a national Opioid Safety Initiative. It convened a multidisciplinary group of pain experts and formed a national task force that has tool kits so that clinicians can make wise decisions based on evidence when treating patients with chronic pain.[6]

At Fort Miley, Tauheed Zaman is the medical director of the Prescription Opioid Safety and Addiction Consult Team. In 2015, after completing a fellowship in addiction psychiatry at the University of California, San Francisco (UCSF), the soft-spoken addiction psychiatrist took over as the leader of a multidisciplinary team that includes clinicians in addiction psychiatry and psychology, as well as nurses and pharmacists. They treat veterans who have chronic pain, PTSD, and substance abuse issues and who are at a high risk for opioid overdoses. These patients, Zaman explains, are some of the sickest and most complex patients in the medical center. "We feel like we're an intensive care unit for outpatients," says Zaman. "Our patients are between a rock and a hard place—between use and overuse."

Three kinds of patients are referred to Zaman's team. Some have chronic pain issues and are on very risky opioid medications. Zaman describes a typical patient in this group. "He comes in and says, 'You know, I've been on opioid pain meds for fifteen years for my back injury, and I keep taking more and more. But my pain's not getting better, and I'm getting too sleepy and having side effects. I feel desperate about how to manage pain and get off these meds.'"

A second group of patients are taking risky benzodiazepines—medications they take for anxiety, insomnia, muscle spasms, or PTSD. These medications may work well in the short term but are highly addictive, putting patients at high risk for overdosing, particularly if the patient is also using opioids. It is very hard to taper them off medications, Zaman explains, because when patients try to reduce the medication, they experience the typical withdrawal symptoms of increased anxiety, more insomnia, and more muscle spasms. Some patients may also be at increased risk for seizures. All of this may create a cycle of continued risky medication use. Breaking the cycle in a safe way is thus part of the team's job.

A typical veteran in this group will come in, Zaman says, complaining that his anxiety from PTSD got better when he first started taking Valium, but now it's worse. He will explain that his VA doctor thinks he's addicted, but the patient is worried he could have a seizure if he stops taking the medication too quickly. The veteran is at a loss, and says: "Help! What should I do?"

Finally, the team also sees a wide spectrum of patients who have more generalized addiction problems with, say, alcohol, methamphetamines, cocaine, or marijuana. This group includes patients like the young Iraq vet who recently came into the clinic explaining that he started shooting methamphetamines and is now hearing voices, seeing things, and getting paranoid. He is finally convinced that he needs help getting off meth. Some of the team's patients have tried to kick their habit hundreds of times. Some have never tried and want to do so when they come in. All clearly need a lot of help.

"Anyone who wants to fast-track a patient into treatment for general addiction problems can refer them to us," Zaman says.

When patients are referred to the clinic, the multidisciplinary team evaluates them in person, through telehealth, or in visits to all outpatient clinics in the area. Patients are given a complete pain, mental health, and addiction evaluation. These evaluations are then brought back to the entire team, which collaboratively figure out a plan of care. Because this is a consultation and not a treatment team, 90 to 95 percent of patients are seen only a couple of times and then sent back to their primary care physician, psychologist, or psychiatrist with recommendations for a treatment plan. If patients want to enter into a program of talk therapy, they will be referred to individual or group therapy conducted by a psychologist. If they want to deal with a chronic mental health problem that requires medication, they will be referred to a psychiatrist. For pain issues, they will be referred to a pain clinic. Pharmacists provide consultation on all complex medication issues.

One Monday morning in July 2017, I sit in on the team's discussions of the variety and complexity of their cases. The meeting includes Tessa Rife, a pharmacist and academic detailing manager; Mapara, who works in the pain service with rural veterans over V Tel to improve access to care; and Taylor Castanetta, a registered nurse in primary care–mental health integration. Reflecting the VHA's teaching mission, the group also includes Brad Zicherman, an addiction psychiatry fellow, and two nurse-practitioner residents, Julie Tea and Jen Jones, as well as Matt Tierney, who is from the UCSF School of Nursing and supervises these nurse-practitioner residents.

Because, as Zaman said, the group works with such difficult patients, every team meeting begins with affirmations and what are called "service moments," things that went well in the team's efforts to serve veterans. In this case Rife talks about appreciating staff who helped a patient taper off risky benzos. She also applauds the patient who, although not present, began a journey of recovery he had avoided for decades. Zaman thanks Zicherman and Tea for going to see a patient in the hospital when Zaman himself was incredibly busy. The group, which bears a heavy burden, seems enlivened by beginning on the positive.

The next hour and a half is spent discussing various patients who have for decades used and abused a variety of substances to deal with their many physical and emotional problems. Tierney describes a patient who is in his seventies and moves in and out of Fort Miley's Community Living Center, or nursing home, and who is now dealing with lung cancer. He is, Tierney says, profoundly ambivalent about whether to stop using amphetamines. When he was told that the police might search his room in the CLC and he could face eviction, he suddenly expressed interest in doing something about his addiction. But, Tierney cautions, he has said that many times before. Over the weekend he left the CLC against medical advice, and, Tierney tells the group, it's anybody's guess when—or even if—he'll come back.

Mr. J. is another patient who has had opioid-use disorder for years. He is taking methadone and is in the psychiatric intensive care unit because, Zicherman reports, "he became very psychotic." He was started on an antipsychotic, risperidone, but this will affect his methadone dosing. The team worry that treating his psychosis could trigger opioid withdrawal, and they strategize about how best to treat him.

Rife describes a seventy-five-year-old veteran who has struggled with alcohol-use disorder and smoking. When he stopped drinking thirty years ago, he took up methamphetamines and cocaine to deal with chronic pain as well as to get an energy boost. At first he sniffed or smoked the cocaine. Then a friend gave him a helpful tip: if he crushed it in his tea, it would last longer, and he could avoid nasal bleeding. He has been drinking cocaine-laced tea for many years. Finally, he has decided to cut down.

With the team's help, the veteran has decided to learn other ways to manage his pain and to cut down from smoking two packs a day to half a pack. He has also cut down on his cocaine intake. The group discusses harm reduction and motivational interviewing, as well as trying the antidepressant Wellbutrin, which doesn't have much impact on substance abuse but may help boost his energy.

Zaman and his colleagues believe this kind of collaborative approach not only helps patients but makes it possible for the team to maintain the energy necessary to continue to work with patients who have tried—and too often failed—to change their lives over and over again. From the personal and professional point of view, they believe their approach helps, not overnight but slowly and surely. This is not simply a subjective assessment but is documented in research the VA has undertaken.

"The VA has started tracking safety measures, which include numbers of patients who are on a combination of opioids and benzodiazepines, which doubles or triples the risk of overdose," says Zaman. "Over six months we've reduced the number of people on these meds by over 30 percent, which is a huge number."

News about the model's success has percolated outside the VHA, and Zaman and his colleagues have been asked to help institutions like Kaiser develop similar teams. It's another example, Zaman says, "of how VHA practice and research are helping outside institutions that want to help risky patients. What we are doing overall is, hopefully, playing a productive role in addressing the opioid epidemic that has hit veterans so very hard. So many veterans with addiction issues really need to be connected to competent, compassionate clinicians, and we provide all this in one service."

Just as I was concluding this chapter, an Office of the Inspector General (OIG) report compared opioid prescribing to patients being treated in the VA and those treated by Veterans Choice providers outside the VA. There was an increased risk of overdose deaths among veterans prescribed opioids by community providers. Veterans with chronic pain and mental health disorders are at particularly high risk. Veterans treated in the community were more at risk because the VA's prescribing and monitoring guidelines were more stringent, and there was little information-sharing between the VA and community providers.

The OIG recommended that all non-VA providers be held to the same Opioid Safety Initiative guidelines and that all requests for care in the community include a medical history and a complete and current list of medications. It also recommended that community providers submit opioid prescriptions directly to a VA pharmacy for dispensing and recording in the patient's electronic health record.[7]

The Martinez Pain Team

Initiatives to manage the kind of chronic pain from which veterans suffer take place all over the country. The large Community Outpatient Clinic in Martinez, California, about forty-five minutes across the bay from San Francisco, also runs an impressive integrative pain program. As members of the pain team, chiropractor Jeffrey Chan and clinical psychologist

Crystelle Egan work with veterans to ease their pain and try to wean them from opioids. They do this with group and individual therapy and in a six-session course that explores, with veterans, the complex system that makes up our perception and responses to pain.

Chan has been working on pain issues with veterans since 2011. Pain, he understands, has become almost a way of life for veterans, from the time when they were in the military and continuing after they left it. "Given their duties and what's involved in deployment, or even in non-combat roles, a lot of them have musculoskeletal injuries—problems with their necks, and backs, and knees, and shoulders, and joints, anywhere and everywhere." In fact, Chan tells me, they may not be aware of a lot of these injuries until they actually come home.

If the pain persists, so do the lessons they have learned in the military about responding to pain. "In the culture of the military, you learn to tough it out," Chan says. "Obviously, when you're in combat, that attitude is an advantage. It keeps you alive. But when you're discharged, that mind-set lingers and becomes a barrier to care. When they finally go to the doctor, they often get pain medication that takes the edge off."

In our culture, Chan adds, taking a pill that gives temporary relief may even seem like a more acceptable way to treat chronic pain than dealing with the complexity of how mind and body, muscle, cell, and psyche interact. The problem is that the medication provides only short-term relief and also becomes addictive and has multiple side effects.

To avoid the inevitable cycle of denial and self-abuse, Chan and Egan work with primary care providers and physical therapy staff to educate their patients about chronic pain. "We are trying to help our patients understand that pain is multifaceted," Chan says. "There is an emotional, cognitive aspect to pain. Like adding gas to a fire, stress, for example, intensifies pain. One of the worst things about pain is that veterans may catastrophize. They may get a back flare-up and feel, 'Okay, this is going to be it. I'm never going to walk again.' They isolate themselves, avoid activity, and all this does is amplify the pain. When you add PTSD and other variables, sometimes guys don't leave the house for weeks.

"Research has documented," Chan continues, "that the more educated people are about chronic pain, the more functional they are and less disabled.[8] We try to work with patients to give them that education. We talk with patients. We show them the concrete benefits of physical activity and help them to avoid catastrophizing about their condition."

To alleviate the pain and wean veterans from addictive medication, Chan and his colleagues use, among other things, physical therapy, chiropractic services, soft-tissue therapy, exercise, and stretches. Veterans see an orthopedist and pain specialist and primary care provider, all of whom work together to change their medications and dosages. Chan and his colleagues also try to get veterans moving in a way that is appropriate to their current conditions. "These guys," Chan says, "were elite athletes. They were used to extreme exercise. They can't do that now. But that doesn't mean they can't do anything. The goal shifts from training for deployment to being able to play with your children or go on a fishing trip."

As part of this educational effort, Chan and Egan also run a six-week pain class, which, Chan says, is a "place where veterans get to really talk about what's going on. They get to vent their frustrations with pain. A lot of their spouses or kids don't really get it. They are irritated and frustrated because Dad can't go for a walk, or their husband can't do any heavy household lifting. They can't see the pain, and so they think people are faking or just trying to avoid doing household chores."

The day I attend the class is the penultimate session for a cohort of six men—white, African American, and Latino—all in their fifties and sixties. These men, who are hardly sensitive New Age guys, were learning how to share and reflect in ways they hadn't done before, as is clear when Egan begins the session by asking the participants how their thoughts were affecting their behavior.

One of the veterans acknowledges that if he exercised, his back would be stronger.

Another says that if he got up off the couch and just moved, his quality of life would improve.

A third admits that he needs to stop snapping at his family just because he's not feeling well.

A Vietnam vet who was in the process of moving house explains that he had been packing day in and day out and was exhausted, so exhausted that he didn't even want to come in for the class. "But I pushed myself," he says proudly.

"You should give yourself a lot of credit for coming here today," Egan congratulates him.

When the group members finish catching up on their pain journeys, Chan pulls up some slides to talk about the psychology and physiology of pain. Pain, he explains, isn't just about actual physical damage. It's a multifaceted phenomenon that involves some of the oddest and most mysterious forms of perception. To illustrate, he displays a slide of a normal spine. The vertebrae, he explains, pointing to the MRI image, all look great. The nerve canal is in stellar shape. Looking at the MRI, you would say nothing is wrong with the person whose spine is displayed here. It just so happens that this veteran is in incredible pain, he tells the group.

Then he contrasts this MRI with another of a veteran with terrible scoliosis. The spine snakes in an S curvature. Wow, people exclaim, the person who owns this crooked back must be in excruciating pain. But no, Chan says, he has no pain at all in his back but instead complains of pain in his neck, which on the MRI is perfectly fine.

The point he is trying to illustrate is that pain is a combination of sensory, emotional, and cognitive factors. The sensory component, he explains, is what happens when we feel something. The emotional component is how we respond to that feeling, and the cognitive component involves the meaning we attach to it. Chan then explains that thoughts and emotions can influence pain perception and physical function. Exercise, for example, can be as effective as medication in managing pain. "You can walk for twenty minutes, go up a couple of flights of stairs, and your fitness increases. Exercise also produces endorphins that calm the brain and reduce muscle tension."

Chan lists the hormones norepinephrine, dopamine, and serotonin, and he notes that exercise naturally increases the levels of all of them. He cites a 2001 study comparing exercise and the antidepressant Zoloft. For every fifty minutes of exercise performed in a given week, use of medication was decreased by 50 percent.[9]

He asks the group what they notice when they exercise.

"I get distracted," one chimes in.

"My mind clears up," another explains.

"It's hard to start," another confesses, "but I feel better at a certain point after doing it."

"That's a helpful thought," Egan interjects. "It's going to hurt when I go, but I will feel better after." Egan then reminds the men, "Do it, but don't overdo it; add a little bit at a time." She adds, "When you increase your exercise, you should only increase it by about 10 percent, not 50, not 100—10."

Every session includes a walk—a loop on the sidewalk around the facility. Today there's a slight drizzle, but that doesn't stop the group from moving. Ever so slowly, the six men and two caregivers walk around the Martinez campus. As we move, I talk with Vietnam veteran David Sanderson.

"It took me forty years to get in here," Sanderson tells me. For years, he says, he had been living with both physical and psychological pain. "I was a welder in the Navy during Vietnam," he recounts. "I worked with all kinds of stuff, lifted all kinds of weight. When you got hurt out there five hundred miles from shore, you couldn't do anything but carry on, which is what I did for the last forty years or so." His second wife finally had enough and insisted he get help.

When they return to the class, Egan asks how they feel. They all agree that exercise helps. They feel better. "So what can you do to make sure you keep walking?" Egan asks. "What would help you keep up with exercise and activity once you leave this class?"

One veteran says he will go to a class at the Mare Island CBOC.

Another suggests finding a walking group.

A third says it'll be useful to walk the dog.

Making a schedule, with specific times and days and hours—say, between nine and ten forty-five, someone else suggests.

Egan proposes that people in the group could team up with one another.

She then asks what could get in the way of exercise.

"Pretty much everything," one veteran admits.

"It's critical to prioritize exercise when your schedule changes," Egan advises.

What about thoughts that could get in the way? Chan asks the group.

"You're cold, it's wet, the weather."

Egan suggests that people could walk in the mall or even in Home Depot.

In an insightful comment, one veteran reveals a negative thought that gets in the way: "You can also feel defeated because you haven't done enough. A real workout has to involve working up a sweat, exhausting yourself. Now I realize I don't have to feel bad about just walking."

Yes, Egan agrees, any amount of movement is important.

Another veteran expresses frustration that people claim his pain is all in his head, that he's somehow faking it. To which Egan immediately responds, "I never think of pain as being in your head. Your brain is part of your body too. You may not have control over it, but it influences it."

As the class ends, one veteran raises his hand. "So what you're saying is that we may not be able to stop the stimulus, but we can change the response."

Chan beams his delight. "That's just what we want you to take from this class."

After observing the kinds of programs described here, it was hardly surprising that the RAND Corporation reported that VA pain management is superior to that provided in the private sector. "Interdisciplinary pain management continues to grow in the VA (as well as internationally) but is rare in the U.S. private sector where health care tends to be fragmented and truncated. VHA accounts for 40% of the U.S. interdisciplinary pain programs even though it serves 8% of the adult population," the RAND report noted.

"The VHA's superior quality of care results in part from its organizational ability to implement and monitor adherence to standards," it said. "When care is diffused across the community, quality lessens. Because the VHA is a single health care system . . . it has the advantage of a unified organizational structure, a single set of clinical practice guidelines, and policies and procedures that likely contribute to reducing variation across VISNs."[10] The private-sector health care system, constructed as it is of disconnected and competing insurers and providers, is incapable of providing this kind of oversight, accountability, and care coordination.

One day, just as I was about ready to conclude this chapter, I was walking down the hall at Fort Miley, heading for the canteen, when I overheard an older woman talking with what turned out to be her husband and her son, an Iraq veteran. "So you learn to relax every part of your body and just let the pain drain away? I wish I could learn to do that."

Curious, I stopped them and told them I couldn't help overhearing their conversation and that I was writing a book about VA health care. I asked the veteran if he was talking about the VA's integrated pain program.

"Yes," he said. "I feel like I'm finally getting out of pain, getting my life back. I feel like there's finally hope."

When Wounded Warriors Are Women

Caring for Female Veterans

Once a week, about ten women veterans gather in the Sacramento VA Medical Center for a yoga class and a group discussion led by social worker Rebecca Stallworth, who provides mental health services in the medical center's Women's Clinic. The women who come for yoga and conversation range in age from their early thirties to late sixties. They have served in Vietnam, in the United States, in Iraq, as nurses, clerks, secretaries, and mechanics in the Army, Navy, and Air Force. Many went to private-sector providers before they tried the VHA. "I went to one doctor, and he wanted to know why I didn't do my back exercises," Joan* says.

"They just don't get it," she adds. "In the military you learn to just suck it up—pain, emotional problems, whatever. Here, people get it; it's like there's an instant connection. We've all been down the same road, no matter where we started."

Maureen* says that when she came to the group, she was practically suicidal, a "real mess."

"This group," she says, "helped me get my life together. It helped with the PTSD I didn't even know I had."

Ellen* finds that yoga increases her bone density and helps her osteo-porosis.

Brenda* says the group and various other therapies keep her centered when she encounters someone who reminds her of the guy who raped her over and over again when she was in the service. Lily,* the youngest woman in the group, says equine therapy teaches her how to cope with other human beings after the sexual harassment she experienced in the Navy.

Many of these women also do individual and group therapy as well as mindfulness or walking meditation, massage, and empathetic touch, all of which help them manage stress and anger and control PTSD symptoms. They all say they could never afford these services if they weren't available at the VHA. Nor would they have the time to travel from one class to another across the Sacramento region. Here, they say, it's one-stop shop-ping: a therapy or group appointment, a medical exam, seeing a specialist, doing yoga, massage—all in one place, sometimes on the same day.

As they discuss their progress, Stallworth asks how many will be com-ing to the all-day retreat that will be held in several weeks in Placerville. The VA will hire a bus and transport the women to the site an hour away from the hospital where they can socialize and enjoy a variety of different spa-like services. When one of the women worries about how much it will cost, Stallworth explains that it won't cost them a cent. "Zero," she says. "You already served your country."

This is why, Maureen comments, "this group is more than just a group—it's the putty that makes it all stick together. We take care of each other, just like we did in the military."

Women's health has become another hot-button issue raised by crit-ics of the VA. The Iraq and Afghanistan Veterans of America (IAVA), for example, has assailed the VA for its failure to adequately serve women vet-erans.[1] In an op-ed in the *Philadelphia Inquirer*, Allison Jaslow, executive director of IAVA, slammed the VHA because "the very agency meant to acknowledge and serve veterans—falls short. At IAVA, we often hear from women who are 'welcomed' at their local VA hospital by staff addressing their husbands first. We hear from women who have to drive more than 40 miles for a medical checkup because one-third of VA medical centers don't have a gynecologist on staff."[2]

Jaslow's op-ed left the impression that the VHA has done—and con-tinues to do—little or nothing to provide health care to women veterans.

While it may be true that the VA could do more, as IAVA argues, it is certainly doing a great deal to catch up with the fact that the percentage of women in the military is growing. Rather than concentrating only on what the VA lacks, we also need to consider the progress it has made in caring for women veterans and the systemic obstacles it has to overcome as it attempts to reach them.

"Healthcare for Women Military Veterans," an article in the excellent four-volume series on the VA published by Praeger, reviews the history of women in the military dating back to the American War of Independence. Over the past two centuries, women have served in various capacities and conflicts. In 1943, with 280,000 women serving in the military—mostly as nurses and in clerical positions—Congress established the Women's Army Corps (WAC). The Navy established the Women Accepted for Volunteer Emergency Service (WAVES). Added to these were the Marine Corps Women's Reserve, the Coast Guard Women's Reserve (SPARS), and the Women Air Force Service Pilots (WASPs). This was followed by a push to recruit more women into the military in the Korean War and an even bigger push for the Vietnam War, where nearly seven thousand women served in Southeast Asia, mostly as nurses. Even though there were efforts to recruit and integrate women more fully into the military, it wasn't until 1979 that women who were in the WAC in World War II were granted veteran status.

After the Persian Gulf War, the Department of Defense opened up 90 percent of military occupations to women.[3] By 1994, when the United States instituted a ban on women serving in combat roles in the military, 14 percent of military personnel were women. President Obama officially lifted that ban in January 2013.[4] About 280,000 women served in Iraq and Afghanistan, some in combat roles. Today women make up 14 percent of the active component of the armed services and 18 percent of the reserve component. By the year 2020, it is estimated that women will account for 11 percent of the veteran population. As of 2015, five hundred thousand women had enrolled in the VA health system.[5]

Because of the huge changes in the number of women and roles they play in the military, the VHA has had to both fundamentally change and catch up. It has also had to provide for the needs of women veterans in spite of the fact that the system still serves a vast majority of men. The questions it has to cope with are ones like the following: If female veterans are only 14 percent of your patient population—not 50 percent, as is true in the private sector—does it make sense for VA hospitals to deliver babies or have expensive mammogram machines or even a full-time gynecologist on staff, particularly when half of women veterans live in nine states (California, Texas, Florida, Virginia, New York, Georgia, Pennsylvania, Ohio, and North Carolina)?[6] Or does it make more sense, at least in facilities that serve few women veterans, to pay for those services in the private sector? While it is beyond the scope of this book to answer these questions, let's look at how the VHA is dealing with women's needs today.

Over the past several decades, the VHA has created special women's health programs to accommodate women's primary care and mental health needs and accommodate others by paying for services in the private sector. Moreover, it has devoted a great many resources to trying to figure out how to do more outreach to women veterans and understand why women veterans may not make use of VHA services. For example, the VA recently began to explore the barriers to care for women veterans. Its 2015 report found that many of the women veterans who did not seek VHA care had little information about the system and were concerned about lack of female providers or female-only services beyond those offered by obstetricians and gynecologists. It is interesting, but perhaps not surprising, that many women veterans shared the same reluctance to seek care for mental health conditions as male veterans. Women veterans who had experienced military sexual trauma were much less likely to use the VHA than those who had not.[7] Like male veterans who have not been in combat, many female veterans feel that the VHA is for combat veterans only.

One of the most vexing problems in the provision of women's health care is the fact that, as we saw in chapter 2, so many women in the military have experienced military sexual trauma and do not want to be in a health care setting where they will encounter men who have served in the armed forces. Like many victims of trauma, these women are triggered by the sight of a bunch of guys whom they view not as patients but as potential perpetrators. In her comments at a mental health summit sponsored by the San Francisco–based veterans' advocacy organization Swords to Plowshares, Nidia Y. Holmes adamantly expressed her resistance to even stepping into a VHA facility. Holmes had been raped when she was in the Army.

In 2017, I spoke about the challenges facing the VHA at a Veterans for Peace Conference in Chicago. During the question period, a woman veteran who had clearly experienced some form of military sexual trauma spoke about the VA in a voice trembling with rage, fear, and anxiety. She said she wanted nothing to do with the military, with war, or with men. The VA owed her, she insisted. But she did not want to step into a VA facility to collect that debt. In fact, she wanted the assurance that she would not encounter any men when she connected with the health care system, inside or outside the VHA. Her demand? That she encounter only providers who are women, who only take care of women, and who guarantee that she will not encounter men in a medical waiting room.

All the women veterans I talked to wanted to be recognized as women. They were displeased, if not infuriated, when a clerk in a waiting room summoned Mr. Jones for the appointment of Ms. Jones or assumed that they were the wife, daughter, or friend of Mr. Jones. Not all, however, wanted to go to a gender-segregated women's health clinic or insisted on being cared for by a female provider. Representative of the myriad views on gender issues in the broader society, some women veterans scoff at those who want special treatment in what they describe as a female-only bubble, while others find that bubble a great source of comfort. I met one woman veteran sitting in the pleasant waiting room in Sacramento who had served as a secretary in Vietnam. She had gone to the VHA for many years and appreciated the fact that "it's like you are in your own little world. It's very calming."

Diane Reppun is a sixty-year-old retired lieutenant colonel in the Army who served in Iraq in 2009 and 2010, lives in Palo Alto, and works at the San Francisco VA Medical Center as a program analyst for the Office of Education. She is very pleased with the care she gets at the VHA in Palo Alto but does not use the Women's Clinic in any VHA facility. "I totally understand why women with military sexual trauma would choose to use gender-segregated services," Reppun says. She herself did not have that experience and was comfortable working in a unit with fifteen people, only two of whom were women. "If I was going to be segregated with only military women, that would seem to me to be an odd idea. I went through all of my pre- and in-country training basically living with thirteen men. Going to a hospital where there are mostly male veterans doesn't faze me at all. In some ways I still have that shared experience with them. What I find in the VA is the same kind of camaraderie I found in the military. You are in a waiting room or walk down the hall and see other veterans—sometimes someone you know—and you have a great time sharing stories with them."

Whether they want to use them or not, women veterans now have a choice—pun intended—within the VHA when it comes to their health. Each major medical center has dedicated and separately located women's primary and mental health clinics. In 2010 the VA set up a call center to urge women veterans to enroll in the VA. In 2013 the VA launched a special Women's Health Hotline, 1-855-VA-WOMEN, to answer information women might have about services, benefits, and other needed resources. Each major medical center has dedicated women's health outreach coordinators and a women veterans program manager.

When I visited the San Diego VA Medical Center in 2015, I met with social worker Jennifer Roberts, who told me how far the VHA has come over the past two decades. "Until recently, the population of women veterans was so small that there was just one person, a nurse-practitioner, in primary care who sort of did it on the side. There were special days when women were seen in primary care and they were the only ones in the waiting room."

That has all changed, Roberts was happy to report. "There are now three models of care VAs can adopt. Model 1 is a completely separate space, with separate brick and mortar. You get mammograms, gynecological appointments, primary care, mental health care. It is a haven for women's health, and there are no men at all.

"Model 2," Roberts continues, "is a separate but shared space, a special women's clinic in a separate wing, where women receive primary and mental health care as well as gynecological care. They walk down the same corridors as men, but they do not share waiting rooms or exam rooms with male veterans."

Then there is Model 3, where women's health is integrated into primary care, just like in any primary care practice. Female patients sit in the same waiting room and use the same exam rooms (although obviously not at the same time) as male patients. Every woman veteran is, however, assigned to a designated women's health care provider (who may be male) who has special training in women's health. (In VA CBOCs, one health care provider is required to have training in women's health.) Those providers learn how to do a Pap smear on a survivor of military sexual trauma. They are also trained to understand the special problems women veterans encountered in the military. "They have bladder issues because they had to hold their urine when on convoy and didn't have sanitary napkins or tampons on convoy," Roberts cites as only one example.

In San Diego, where there are many military bases and active-duty service members, Roberts also does a great deal of outreach to encourage women veterans to prepare to sign up with the VA before they even leave the military. Roberts goes to a variety of meetings like Individual Ready Reserve musters or Yellow Ribbon events for families who have a service member deployed or coming back and need resources. Her goal is to find active-duty service members or reservists who might not identify as veterans when they leave the service. They think you have to be a guy to be a veteran, or in combat, or in combat and injured, she tells me. These women may not know that all post-9/11 veterans get five years of care at the VHA, no questions asked.

When I spoke with Megan Gerber, medical director of women's health in the Boston VA Healthcare System and lead in women's health for VISN 1, she explained that in 1994, the VA was one of the first systems in the country to develop women's health centers that gave gender-specific care from mostly female providers. The VA has a national mini-residency to train or retrain providers in women's health. This is usually held in Orlando, Florida, but is also available through the VA's virtual learning eHealth University, or VeHU. The VA, she went on to explain, has developed a military culture training requirement that tries to find out where veterans served and what major medical challenges patients are experiencing. Many women in the conflicts in the Middle East suffered from Gulf War syndrome. Before the combat exclusion policy was lifted, of course, they were not allowed into combat positions. Even before the ban was lifted, she points out, women served in those positions in Iraq and Afghanistan because there were no clear frontlines. "Women who were driving trucks were in combat zones. I have seen patients who had to clean body parts out of trucks, which is no different than being on the front lines."

The women seen in her clinic, Gerber says, are mostly between the ages of forty-five and sixty-four. The VA also sees patients who are eighteen to forty-four years old. For women veterans of reproductive age, the VA provides maternity care, contraception, a week of newborn care after delivery, and breast pumps. Since 50 percent of all pregnancies in the United States are unintended, the VA also provides preconception counseling.

While maternity care is provided in non-VA facilities in the community, the VA has a maternity coordinator in each large facility or VISN to make sure that maternity care is completely paid for and of the highest quality.

The VA also helps women stop smoking and reviews medications, particularly to make sure that a woman who is pregnant is not on any medications that could harm the fetus. Gerber believes that the VA is good for women not only because of its dedicated, gender-specific attention and services but because VA primary care and mental health providers have smaller patient loads and thus can devote more attention to the problems of female veterans, with which they are far more familiar than providers in the private sector. "Veterans get more time with us because our patient panels are smaller. We have follow-up visits of thirty minutes on a routine basis, rather than ten or fifteen."

The problems the VA has to overcome are those that also pertain to male veterans: reluctance to seek help and misperceptions about who is and who is not a "real" veteran. Added to these are ones specifically created by military sexual trauma. Gerber goes to great lengths to explain that military sexual trauma is not a percentage service rating—it's a yes. Yes, you are immediately service connected and at 100 percent. It's an exposure, like Agent Orange, she explains to women veterans, which they should acknowledge and for which they should seek treatment. "Many women veterans screen negative for MST or PTSD because they suppress their feelings," she says. "They choose not to report it. Women in the military have been socialized to be tough, to be even tougher and better than men. This is so widespread that they may feel they have to accept MST. They don't realize it's not just a mental health condition. It's the result of a crime. Our problem isn't overreporting—it's underreporting."

This is why, Gerber says, it's so important for women veterans to be seen by VA primary care providers who are expert in their problems and have the sensitivity to ferret them out. When people are reluctant to admit to a mental health problem like PTSD or military sexual trauma, they aren't going to bop into a mental health provider's office and begin to talk. "We PCPs may be the first person to hear their story. That's why we have to be trauma informed. It's almost like taking the kind of universal precautions you use when cleaning your hands. We have to provide trauma-informed care, never rush through a pelvic exam, always be attentive."

Gerber, who worked for fourteen years outside the VHA in the Cambridge Health Alliance, smiles as she concludes, "I have never seen anything like this. I have never seen such attention to privacy. It is way better for women."

According to a 2018 article in the *Federal Practitioner* by VHA psychologist Russell Lemle, "Each VA facility has a dedicated MST Coordinator, mandatory MST training for all primary and mental health care providers, free MST-related treatment and MST outreach efforts. All veterans enrolled in the VA are screened for experiences of MST, and tailored treatment plans are created for survivors in need of care. Over 1.3 million outpatient MST-related mental health visits were provided to veterans with a positive MST screen in FY17, a 9% increase from the prior year."[8]

When I met with Women's Health providers in San Francisco, Sacramento, and Las Vegas, they outlined their own commitment to the special needs of women veterans. In Las Vegas, for example, primary care providers and a urogynecologist escorted me around the beautiful new Women's Health Clinic with its serene exam rooms and beautifully decorated waiting room. Charu Gupta, a urogynecologist, and Sarah Zinati, a family medicine physician, told me about the military sexual trauma specialist who works in the clinic two days a week, the therapist who specializes in pelvic pain, and the cancer specialist who comes to the clinic once a week. Since 50 percent of women veterans (compared to 30 percent in the private sector) have mental health diagnoses, the clinic also employs two mental health professionals and a full-time pharmacist. Gupta was proud of the fact that the VA employs a number of urogynecologists like herself who can specifically target the kind of pelvic-floor disorders from which many women suffer. They are experts in problems with bladder control, bladder prolapse, and other conditions. Gupta herself has done special training in reconstructive surgery.

Stallworth, the social worker who guided me at the Sacramento VA medical center, pointed out how carefully the Women's Clinic in Sacramento, with its soothing décor and calming art, was designed. "We have women with MST," she says. "So sometimes a routine pelvic exam can trigger something. The majority of [Operation Enduring Freedom, Operation Iraqi Freedom] veterans have MST but won't tell you about it. Many of them just want to put it all behind them." This understandable impulse does not, however, make military sexual trauma disappear, and one of

Stallworth's main concerns is helping women talk about their problems and get treatment for them. The Sacramento VA Women's Health program is, in fact, conducting research to do outreach to the many women veterans who live in the surrounding rural areas.

Many of the women veterans I spoke with said they were impressed with the efforts the VA has made to deal with their specific concerns and special problems. Although Reppun does not use the women's clinic and sees a male primary care physician, she says she has gotten great care as a woman and a veteran from the VA. In 2010, while still on active duty, she came back from Iraq with a shoulder injury. She spent six weeks in what is called a Warrior Transition Unit at Fort Dix, New Jersey, and then another in the Seattle–Tacoma area. Then she was sent back home to California via a community-based transition unit out of Sacramento. She eventually had shoulder surgery that was paid for through her Tricare military insurance.

"As soon as I was off active duty, and after my surgery was completed and rehab finished, I immediately went to the VA for my care. In fact, before I was even off active duty, I had my VA medical evaluation, and they rated my combined service-connected disabilities at 60 percent. This made me eligible for complete care at the VA, not just service-connected injury care," Reppun recounts.

"I was screened for PTSD. Although I was asked about any blasts or blows to the head, I was not screened for TBI because I had nothing to report."

Reppun is being treated for asthma, which was a result of atmospheric conditions in Camp Victory, where she was billeted on the outskirts of Baghdad, near the airport. She also suffers from multiple joint issues from thirty years of running and marching. She just got a knee replacement at the VHA.

"I have a primary care physician," she says. "He treats me like every other primary care physician I've had. He tells me when I am due for a mammogram or Pap smear and puts it in the computer, and I get a call to schedule an appointment. Originally, when I started with the VA, I could call Stanford, schedule an appointment for a mammogram. They would send the result to my primary care physician. The last time he said I needed a mammogram, the doctor told me I'd have to go through Choice program. I had to wait to get a phone call from TriWest [the program's West Coast third-party administrator]. They spent a lot of time questioning me about when I was free for an appointment and said they'd have to call me back when [an] appointment was available in my area. I explained that I always got my mammogram at Stanford. Well, they told me, maybe I could get my mammogram at Stanford and maybe not."

Reppun decided to take matters into her own hands and call Stanford, and she was told to come in the next day, which she did. She then went on vacation and came home several weeks later, only to receive a call from TriWest telling her a mammogram appointment had been scheduled for her in San Jose for several weeks later. She said thanks, but no thanks. She was never sent a bill. The next time she had her mammogram at Stanford, she received a bill for $269, which she has been fighting for the last eight months.

Her experience with the Choice program, she says, has not been reassuring. She is also worried that she will not be able to receive care at the VHA for her newly diagnosed sleep apnea because the test used to diagnose her specific version of the problem and the equipment needed to solve it are not available there. Stanford again is the fallback. Under Choice, however, she has been informed that, once tested at Stanford, she will have to stay at Stanford for her treatment and sleep apnea device (CPAP machine), even though that treatment and device are available at the VHA.

More disturbing, she said, is she was not able to get an appointment at Stanford before her knee surgery, in spite of the fact that her recovery would have been enhanced if she had had the device before, not after, the operation.

"I couldn't get the test in the private sector until after the surgery. So I risked not recovering as well. None of this makes much sense to me. Why San Jose for a mammogram?" she asks with surprise and frustration. "I've never been there. It's crazy. Why is Congress so intent on sending us to the private sector when the answer should be to increase the services and capabilities of the VA, not ship me out to a bunch of disconnected providers who never talk to each other?"

Gwen Shepherd is a fifty-five-year-old African American veteran who was in the Air Force Reserve and did her military service from 1980 to 1989. She was also commissioned in the Navy Reserves as a civil engineering officer. In Iraq from July to November 2003, she officially retired from the military in 2009. She went to the Clement J. Zablocki VA Medical Center in Milwaukee because she was having memory and eye issues as well as a lot of joint pain, she tells me as we talk over the phone. The biggest problem, she says, was her memory. "Here I was, forty-two years old, and I didn't think I should have these memory issues like I was having. I was leaving food in the oven and burning up my dinner. I was forced to write everything down, or I would forget."

Given her engineering background, this was, she recounts, very unusual, and she did not like it one bit. "I was dealing with a lot of computer coding in my civilian job." The VA set Shepherd up with a neurologist who found out that she had a disease whose name she can barely remember or pronounce. But, she tells me, the long and short of it is that her brain cells are dying. She is now classified as having Gulf War syndrome. She also had an episode of total left-side numbness and bad vertigo. She was hospitalized at the Milwaukee VA medical center, where she was diagnosed with cervical spinal cord compression. She was also diagnosed with a rare form of lupus, which may have been a result of toxic exposures to the burn pits in Iraq. None of her care is given in a women's clinic. No way, she says, does she want to go there.

She is also getting therapy for mental health issues "When I came back from Iraq, I had a lot of anger issues," Shepherd tells me. "I was basically pissed off at the world because of my declining health. This was ending my career in the military. Also, a lot of stuff happened in Iraq, so there was just a lot of stuff piling up." Shepherd began doing therapy with VA psychologist Catherine Coppolillo and then joined a group the therapist runs. She does sports with the Wounded Warrior Program. "I won't say things are perfect," Shepherd concludes, "but they are so much better."

"When I started at the VA, I couldn't stand it. I didn't feel they were doing enough taking care of me, one, as a woman, and two, as a combat vet. They would call me Mr. Shepherd, and I would think, 'How can you take care of me if you can't read on my chart that I'm a female?'"

Then, Shepherd says, she got hooked up with a fantastic primary care physician and was correctly diagnosed. "It was like a lightbulb switched on. This place ain't that bad; you have to know how to work the system. As I look back on it, there's no place in the civilian world other than the VA that can give me the integrated care I need. Trust me," she says, and I do. "I have screamed bloody murder about the VA and how it sucks. But it works because I am so pushy."

In spite of any problems she has had at the VA, she is totally opposed to privatization. "Even though people are pissed off, you can get what you need at the VA. Here's why. I can go to the VA and go to the canteen and sit next to a buddy. A buddy will come up to you and start talking, and sometimes that is more therapeutic than going to a mental health appointment. That vet sitting next to you is sometimes a Vietnam vet. They've been there, they've done that, they know things to say and not to say, what will keep you calm and keep you going. They will give you advice, help you negotiate the system. You are not going to have that in a civilian hospital."

7

Mental Health
the Way It Should Be

I met Lanier Summerall, a psychiatrist who is now deputy chief of staff at the the Ralph H. Johnson VA Medical Center in Charleston, South Carolina, in the summer of 2014, when she was head of mental health at the White River Junction VA Medical Center in Vermont. The main hospital there is a brick building that sits on a hill above the junction of Interstate Highways 89 and 91. The entrance boasts imposing white columns that seem to come straight out of *Gone with the Wind*. Summerall, a trim woman in her late forties with shoulder-length blond hair, has worked for the VHA for several decades. As we sit in her office in the back of the hospital's main building, she says she is consistently astonished and disturbed by the kind of press the VHA now receives. She outlines facts that are so often lost in the current political and media narrative.

"We have a breadth of psychosocial services under one roof that is unequaled even in the most well-resourced private-sector environment," she notes. "If a person is homeless, they can get help with a variety of agencies to get housing. If they are having trouble getting a job, we have supportive employment and compensated work therapy. We have residential programs for PTSD and substance abuse and for chronic, hard-to-treat psychiatric illnesses like bipolar disorder or schizophrenia."

This integrated system of services, Summerall continues, is critical because of the various issues VHA patients face: "Our patients have lifestyle problems, relationship problems, work problems." A lot of the patients, she explains, cannot possibly coordinate their own care or take responsibility for self-care, which is the mantra in the private sector. "The paramount thing for these people is that everybody here knows each other," she says. "We are all on the same team in the same place."

She gives me a typical example of how this integrated care works. "A thirty-three-year-old veteran comes in after two tours in the National Guard in Iraq and Afghanistan. He lives in a remote cabin in the woods of Vermont or New Hampshire. He is preoccupied with intrusive thoughts and flashbacks, is having trouble with his marriage, and has firearms in the home. When he gets into a fight with his wife, he pulls out his gun and is threatening to her and his kids."

He is not, however, enrolled in VA services, Summerall explains. He thought he didn't need it. He heard all the bad press. He feels that he shouldn't hog the benefits because other vets—the ones with no arms or legs or with TBIs—are much worse off. You name it, Summerall says, he has an excuse.

"But finally," she continues, "because the VHA in Vermont has a unique program with the National Guard, he is contacted by an outreach worker and admits that he needs help. Within a few hours of coming to the VHA, he sees a primary care physician, who immediately refers him to a mental health practitioner who is just down the hall. He does not need to get a referral to a psychiatrist or psychologist from a PCP, which he would probably just throw away.

"In this case the veteran needs to be hospitalized on an inpatient psychiatric unit. He also needs evidence-based therapy for PTSD. He is immediately hospitalized with no dictates—the kind that are notorious in the private sector—about the length of his stay. When he leaves the inpatient psychiatric unit, he can also go to a residential recovery unit. And if he has a problem with substance abuse, he can be admitted to a drug-and-alcohol program. We have the only system of integrated mental health and primary care in the country."

The VHA System

This unique integrated system provides not only discrete clinical services but embeds patients in a community of care. This community of care does more than connect patients to clinicians and then to the appropriate treatments and facilities. It also connects patients to one another as well as to the services, resources, and groups that will help them live better and more fulfilling lives. And it connects caregivers with one another so they can learn, teach, research, and care for the broader community of VHA patients as well as each other.

As Harold Kudler, the VA's chief mental health consultant, explains, "In our programs veterans don't only see doctors or therapists. We make sure that they have resources outside of hospitals or clinics or mental health programs. We also make sure their families have the resources, jobs, and housing that support a healthy family. This is instrumental to ensuring healthy outcomes whether or not they end up in a formal mental health program."

Mental health providers make sure that a veteran's physical problems are also addressed. "I remember years ago taking care of a World War II veteran," Kudler tells me. "With his PTSD foremost in my mind, I asked him how he was." The seventy-five-year-old gentleman, Kudler says, barely mentioned his PTSD, which he said was under control. What was really driving him crazy was the excruciating pain he was feeling from a tooth that was crumbling. "So I got on the phone and called some dentists and some county dental programs and finally found out that we had a mobile dental program in the VA. I called and made an appointment for him and made sure he got there. Some people wouldn't consider that to be 'mental health care' or the job of a psychiatrist or doctor. But to me that was the essence of mental health and health care."

And it's not just a matter of serving individual veterans; it's also about serving their families, Kudler says. Kudler and Army colonel Rebecca I. Porter recently wrote an article titled "Building Communities of Care for Military Children and Families." Colonel Porter, former director of psychological health for the Army, is now commander of Dunham US Army Health Clinic in Carlisle Barracks, Pennsylvania, which provides primary health care for approximately twelve thousand students at the US Army War College.

In their article, they note that "57 percent of active duty troops who served in 2011 were the children of current or former active-duty or reserve service members."[1] Their current problems may have been connected to the fact that their father, mother, grandfather, uncle, brother, or sister had unaddressed mental health problems. More important, if their current mental health problems aren't dealt with, this can have a serious impact on their own children.

"From a humanitarian point of view, it's important that we help our veterans," Kudler says. "From a societal point of view, it's critical that we honor their service by serving them. And from a purely instrumental point of view, if so many military families produce the next generation of service members, we really want them to have a good start in life."

To do this, the VHA provides a vast array of mental and behavioral health services. As of this writing, the VHA has over eight thousand beds in short-term residential programs. These programs for people having serious difficulty with mental or behavioral health issues are the descendants of the old post–Civil War soldiers' homes.

The VHA mental health system is particularly known for its use of evidence-based therapies, gold-standard treatments whose effectiveness is confirmed in a variety of scientific studies. These treatments include the use of traditional psychiatric medications, individual and group psychotherapy sessions, methods like prolonged exposure therapy and cognitive behavioral therapy for PTSD, and a variety of other treatments proven to be of help for mental and behavioral health problems. In 2014, RAND conducted a study comparing VA mental and behavioral health programs with those in the private sector. To find out whether private-sector providers were, in fact, "ready to serve" the nation's veterans, the study focused on two common problems from which veterans suffer: PTSD and major depressive disorder (MDD). In a startling finding, RAND documented that only 30 percent of private-sector clinicians (including social workers, psychologists, and psychiatrists) reported using evidence-based therapies to treat their patients who suffered from PTSD and MDD, compared with 75 percent of VHA clinicians who used them. To put it another way, VHA clinicians were two and a half times more likely to use evidence-based therapies than those in the private sector.[2]

The VHA is also using and researching integrative therapies, like yoga, mindfulness, therapeutic touch, and massage, among many others.

Although one doesn't necessarily imagine veterans using the kinds of therapy associated more with Berkeley hippies or power yoga–crazed millennials, in every VHA medical center or CBOC that I visited, I found groups gathering to do yoga or meditation. At the Sacramento VHA Medical Center, I attended a yoga session with nine female veterans from the ages of thirty-one to seventy who had been deployed in conflicts from Vietnam to Afghanistan. These were gritty, working-class women who said they would have never considered taking a yoga class outside of the VHA, even if they could have afforded the fifteen-to-eighteen-dollar price of admission. Yet here they were, doing downward-facing dog, if they could, or adapting postures if they couldn't.

Not only were they enrolled in yoga; some were doing therapeutic touch and massage. One African American thirty-one-year-old who had served in the Navy, where she was a victim of constant sexual harassment, was going to equine therapy. The VHA wasn't paying for the treatments because they had not been officially vetted but had linked the veteran with a community group that provided funding for the therapy. "Because of my family background and what happened in the military, relationships are very difficult for me," the woman told me. "I have to learn to deal with boundaries and do things differently." Working with horses rather than with people, who "are constantly in my face," she said, is helping her learn to cope.

These various VHA therapies are increasingly delivered via telehealth, which is of particular help to those veterans who live in rural counties that are mental health deserts. As we will see in a subsequent chapter, the VHA has a robust suicide prevention program in all its major medical centers and trains every VHA employee to recognize and respond to the signs of suicidality in veteran patients. Its national Veterans Crisis Line responds to thousands of calls a year and, although it is still growing, has successfully prevented the suicides of thousands of veterans.

In a community-of-care model, mental and behavioral health problems cannot be segregated from physical and social ones, and one of the VHA's most significant innovations is its extended care program that targets aging veterans through geriatrics, home-based primary care, VHA nursing homes, and palliative care. For younger veterans, VHA mental health programs also connect them to employment support and help with housing and the kind of readjustment problems that veterans have when they return to higher education following separation from service.

Whereas private-sector mental health care often comes with strict limits on availability, access, and duration, the programs available in the VHA may continue over the course of the veteran's lifetime. Some mental health services include family members if the veteran's behavior has a significant impact on his or her family or if family problems significantly impact the veteran patient.

The VA has a Comprehensive Assistance for Family Caregivers program that provides help for caregivers of seriously ill post-9/11 veterans. In 2014, when the RAND Corporation conducted a systematic study of those who provide care for current or former members of the military, it found that of the 5.5 million military caregivers in the United States, over 19 percent were caring for people who had served after 9/11. Unlike caregivers of veterans who had served earlier, these caregivers were younger—sometimes much younger. They were also providing less assistance with activities of daily living and more help with emotional and behavioral problems. That's because so many post-9/11 veterans had problems with PTSD, TBI, or substance abuse.

The program now provides these caregivers with financial stipends, health care insurance, training needed to provide effective and safe care, respite care for themselves, and mental health services and counseling.[3] The program helps caregivers like thirty-five-year-old Deborah Ramirez,* whose husband Doug was thrown out of his Humvee in Iraq and suffers from a traumatic brain injury and PTSD. Doug has since coped with intense anger, been cuffed and jailed after getting into repeated fights, and is constantly assailed by suicidal feelings. To blunt all this, he has resorted to the usual toxic brew of drugs and alcohol.

Although Deborah told me she swore she would never date someone who had a drinking problem, she confesses that she violated her golden rule because she felt so connected to this wounded warrior. The caregiver support program has helped her survive what she realizes may be a lifelong commitment to caring for her husband. She says she learned a great deal about how to provide needed care to her husband. More important, "I learned that I have to care for myself," and how to put theory into practice over the long term.

Most impressive is the way the VHA has, for many veterans and family members, destigmatized mental illness through its integrated model, staff training, and Make the Connection program.[4] This national mental health

awareness campaign, with its own Facebook page and website, has produced over four hundred videos of veterans talking about their experience
of mental illness. Each story is unique, but their take-home message is the
same: do not be afraid to get help. Seeking help is not a sign of weakness,
cowardice, or failure; it is a sign of strength.

When the message takes and veterans do come for help, the results,
which have been well documented, are impressive. Between 2000 and
2010, suicide rates for veterans using VA care decreased, whereas rates
for veterans not using VA care increased. By 2010, veterans using VA care
had much lower rates of suicide than those not using VA care. Veterans
with serious mental illness who get VA health care (not just mental health
care) live longer than persons with serious mental illness in the general US
population. Here are some of the reasons why:

- The VA practitioners were more likely than non-VA practitioners to
  follow recommended care guidelines for depression.
- The VA outperformed the private sector in adhering to quality guidelines for prescription of antidepressants during the initial, early, and
  maintenance phases of treatment.
- Compared with individuals in private plans, VA patients with a major
  depressive disorder were more than twice as likely to receive appropriate initial medication treatment and appropriate long-term treatment.
- VA patients with schizophrenia were more likely to receive an antipsychotic medication than those in the private sector and were more than
  twice as likely to receive appropriate initial medication treatment.
- Compared with non-VA facilities, the VA's women's substance use
  programs offered a significantly greater number of testing and assessment services, addiction pharmacotherapies, and recommended
  key ancillary services, including assistance obtaining social services,
  housing, and transportation.[5]

Understanding Military Culture and Socialization

If the VHA has produced such stellar results, it's not only because therapists have mastered the latest evidence-based treatments. VHA therapists have also mastered what is known as "cultural competence":

understanding and being sensitive to the cultural context and real-life experiences that have shaped their patients. As the RAND study *Ready to Serve* states, "The degree to which providers are sensitive to the unique needs and relevant issues of concern within the veteran population . . . can facilitate provider's ability to deliver patient-centered care and develop effective therapeutic rapport."[6]

When RAND assessed cultural competency and sensitivity in VA or military staff, it found that 70 percent had high scores in this area. When it came to private-sector therapists in the TRICARE network, the score dropped precipitously (to 24 percent) and plummeted even further (to 8 percent) for those private-sector mental health providers with no military or TRICARE affiliation.[7]

VHA clinicians are unique in their ability to navigate the tricky psychological and social dynamics that may produce a complex constellation of anger, hostility, alienation, and immense need—accompanied by a terrible fear of vulnerability—that is common in the population of veterans the VHA serves. Kudler's contributions to the volume on military children and families are only one example of decades of research into the realities of veterans, active-duty service members, and their families.

Another example is *Fields of Combat* by Erin Finley, a medical anthropologist who works at the South Texas Veterans Health Care System in San Antonio. Using research that was conducted with veterans at the South Texas VA, Finley considers the impact of culture, ethnicity, and gender on patients'—and their families'—experience of, and willingness to seek, treatment for PTSD. She illuminates "how veterans and family members understand early symptoms—as illness, moral failing, or bad behavior—influences what they do about them, whether demanding behavioral change, seeking treatment, or falling into negative cycles of conflict, self-blame, or substance abuse."

Explaining why anthropologists are so important to health care, Finley observes, "As healthcare delivery becomes increasingly complex, pulling in social scientists trained to think about how individuals, teams, and organizations work together only makes sense. Anthropologists in particular have wonderful tools for examining how people work together (or don't!), why and how change happens (or doesn't!), and what the implications of change are likely to be for all the stakeholders involved. It also turns out that qualitative methodologies like interviewing and observing individuals and groups can make a world of difference in explaining what all the big data findings actually mean. We are awash in performance measures and other metrics describing care and quality and access, but it's often difficult to understand their implications without solid grounding in what's happening in real time on the ground."

Unlike most private-sector health care systems, the VA employs about sixty anthropologists.[8] These social scientists do research on everything from why veterans may not take prescribed medicines to how effective teams function or how veterans with spinal cord injuries form social networks that help them find employment. The VA plays such an important role in utilizing the knowledge and skills of medical anthropologists that *Annals of Anthropological Practice* did a special issue on anthropology at the VA in 2014. As Elisa Sobo explained in an article, "Anthropologists employed by the VA are responsible for some of the most important and actionable anthropologically informed health research today. Far from being a marginal pursuit, VA anthropology is in fact a generative force for medical anthropology and, indeed, the discipline as a whole."[9]

Anger Management

Every health system has its problem with angry patients. In the VHA the problem may be even worse. That's because the VHA cares for more mentally ill patients than the average private-sector provider. Because of the wars in Iraq and Afghanistan, with their signature injury of TBI, often coupled with PTSD, veterans may have more difficulty controlling their behavior. In a recent study of 889 patients who were referred to the Prevention and Management of Disruptive Behavior (PMDB) program, examples of this kind of behavior included "setting a hospital bed on fire, pulling a fire alarm, throwing a chair through a window, threatening lawsuits or to have people fired."

In March 2018, a veteran of the conflict in Iraq who suffered from severe PTSD was told he could no longer remain in a community-based, not-for-profit program called Pathway Home, in Yountville, California. In retaliation he shot and killed three women who worked for the program before also killing himself. One of the victims was a thirty-two-year-old VA psychologist, Jennifer Gonzales, who was six months pregnant.[10]

This was sadly not an isolated incident. In January 2015, a VA psychologist was killed by an angry veteran employee in El Paso.[11] The following December, a seventy-seven-year-old veteran went for an appointment with a nurse-practitioner at the Denver VA Medical Center. As soon as he entered the room, he pulled out a handgun and threatened the nurse, holding her hostage in the small exam room. Fortunately, the nurse—as well as VA security—de-escalated the situation, and no one was hurt. A subsequent investigation revealed that the veteran, who brought extra ammunition with him, planned to shoot at the ceiling and had hoped that the VA police would come and shoot him, a phenomenon known as "suicide by cop."[12] The fact that no one was hurt was not a happy coincidence.

As Kathleen McPhaul, then chief occupational consultant at the VA, told me, both the nurse-practitioner and VA police involved in the incident had been trained in a nationwide VHA program designed to teach health care staff at every level how to deal with angry, aggressive, and potentially dangerous veterans. When I was recently waiting to talk to a physician at Fort Miley, I heard a loud noise—a chair being thrown across the room—and a veteran shouting a barrage of unprintables at a provider who seemed to be desperately trying to help him. This very large man stormed down the hall, continuing to curse just like what he had been—a Marine. Like all health care personnel, VHA employees wear a lanyard holding their name tags. The VHA lanyard has a plastic clip on the back of the neck so that if pulled by an angry patient, family member, or even employee, the lanyard will unclasp and cannot be used as a weapon.

Although more hospitals and health care institutions are taking violence against the workforce more seriously, the VHA's approach to this problem is both systematic and system-wide. That is in part because, when dealing with what is now referred to as disruptive patients, private-sector institutions have an option that is unavailable to the VHA. Private-sector providers—whether hospitals or physicians and other clinicians—can and do routinely "fire" patients who are uncivil, threatening, or physically violent. A federal regulation prohibits the VHA from firing or refusing to care for veteran patients. The VA can "limit the time, place, and/or manner of providing services to violent and disruptive patients," but it "must continue to offer the full range of medical services to which a Veteran is eligible."

Because of this, the VHA has tried to develop consistent standards across the system to define exactly what constitutes disruptive behavior, as well as programs to prevent and manage it. The result is the PMDB four-level curriculum and train-the-trainers program that helps people to understand the kinds of stressors that produce violent behavior and to develop a keen awareness and sensitivity to the kinds of situations that would produce and exacerbate such behavior. All VHA medical centers have Workplace Violence Prevention Committees and coordinators.

Michael Drexler, a psychologist who is coordinator for the Workplace Violence Prevention Committee at the San Francisco VA Health Care System, described how the program works not only at Fort Miley but throughout the country. As we sat in his small office in Building Eight, which houses the system's behavioral health programs, Drexler, a white-haired man in his late fifties, outlined the particular problems he and others deal with.

"At the VA," he says, "we don't deny care. We have to make sure that veterans aren't the only ones who are safe. Staff have to be safe as well. We have a Disruptive Behavior Committee to which veterans who exhibit challenging behaviors are referred. The committee has conducted surveys of employees to ascertain staff perceptions of threats and contributors to threats and is currently adding surveys and interviews of veterans to determine the same thing." This could include not only the obvious physical assault but sending threatening letters or e-mails, leaving thirty to forty intimidating voice mails, and being verbally abusive or in other ways threatening. The group uses an evidence-based threat assessment to evaluate static (a history of incarceration) and dynamic risk factors, which could include homelessness or recent history of assaultive behavior. The system also collects information on the number, location, and nature of behavioral incidents throughout the catchment area. Based on this data, the workplace behavioral risk assessment determines the upper level of PMDB needed.

Drexler says that, in his experience, the VHA is ahead of the game when it comes to preventing and managing workplace violence in several ways. "Every intervention is carefully coordinated," Drexler says. "The level of training [that] staff need is logically determined. Moreover, everything is subjected to ergonomic analysis and testing to make sure every move and activity is safe for both patient and staff."

Points of Entry

As we shall see in the next three chapters, through years of research and practice, VHA therapists have developed many ways to do their complex work, which veterans can access through multiple points of entry. A veteran who decides he wants to seek out mental health treatment can call Behavioral Health Services directly. He will then be referred to the mental and behavioral health access clinic, where he will be evaluated and referred to the appropriate services. Another veteran can go to a primary care provider for help with physical problems, where she will be screened for PTSD and depression. As I have mentioned earlier, the veteran can talk to a primary care provider who will provide a warm handoff to a mental health provider embedded in the clinic. If the problem is more serious, the veteran will be referred to an access clinic and sent to General Outpatient Psychiatric Services for ongoing treatment.

At Fort Miley, for example, I sat in on a meeting between a psychiatric resident and a Korean War veteran who had suffered from schizophrenia for years. The resident, who was being supervised by his colleagues, had finally succeeded in getting him a spot in the California state veterans' home in Yountville. The veteran, stooped over from age and weighted down with decades of hallucinatory imaginings, said that he was eager to go to the veterans' home but at the same time indicated he was terrified that any move toward the positive would trigger an attack in which North Koreans would swoop in and carry him off and hold him hostage. Over countless sessions his therapists tried to help him overcome his fears so that he would be able to live out his life with some semblance of serenity.

Veterans can enter the mental health and primary care system through the emergency room if they are experiencing a crisis. If that crisis requires hospitalization, many large VA medical centers have psychiatric inpatient units where the veteran can be treated. Once discharged from the hospital, the patient will be given a speedy appointment with a mental health practitioner and intensive monitoring. Psychiatrist Thomas Neylan at the San Francisco VA Health Care System says that this kind of immediate follow-up is very important.

"People who are discharged from an inpatient setting are very vulnerable," says Neylan. "Epidemiological studies have documented that during this transitional period between hospitalization and seeing an outpatient provider is a time when suicides can occur. So we have people who call the patient very quickly after discharge to remind them about their upcoming appointments and make sure they are all right."

As we've seen in the last chapter, female veterans, whose numbers are increasing, also have special mental health programs located in the women's health clinics or as part of other programs that the VHA has opened. These programs are particularly important for women who have suffered military sexual trauma and find it difficult, if not impossible, to sit in a waiting room with a group of male vets.

And finally, since the 1970s, the VA has funded Vet Centers that function as an alternative mental health service within the VA. Vet Centers were formally established by Congress in 1979 to help Vietnam veterans who had readjustment problems. Today the VA funds three hundred Vet Centers across the nation. These are part of, but not located on, VHA campuses, and the same eligibility requirements that govern VHA enrollment don't apply to Vet Center patients. Any veteran who served in combat, experienced military sexual trauma, delivered medical or mortuary services in a combat zone, or "served as a member of an unmanned aerial vehicle crew that provided direct support to operations in a combat zone or area of hostility" is eligible for services at Vet Centers, regardless of VA status. Vet Centers also provide counseling for family members if this will help with a veteran's readjustment. Both immediate and extended family members of a service member who is killed while on active duty can also get bereavement counseling at Vet Centers.[13]

As Venia Honick, a veteran and a team leader at the Honolulu Vet Center, explained to me when I visited in 2014, the Vet Center specializes in readjustment counseling for combat vets as well as their immediate and even extended families in cases of bereavement. Veterans can go to a Vet Center, which are mostly staffed by veterans themselves, if they have marital conflict, sexual trauma, or other problems.

Vet Centers can access the VHA's electronic medical records, but the VHA cannot access the Vet Centers' medical records. Because Vet Centers are connected to, but set apart from, VA clinics and medical center campuses, veterans who are wary of the VA or the government, or both, often feel more comfortable going to a Vet Center than to a VHA mental health facility. This distrust is particularly acute with Vietnam veterans who had bad experiences at the VA when returning from the war and connect the modern VHA with the VA of fifty years ago.

"You have Vietnam vets who never wanted to go on sick call when they were in the military and who, when they got out, just suffered through it and tried to constantly outrun it," Honick told me. "They go through their whole lives and just keep pushing through, and then suddenly they are facing retirement or have retired, and it just hits them because they are no longer working, and the sadness, or depression, or recognition of PTSD finally surfaces. They find caring and help at the Vet Center, which opens the door to VHA treatment as well." Honick recalled a veteran she cared for who had hypertension and heart problems and type 2 diabetes on top of his mental health problems. "I encouraged him to go up to the VHA to be evaluated, and he reluctantly did," she said. "He came back and reported that the doctor there could not have been more caring."

For veterans with mental health problems, the VHA offers not only accurate diagnosis and treatment but is literally a haven in what many perceive to be a heartless world. "When you go into the VHA, it's like you're returning to military culture. You know that people understand you, that they know who you are and how you think," Jerome Serdinsky explains. "My doctors know who I am. I go with my wife to the private-sector doctor, and sometimes it's like she has to remind them of who she is. We've been asked to go up to the Medical College of Wisconsin and sit with these medical students in classes, and it's all so robotic. Patient A has Problem B, and for that you do C or D. But Patient A is a person. They ask us to remind them of that, that we are people. At the VHA you go in, and you feel more at home. It's the only place I feel safe."

8

Unpacking PTSD

From Diagnosis to Effective Treatment

In 1966, when Louis Kern turned eighteen and got his draft notice, he knew exactly what that meant—ending up in the Army and going to Vietnam. Born to an Iowa farm family, Kern wasn't interested in becoming a grunt and knew he could choose his branch of service if he enlisted. After talking to Navy and Air Force recruiters, he chose the Marines and volunteered to be part of Force Recon—one of the special operations units that provided intelligence to the Marine command in Vietnam.

When he arrived in Vietnam in 1968, his Force Recon company was divided into teams of four men who "ran the bush"—finding out "whether the enemy was moving, how they were armed." They spent much of their time in the jungle where the soldiers from North Vietnam and armed supporters of the National Liberation Front sought shelter from the immense airpower of the US military. "If we spied enemy and observed them, we would call our mission, and they would bring in B-52s, or Phantom jets, or napalm," Kern explained.

"We were always in camouflage," he continues. "Our faces and hands were painted. Nothing made noise. Everything had to be taped, padded, tightened down. Nothing could reflect light. We covered our rifles with green rags or greasepaint. The goal was to melt into the jungle so the enemy had a hard time knowing you were there. I had enemy soldiers within six feet of me, and I thought they looked right at me and didn't see me. This was a common experience."

There's a lot of talk about the way members of the Marine Corps or Special Forces bond with one another. Kern describes it as a minute choreography executed across the endless silence of waiting, watching, and fearing.

"You get real close to guys when you tune in very finely and watch their body language: how he moves his hands, where's his thumb? Do I see his thumb move up to his safety? He's the point. If he stops, we squat slowly, and I watch, and if his thumb doesn't come up, then he doesn't really think it's NVA. Maybe it's a lion, or a deer, or a flock of birds. This goes on constantly; you watch, stop, don't make a noise, don't move for five, six minutes, just listen, then move again. If you didn't check in on your environment constantly, it'd get you for sure."

"The jungle is like a giant compost heap," he continues. "You take a step, and you break through a crust that is six or seven inches deep, and the jungle exhales. It releases an unmistakable aroma when people are walking over it. It's a smell I still remember. The jungle is a beast; you have to make your peace with it because it's always trying to eat you."

His team usually went on three-day missions, as long as they could last without restocking food and water. Some of their intelligence gathering forays were longer. During the siege of Khe Sanh, Kern and a fellow Marine spent eleven weeks on radio relay, without showering or shaving, on Hill 950, thirty-five hundred feet high. "Field radios had limited range and were line-of-sight, so radio waves wouldn't travel through a hill. Hill 950 had a sheer drop on three sides. If we wanted to be in contact with teams scattered around mountainous territory, we had to be up high. We were the umbilical cord for these teams and called in the helicopters or artillery if they got into trouble."

One of only two photos he has of his time in Vietnam is a picture taken after his mission on Hill 950 was completed. In it we see a bare-chested twenty-year-old, his body buffed by training and months in the field, his arms raised in an ecstatic gesture of pride. "It was late May '68; for the first time in weeks, you could stand up without fear of an enemy sniper or mortar or artillery round coming in, and I'm proud. Yeah, we lived through this. That was a big deal."

When Kern got out of the military in the spring of 1969, he used his GI Bill to continue his education at Drake University in Des Moines. There he began to experience problems the significance and impact of which he would understand only decades later. In high school Kern was known for his great memory, something that helped him excel. "How can you remember all that?" his buddies would constantly ask in wonder.

When he got back from Vietnam and entered university, his knack for remembering things was gone. "I didn't do well in school because I couldn't memorize stuff. I didn't connect it to the war. I went to a college counselor, and he said, 'Well, you're older.' I was twenty-one. But now, looking back on it, I had a concussion, which was pretty severe. I was out for, who knows, maybe two or three hours. But there was no concussion protocol then. The corpsman just took care of me. I later found out I have a cracked skull and deformity, and my left carotid artery is 100 percent occluded."

Drake provided a bucolic setting. It was as far from Vietnam as you could possibly get. "You would have thought it would be therapeutic. But it wasn't," Kern recalls. That was because he was also suffering from the symptoms of what no one then recognized as PTSD. He was irritable and had trouble sleeping. Far from the jungles of Southeast Asia, in a classroom in the middle of cornfields, he would be startled at the sound of a book falling to the floor or scan the perimeter of the classroom to detect any sign of imminent danger.

He was also assailed by a permanent sense of separateness. He was no longer a young kid. He had become a Marine—a member of a branch of the service known for its warrior ethos. The military may be a band of brothers, but it is a club with a very distinct pecking order. Marines are taught that they are more courageous, more honorable, more selfless than those who serve in other branches of the service. As former Marine Steven Pressfield writes in his book, *The Warrior Ethos*, the Marine tradition has its roots in cultures that go as far back as Sparta. In those cultures, he notes, "the ability to fight was of paramount importance. Tribes and nations prospered or were conquered by the strength of the warrior culture existing within a warrior society—a far cry from today when the military is just a tiny fragment of a civilian society."[1]

In Force Recon Kern had become part of an elite within an elite. At Drake he was not only older than most other freshmen; he felt they had no knowledge of what the world was really like and could never understand what he had been through. "It felt like I was watching some sitcom where kids were worrying about trivial shit," he recounts. "What they were concerned about just seemed silly."

There was no way he could connect to them or anyone else—particularly girls. "You'd be in an introductory course and meet some girl, and she'd notice that you were older and ask about that. If you said you were in Vietnam, she would ask you if you'd killed someone. That was the first question, like we were all baby killers. After a while, you just lied, said you'd been in the military working in an office."

He left Drake after a year, transferring to the University of Wisconsin at Milwaukee. He left there after two years and completed his degree at New College in Berkeley, California. He made it through school, but with little help from anyone. Back then, nobody connected his failing memory and sense of social isolation with concussion or PTSD or problems with reintegration or readjustment. These concepts and terms had not yet been invented. Moreover, Kern and his fellow veterans never talked about these things. "You just closed one door—military service—and opened another," he recalls. "You didn't go for help, and none was offered to you."

After he came back from Vietnam and graduated college, he worked as a technical writer for a year and then in sales. "I knew," he acknowledges, "that I didn't make people around me comfortable. I would work at a run all day. I expected everyone to run alongside me. My employees thought I was a pain in the ass to work for." When he looks back, he now understands that this stemmed from his hypervigilance. As he puts it, "You never know; anything behind you, any little sign in the jungle, could be the enemy."

Kern got involved in pickup basketball. "Continuous physical activity was the best thing I could [do] for myself," he says. There was also a lot of drinking. "You couldn't wait to have that drink after work," he recalls. But he got married, had four kids, and finally got out from behind a desk and got a hammer in his hand. "I got laid off from a sales job and began working in construction, framing houses, and building decks," he says. "I just fell in love with the work." Eventually he moved from working on decks and framing to building interior staircases. In the San Francisco Bay Area, he is known as the go-to guy when a hotel or a fancy house needs to replace one of its majestic original staircases.

Although his work was going well, there was trouble in his marriage, which ended in divorce, and he had nightmares of increasing severity. There were also moments when he acted in almost unrecognizable ways. Once, in Portland, he was driving down the road and witnessed a two-car crash. "I put on my brakes and saw one of the other car's headlights come rolling by me," he recounts. "My instinct was to jump out of my jeep, just like in Vietnam. I would have known who was going into shock and how to pinch off an artery. But I kept on going and didn't stop. I didn't know that person who didn't stop, who just drove away."

This was in the early '80s, and Kern eventually went to a therapist in Portland who helped him cope. But at that time, no one mentioned PTSD. Kern never considered going to the VA for help—with anything. He knew how Vietnam vets were treated in the 1960s and '70s. Of course, the VA had changed since then. There was, however, still the problem of wannabes. "You know when someone's been in the shit and when they haven't," he says bluntly. He had no intention of sitting in a waiting room listening to a bunch of Vietnam vets trading war stories when they really hadn't been in the war—at least not in his kind of war.

Kern's second wife had good insurance, which also covered him, so he didn't need the VA's help with that. When the first of his children approached college age, he learned that, in California, the VA provided financial help at state universities to children of veterans with a 10 percent service-rated disability. Okay, he figured, maybe it's worth putting up with the VHA and the wannabes for that.

He began the process of getting service connected and also checked out a local Vet Center, where he was given a pamphlet about PTSD. "When I got home," he says, "I laid it on [the] coffee table and went to work the next day. When I came home that evening, one of my daughters, who was living with me at the time, was sitting in the living room, crying. She had the pamphlet on her lap and said, 'This is you, Dad; this is you.' I thought it was nonsense up until that point. Denial is denial, but when your kid is sitting there weeping, well," he pauses, sighs, and then goes on. "That's when it first sunk in. Okay, well, maybe this isn't airy-fairy stuff. It's like the mirror's the last to know."

When he began the process of getting service rated, he thought maybe he'd get a 10 percent or possibly 30 percent disabled rating, but he was startled to receive a 50 percent rating. Now he marvels at how long he and his Marine buddies spent ignoring the obvious. "You begin to go to these reunions, and everybody's trying to be macho, and then suddenly you realize we're all like a rubber stamp. Ten of us sit in a group, and there's a loud noise, and we all startle. At the very same time. We're all the same set of psychological profiles—all hypervigilant."

Kern began counseling with Denver Mills at the Vet Center in Concord, California. He took medications and did group, as well as some individual, therapy. He was better—until his son volunteered for Iraq, and it all came back to him.

"I felt helpless. I called Denver and said, 'I can't sleep. I keep making all these foolish decisions.'" There was more treatment, and his disability rating went up to 100 percent.

He's done a 180 on the value of the VA. "You can walk in the VA clinic, which is right here, and unless you walk in with some kind of hard-on about something, if you just walk in and you look around, it will almost bring you to tears," he says. "That staff is so dedicated, and you can just see it."

Kern is just one of millions of veterans who have been diagnosed with PTSD. Here are some of the experiences associated with PTSD:

- Exposure to trauma as a victim or a witness.
- Being seriously hurt during the event.
- Going through a trauma that was long-lasting or very severe.
- Believing you or a family member was in danger.
- Having a severe reaction during the event, such as crying, shaking, vomiting, or feeling apart from your surroundings.
- Feeling helpless during the trauma and that you were not able to help yourself or a loved one.

Paula Schnurr and Matthew Friedman, current and former executive directors of the VHA's National Center for PTSD, explain that those suffering from PTSD also have intrusive symptoms such as nightmares and the recurrence of unwanted memories, flashbacks, or distress upon exposure to reminders of the traumatic experience. And they have avoidance symptoms. People with PTSD try to avoid thoughts of the trauma or real-life situations, individuals, or places that remind them of the trauma. They also experience negative thoughts and moods that lead to social isolation, anger, and irritability, among other problems. Finally, there are arousal symptoms consisting of insomnia, the inability to concentrate, hyper-arousal, and feeling jumpy or on guard.

Friedman says that people with PTSD have a "continued sense of threat that manifests itself in extreme fears. Reminders of the traumatic event can be triggered by literal and symbolic experiences. Someone driving down the road can see a bag of trash lying on the shoulder. That can remind them of an IED [improvised explosive device] attack, which was in a bag of trash lying at the side of the road. PTSD leads people to be hypervigilant—constantly on the lookout for threats to their lives. Sometimes people avoid things that are essentially harmless because they perceive them to be potentially dangerous. People with PTSD also think in particular ways about themselves and the world. They may think of the world as unsafe and think of themselves as being incompetent."

Although most people exposed to traumatic events do experience some or even all of these symptoms, they have them only for a brief period of time. Friedman and Schnurr warn that one has to be careful not to overuse or overattribute PTSD to everyone and anyone who manifests some of these symptoms. "People often use terms that have a very precise clinical meaning in imprecise ways," Friedman points out. For instance, for people who work in mental health, the terms "paranoia" or "depression" mean something very different from what they often mean in common parlance. Like clinical depression or real paranoia, PTSD is diagnosed only if symptoms occur at a severe level and for at least a month.

Scientists have discovered that trauma causes alterations to the body's stress response systems as well as psychological changes that create a spiral in which stress cascades and amplifies. Brain imaging research has shown that people with PTSD have alterations in brain structure and function. The character and duration of the trauma, as well as the length of the recovery period, can also influence the extent of PTSD.

PTSD is, of course, a modern term—and diagnosis—for an ancient affliction. In *Achilles in Vietnam: Combat Trauma and the Undoing of Character*, Jonathan Shay links the experiences and reactions of Homer's heroes to military personnel during and after the Vietnam War.

"What has not changed in three millennia are violent rage and social withdrawal when deep assumptions of 'what's right' are violated," he writes.[2] According to Shay, warriors from Homer's time to ours have experienced not only intense grief that turns to rage, but the severe mood swings between rage and "emotional deadness," withdrawal, suicidal thoughts, irritability, and the other components that are now commonly attributed to PTSD.

In *Fields of Combat: Understanding PTSD among Veterans of Iraq and Afghanistan*,[3] medical anthropologist Erin Finley, who works at the San Antonio VHA, explores shifting attitudes toward these types of injuries over time. She describes physicians during the American Civil War who "classified combat stress casualties into such categories as 'insanity,' 'nostalgia,' 'soldier's heart,' or 'irritable heart.'" The veterans with such broken hearts were "often treated as cowards and malingerers." During World War I, the term changed to "shell shock," but the response did not. World War II, Finley explains, began to usher in a small shift in perspective as 1.3 million men who had served in the military experienced some form of mental illness. And military psychiatrists were trying to figure out why some soldiers were experiencing "war neurosis" or what soon became known as "combat fatigue"—as if you could just sleep it off.

In 1947 the VA gave out pensions to nearly half a million veterans for "neuropsychiatric disabilities," which indicated that a slow process of destigmatizing these problems was at least beginning. In spite of the fact that World War II and Korean War veterans had an array of symptoms that would probably be classified as PTSD today, many of these service members did not talk about their experiences or seek treatment for them.

Consider Mr. James Harvey,* a ninety-year-old veteran who talks to me after his primary care appointment at the Medical Practices Clinic in San Francisco. The neatly dressed former Marine with a mane of thick white hair, who served in World War II and then Korea, told me that he was plagued by "horrendous nightmares" for decades. He never talked about it, not with his wife, children, or Marine buddies. "I thought it was a weakness of character," he says. "Then, six years ago, I began to talk with my VA cardiologist. He sent me over to Building Eight, and I took a test, and there it was—PTSD." He finally began treatment and can now sleep through the night.

In Honolulu, in the spacious, sun-filled atrium of the VA Pacific Islands Health Care System, located at the crest of a low mountain overlooking the ocean, I meet Herb Schreiner. An eighty-five-year-old Korean War veteran—part of what is often referred to as a lost generation of veterans—Schreiner was dressed in black jeans and a black T-shirt and wearing a Korean War Veteran baseball cap. During the war, Schreiner served as a mechanic repairing planes that flew over what was called MiG Alley, in the northwest part of North Korea, to protect the ground troops.

"Us Korean War veterans were not notified that we were eligible for benefits," he tells me. "I didn't find out till six or seven years ago."

When he finally found out about the possibility of getting services at the VHA, he was asked to submit his DD214 and other documents to prove eligibility for hearing loss, tinnitus, and problems he didn't even realize he had—like PTSD. Unfortunately, his paperwork had been lost in a fire years earlier, and the only thing he had was a partially burned DD214. He has been trying to get benefits and compensation ever since.

When he was finally able to visit a primary care physician, he got what he believes is superior treatment for his type 2 diabetes. He was also screened for PTSD. He suddenly had a cogent explanation for decades of mental health problems that began with a hospitalization in the 1950s, when, of course, there was no such thing as a diagnosis for PTSD.

"I've had bad dreams since I returned from Korea," he tells me. "Dreams of people in an airplane hanging on to me, grabbing me. 'Help us, Herb,' they shout. But there's nothing I could do to stop us going into a black hole." He's also been plagued by the smell of burned bodies, which is why, if he goes to a barbecue and smells grilled meat, he has to leave.

He has also learned why, since his time in Korea, his temper has been so explosive and why he lost his first wife and was alienated from his five kids. "I thought for years it was because I'm Portuguese. I thought it came naturally—fighting, arguing, yelling."

Thanks to the program he is in at the VHA, he says, he can now deal with what he understands to be an illness rather than a series of ethnic traits. This has made it easier for him to cope and has certainly, he says, helped his second wife of thirty years, who, he adds, has lived through hell with him.

"I go to a group of Korean War vets twice a month," he says. "I know what to do when I want to scream when she asks me to take out the garbage or bugs me in some other way. With the help of people at the VHA, my wife will tell me, 'Herb, it's time-out,' and I grab my cane and walk out the door. My wife was told by my psychiatrist to not let me watch the news. I can't watch violence and murders. This center here is concerned about your health and how they can improve you to become a better person—the doctors, psychiatrists, all these people are concerned."

Just as these older veterans waited decades for treatment, newer veterans from the Iraq and Afghanistan wars may be equally reluctant about going to the VHA to seek help or equally uninformed about the problems that they experience. Jerome Serdinsky walked me through his journey to treatment. No amount of training could have prepared him for what he found in Iraq. Although I have promised him that I would not go into the details of his deployment, he has allowed me—for which I am deeply grateful—to say that the number, persistence, and deadliness of the attacks to which his unit was subjected changed him forever.

As we talk over the phone, he pauses, and I hear silence on the other end and begin to worry that I have pressed too hard and jeopardized his hard-won sense of balance. "Are you all right?" I ask him.

There is a silence and then a quiet but firm, "Yes, I just get emotional. But you know, I have learned that emotions are okay."

For twelve months, the mortars and shelling, the lack of sleep, and the hour-by-hour, minute-by-minute doses of fear, along with the memories of seeing soldiers and civilians killed, have left him on overdrive.

"You know that fight-or-flight part of you that you have, Suzanne? Well, you can turn it off, but for me, it stayed on and won't turn off anymore."

To turn it off temporarily, Serdinsky used drugs and alcohol. Finally, after putting a noose around his neck, he sought treatment at the VHA—treatment that is now available, thanks not only to research but also to activism on the part of Vietnam War veterans and the clinicians who treated them at the VHA.

Along with other psychologists and psychiatrists studying the long-lasting effects of trauma in the broader population—including Holocaust survivors, women who have been raped, and victims of natural or man-made disasters—the VHA has created a coherent diagnosis of, and effective treatment for, those who suffer from traumatic experiences. Within the VHA two of the most prominent clinicians who led the way were Terence M. Keane and Matthew Friedman.

Keane, a clinical psychologist, is the director of the Behavioral Science Division of the VA's National Center for PTSD. This tall, trim, energetic—almost ebullient—sixty-four-year-old greets me in his office at the VHA building in Jamaica Plain, a few blocks away from Boston's Longwood Avenue medical area, with its world-renowned private-sector hospitals like Beth Israel Deaconess Medical Center, Boston Children's Hospital, and Brigham and Women's Hospital, as well as Harvard Medical School. Advertising and branding for these fancy hospitals clog the Boston airwaves and litter Fenway Park. Like so many older VHA facilities, the VA at Jamaica Plain seems drab and worn, and you will never see millions of taxpayer dollars wasted on ads for its research on PTSD or Alzheimer's or its Million Veteran Research Program. But the place is abuzz with activity, some of it shepherded by Keane, who has worked for the VHA since the late 1970s.

Although Keane was never in the military, he has developed a profound understanding of military culture and socialization, as well as a long-term perspective on the changes in mental health treatment in the VHA. He takes great pride in the way the system of mental health treatment has improved, in spite of its problems.

"We have inched the system forward—sometimes with several steps back, but with steady progress," he says. "It's amazing to see how well people are evaluated and treated today compared to what routinely happened thirty to thirty-five years ago. The same leaps and bounds have not occurred in other psychiatric conditions and in few physical health conditions."

His only lament is that he, as a non-veteran, cannot get his own care in a system where care is actually coordinated. He just had surgery, he tells me, at a world-class hospital down the street. The lack of care coordination and failure to convey basic information from one floor to the next, he says, was remarkable. He muses: "Where are the congressional hearings about this? Why are there no investigations into the closure of private-sector psychiatric beds or wait times in the private sector? Just try to get a dermatology appointment in Boston!"

Keane's introduction to the problems that would soon be understood as PTSD began in 1978, when he worked in the addiction program at the VA Medical Center in Jackson, Mississippi. For more than three years, he listened to veterans of World War II and the Korean or Vietnam War talk about their alcoholism or drug use. Over and over again, he heard the same story. They drank, they said, because it was the only way they could deal with their recurrent nightmares, intrusive memories, anxiety, or depression. These responses, it soon became clear, stemmed from their experiences in combat. Keane began to dig deeper into what he was hearing and tried to "put things together."

In those days putting it together did not involve a Google search. There were, Keane explains, a lot of trips to the library and expensive phone calls in an era when a long-distance call to Indiana could cost sixty dollars or more. All of this led him to an underground movement in mental health that he was determined to join. He asked the chief of staff at the Jackson VA to pay for him to go to Purdue University in West Lafayette, Indiana, to meet with Charles Figley, a psychologist who was developing a treatment program for what became known as PTSD.

"My chief," he quips, "knew that a trip to rural Indiana was not exactly a scam, so he agreed."

Figley, he continues, generously shared his burgeoning knowledge with his junior colleague and put Keane in touch with psychiatrist Ann Wolbert Burgess, who was studying what she then described as rape trauma syndrome. Figley also pointed him to other clinicians and researchers.

When Keane returned to Jackson, he began to create a treatment program for Vietnam vets with PTSD. This involved, he tells me, developing a set of diagnostic criteria to define PTSD, converting old psychological tests so they could be helpful in evaluating PTSD, creating new assessment tools that allow clinicians to see if people meet agreed-upon criteria for PTSD, and, of course, creating treatment programs to help veterans deal with the trauma of combat and military service.

Keane left Jackson for the Boston VA medical center and soon joined forces with Matthew Friedman, also a leader in the field. The two clinicians quickly pulled together a national team within the VHA to continue moving forward on diagnosing, evaluating, and treating PTSD in veterans.

When I asked Keane to describe the change in the treatment trajectory for veterans with PTSD, he tells me what it was like in 1979 or 1980, when a typical thirty-five-year-old Vietnam vet appeared at a VA medical center reporting symptoms of anxiety and depression.

"If you interviewed him," Keane explains, "you would find he would have panic attacks, have trouble with his spouse and his employer, be unable to sleep, and perhaps be getting into fights. He would then be diagnosed with anxiety neurosis, or personality disorder, or his problems would be attributed to his addictions, to the fact that he was an alcoholic or abused drugs. He would be prescribed a wide range of medications and maybe get a little psychotherapy for depression or panic attacks. But he would get no specialized evaluation for PTSD, and no specialized treatment would be available. Most importantly, no one would evaluate his combat experience or history."

Keane pauses and then recollects a transformative moment. "Right here in this building, where we are sitting today, there was an affective disorders, or mood, unit. The chief resident asked me to attend a case conference. The resident and medical student described someone who had reached diagnostic criteria for major depression. They described the patient's symptoms and then brought the patient in and asked me to interview him."

The patient came into the room. "Within only a few seconds, I knew that the man was a Vietnam veteran who had probably served in the Army, where he had significant combat experience. If he was depressed, it was because of PTSD. Instead of asking questions about his symptoms, I asked him questions about his time in Vietnam. Where, geographically, was he located? What months was he there? What was his MOS [military occupational specialty]? I asked him to describe what it was like to be in Vietnam. Had he sustained losses? What were the most difficult situations and circumstances he had encountered?"

Keane pauses, as if he still cannot conceal his amazement. "In this entire audience of students and faculty, no one had ever done a comprehensive history of the lives of these people while in the service," he says. "That may seem incredible now, but that was what was going on all over the country. This diagnosis was new, and people did not have the perspective that traumatic events had long-lasting effects on people's lives." This interaction, and the receptivity of the audience to it, helped to move the unit from an exclusive focus on mood disorders so that clinicians would be "more accommodating to PTSD."

Understanding how their work could transform the treatment of veterans, Keane and Friedman assembled a national group of clinicians within the VHA who met three or four times a year to explore diagnostic and clinical issues. With the Veterans Health Care Act of 1984, Congress mandated the creation of a National Center on Post-Traumatic Stress Disorder that would "promote the training of health care and related personnel in, and research into, the causes and diagnosis of PTSD and the treatment of Veterans for PTSD." It was tasked with serving as a resource center to "promote and seek to coordinate the exchange of information regarding all research and training activities carried out by the Veterans Administration, and by other Federal and non-Federal entities, with respect to PTSD."

When the first National Center was opened, it was located at a midwestern VA medical center in Brecksville, Ohio. It quickly became clear that this one center could not fulfill the congressional mandates. The VA thus invited requests for proposals to consider how best to fulfill the mandates. Keane and Friedman, along with Dennis Charney, Bob Rosenheck, Fred Gusman, and Schnurr responded. They recognized that different components, available at different VA sites, were essential to creating a truly national center that would provide critical expertise and scientific breadth. Their proposal was accepted, and in 1989 the contemporary National Center for PTSD was launched at five different sites in four different locations.

The dedicated pioneers in the field assumed responsible positions at these sites. Keane directed the Behavioral Science Division at the VA Medical Center in Boston. At the West Haven VAMC, Charney led the Clinical Neurosciences Division, and Rosenheck directed the Evaluation Division. Gusman, a social worker, led the Educational and Clinical Laboratory in the Menlo Park division of the Palo Alto VA Medical Center. Until 2014, Friedman was the executive director of the National Executive Division of the center at White River Junction. And in 1993 the center added the Women's Health Sciences Division, then headed by psychologist Jessica Wolfe, located in Boston. The Pacific Islands Division in Honolulu conducts research in cultural diversity and is directed by social worker Ray Scurfield. All of these divisions are now connected to academic institutions, like the Yale University School of Medicine, the Geisel School of Medicine at Dartmouth, Boston University, Stanford University, and the University of Hawaii.

In 2014, when I began writing this book, I went to the White River Junction VA to meet with Friedman and Deputy Executive Director Schnurr, who was soon to become the executive director following

Friedman's retirement. He is continuing to work with the VHA as a senior consultant, which, he jokes, is what retirement means in the VA.

As we sit in a small conference room, Friedman and Schnurr give me a tour of the center's history, accomplishments, and strategy for the future.

"When we started," Schnurr says, "PTSD was a new and quite controversial diagnosis. Some people questioned its validity. Our science, and the science we try to get others to do, has produced a body of evidence that PTSD is a real disorder. Our mandate is very broad. It includes research and education, providing information for all federal and nonfederal entities even though we are in the VA. Although we never labeled ourselves as a translation research center, we are. More than doing research and training, we have influenced how PTSD is assessed, diagnosed, and treated."

"The center," Friedman elaborates, "has helped to change the way people now think of PTSD. When we started in [the] late '80s, PTSD was considered to be something that only happened to Vietnam veterans. Now, because of our research and dissemination, the public understands that PTSD can happen to any man, woman, or child exposed to a traumatic event, which may not necessarily be a war-related one. We are helping to set the scientific agenda for [the] field." Over the last three decades, the center has, for example, worked with many outside the VA. They worked with people who survived the Oklahoma City bombing in 1995, they were called in to help after 9/11, and they assisted those impacted by Hurricane Katrina, to name only a few examples.

One of the many things the center has done is develop the Clinician Administered PTSD Scale, which provides a standardized interview for clinicians and researchers so they can accurately diagnose and quantify the severity of PTSD symptoms.

In 1992 researchers at the center conducted the world's first and largest epidemiological survey of PTSD in wartime veterans—the National Vietnam Veterans Readjustment Study. The findings: 30 percent of male and 25 percent of female Vietnam veterans had PTSD sometime after deployment. Almost twenty years after the war was over, 15 percent of male vets and 8 percent of female vets still had symptoms. In 1995, Friedman says, "one of our investigators used brain imaging to show that the hippocampus was smaller in patients with PTSD. This was the first time anyone had shown that PTSD affected the brain."

Wolfe developed the Women's Military Exposure Scale, which helped clinicians understand that simply adapting the treatment of PTSD in male veterans would not work with women. She also did investigations on military sexual trauma that documented that sexual harassment is a risk factor in the development of PTSD.[4]

PTSD researchers have also discovered that upbringing, home environment, and genetics can influence whether one develops PTSD. Because of research in the field, we now understand some of the risk factors that can lead to the development of PTSD. These include being abused as a child, having another mental health problem, having family members who have mental health problems, suffering the loss of a loved one, having other stressful life experiences, and getting little support from family and friends. Overuse of alcohol, being poorly educated, and even being a woman are, researchers have discovered, other risk factors. What is perhaps most relevant for the military, the ranks of which are filled with people in their late adolescence or early adulthood, is that being younger is also a significant risk factor.

When researchers and clinicians inside the VA and in outside practice make discoveries or develop treatments in the field, the National Center synthesizes the findings and disseminates them to a vast network both inside and outside the VA. Since 1995, the center has kept up to date a bibliographic website of the world's literature on trauma and PTSD, which is available through university libraries. This has allowed people far and wide to access it for treatment purposes and in times of emergency.

"When the Red River overflowed in 1997," Friedman recalls, "we got a call from counselors wanting materials to help people in Manitoba. Now we take things like that for granted, but this was one of the first times we were able to use our website in a practical way."

The VA's systematic research helped lead to the gold-standard treatments for PTSD: cognitive processing therapy (CPT) and prolonged exposure therapy (PE). CPT, which is a version of cognitive behavioral therapy, was developed and tested by Patricia Resick because of her work with women who had been assaulted.[5] John McQuaid, deputy chief of mental health at Fort Miley, who has written an excellent book called *Peaceful Mind* about combining CPT and mindfulness meditation, explains that CPT is based on the idea that we all, as human beings, have some core beliefs about how we work within the world and how the world works. How we experience trauma is dependent on those beliefs.

"Many people believe," McQuaid explains, "that the world is a just place. If you do good things, good things will happen. If you do bad things, you will be punished. Then you go to war, and bad things happen that are completely outside of your control even when you are doing everything right. You lose your buddies. You kill people. A car comes at you, and the protocol is that you shoot first and ask questions later, and you find that you have killed civilians.

"When something like this happens," McQuaid continues, "you have three options. One, you assume you must have done something wrong and you deserve to feel terrible because of the trauma. It was your fault, you failed, you don't deserve to be alive or happy or successful. The second option is that you believe your beliefs were wrong and toss them out of the window. You feel you will never have control over your life, which is shattering. The third option? If people reconcile their current beliefs with the reality they face, they will be able to tolerate the fact that you can do everything right, and bad things happen. But just because bad things happened doesn't mean you deserve it." The core of CPT, he emphasizes, is helping people recognize the meaning they place on the trauma and reconsider how they interpret it.

Over the course of twelve to sixteen sessions in individual or group therapy, patients examine "what they are telling themselves about the traumatic experience and start questioning how helpful or accurate these beliefs are," McQuaid says. "Was it really your fault that your buddy died? Did you really mean to kill a child? Does this mean you really are a bad person? What might be more helpful or constructive things you can tell yourself about this experience?"

Part of delving into the meaning you impose on trauma involves writing an impact statement, a description not necessarily of the event itself but the meaning it had in your life. Through this process patients look for particularly destructive or painful beliefs that arose from the event. Did an assault victim blame herself for being in the wrong place at the wrong time, for wearing the wrong dress, for going out with the wrong guy on a date? Did a combat veteran really fail to protect his buddy or mean to kill a civilian? Does that mean that they don't deserve happiness or success in life?

"This is challenging work," McQuaid says. "Writing a statement about trauma can be scary, and we want to encourage people, to help them learn that they can do it." What is also scary for some people is the idea that CPT will wipe away the valuable memories they are trying to hold on to. "One of the things many veterans fear is that they will forget their buddies and dishonor the memory of those who stayed behind," McQuaid says. "We have to make it crystal clear that whenever we talk to people about these therapies, we are not asking them to forget, but rather are trying to help them be with memories in a healthy way. When this happens, it's very inspiring."

PE is based on similar principles. It was developed by Edna B. Foa, an Israeli clinical psychologist who grounded much of her work on women who had suffered the trauma of rape. Foa is now a professor at the University of Pennsylvania, where she directs the Center for the Treatment and Study of Anxiety.

"PE," Schnurr notes, "had been tested and applied to other populations, but we did the first randomized trial for female veterans with PTSD. These studies helped establish the feasibility and effectiveness for its use in the VA."

Leila Zwelling is the assistant director of the Women's Mental Health Program and the director of the Interpersonal Psychotherapy Program at Fort Miley. She describes the process of taking veterans through these PE sessions. "PE is a therapy," she explains, "where you have the patient talk about their worst traumatic memory over and over again. It's an extremely intense treatment. I've used PE with veterans who've experienced combat trauma and military sexual trauma. The patient closes his eyes and retells the memory in the present tense. For example, a Marine in Iraq will say, 'Now I'm picking up the gun. Now I'm seeing something out of the corner of my eye. I think it's the enemy, and I shoot. The body falls to the ground, and I realize it's a small body—the body of a child.'"

Throughout this retelling, Zwelling says, the therapist is paying very careful attention to a variety of parameters. "Every five minutes, I am checking in to get what is called a SUDS level [subjective units of distress]. The patient assigns a number on a scale of one to one hundred of how distressed they are in the moment while staying with the memory. After the person repeats the traumatic memory several times, there is a period of processing where the therapist talks to the patient about what it was like to go through the memory each time. We start to challenge what we call cognitive distortion—some of the beliefs traumatized people develop about the world. For example, they may think the world is not and will never be a safe place, that they cannot and will not ever be able to trust anyone again."

PE and CPT may be the most effective evidence-based treatments for PTSD, but they may not be routinely used in treatment of people with PTSD outside of the VHA, as the RAND study *Ready to Serve* discovered. The VHA has launched a huge training program to teach these two treatments to VHA clinicians. Resick, who developed CPT and directs the Women's Health Sciences Division, has trained over fifty-nine hundred VHA therapists.

A clinical psychologist at the Palo Alto VHA Health Care System and the director of the National Center's Dissemination and Training Division in Palo Alto, Josef Ruzek explains why these rollouts are so important and so unusual. "There is very little precedent in any health care or mental health care system to systematically teach people how to move best practices into the health care workforce," he says.

In most settings where mental health care is practiced in the private sector, already trained and licensed practitioners are, at least on paper, required to maintain up-to-date knowledge and keep current on the latest evidence-based therapies. In reality, to maintain their licenses, clinicians have to amass a certain number of continuing education credits. To do this, they may sign up to go to a conference or attend a workshop, where they gain knowledge of a particular therapy or treatment. Sometimes the institutions they work for will help pay for this continuing education; sometimes clinicians must pay themselves. Most often, even after an intensive workshop, the therapist will not be well supervised in putting this new knowledge into practice.

"Simply attending a training workshop and gaining new knowledge have been found to have little impact on skill or implementation of practice," says Ruzek. "You have to learn the skills to put something into practice. And then, once you learn the skills, you also have to do the therapy."

To make sure knowledge leads to skills and then to implementation in practice, the VA has produced an educational training program and trained seventeen trainers, who then teach thousands of VHA therapists.

In PE, for example, a training was developed in consultation with Foa and Elizabeth Hembree, who developed the therapy. Seventeen specially educated trainers lead intensive four-day, face-to-face training workshops, where therapists spend seven hours viewing every aspect of the intervention, going over difficult cases, and role playing. After the training, seventy specially trained "consultants" or supervisors spend six months supervising each therapist-trainee, who must complete two cases to the supervisor's satisfaction. The trainee sees the patient and, with the patient's permission, audiotapes the sessions, and then, in a weekly consultation, the consultant goes over each session with the therapist-in-training.

"When we launched this program," says Ruzek, "there was only a handful of people worldwide who could train and consult annually. At the VHA we have more people than anywhere else who are competent to teach and supervise both CPT and PE."

Zwelling herself took advantage of this training and became a certified PE therapist. "The therapist listened to my audiotaped sessions and gave me feedback to make sure I was effectively delivering this complex treatment," she says. "She would, for example, listen to the patient describe the memory and then comment that they sounded like they were reading a newspaper account. She would advise me to ask more questions about the emotions the person was experiencing and to ask the patient about smells or sounds when recounting trauma. Asking a patient about what they were smelling or hearing are powerful tools in making a memory come more alive."

This training and supervision, she says, were critical not only to make the therapy more effective but because of the potential consequences of the treatment. "You don't want someone without intensive training practicing PE," Zwelling says. "That could be dangerous for the patient." Imagine, she says, asking someone to go over the minute details of a rape by a senior officer or the inadvertent killing of a child in Iraq. "All kinds of difficult emotions swell up, and without real guidance the patient could decompensate," which, in lay terms, means really fall apart. In effect, without a very educated therapist who knows how to do the treatment and also understands the contextual issues involved, the treatment could be worse than the proverbial disease.

Zwelling says she would never have been able to get training with such intense supervision in the private sector. First, she would have had to take time off to do such training. Then, she would have had to pay for it herself, and it would have been difficult for her to find someone who would provide such extensive and intensive supervision.

After practicing PE for seven years, Zwelling is now participating as a PE therapist in a large, multisite VHA research study comparing the effectiveness of PE and CPT. The study conducted by National Center researchers will help determine if one treatment is better than the other overall and which may be better for different types of patients—men versus women, older versus younger veterans, veterans with combat trauma versus veterans who experienced military sexual trauma.

The VHA trains about forty thousand psychology, psychiatry, social work, and nurse-practitioner students each year. As we have seen, it also expands the therapeutic repertoire of working clinicians like Zwelling and so many others.

The VHA's reputation for thorough training is drawing attention. When Ben Emmert-Aronson, a thirty-one-year-old psychologist in training, had to choose a place for the last stage of training for his PhD, he applied only to VHA programs. "I had seen the quality of the training at the VHA," he says. "There is so much institutional knowledge built into the system for training. They've been honing their curricula for years and put structures into place for high-quality training. The system at the VA is set up to train people." At the VHA, he says, there is a much higher ratio of supervisors to patients than in other institutions, and that means "more time and attention on each patient."

Emmert-Aronson says he can't believe the VHA bashing he hears daily in the media, which has influenced his friends and family. "Every time I told a friend or family member I was working at the VA, they'd get a concerned look on their face. They'd ask, 'Oh, how's that going? That must be really hard.' There's a real disconnect between stories my loved ones hear and the facts on the ground. When you look not only at my experience but at the hard data, you see the VHA is providing higher quality of care sooner, for less money. Anyone who is interested in helping veterans or in saving money should be in favor of the VA. And that should be everyone."

Profile

Karen Parko

A Special Kind of Professional Development at the VA

I met Karen Parko when I went to observe clinical psychologist John McQuaid and his team at their weekly cognitive behavioral therapy group supervision at Fort Miley. Parko, a neurologist, is the national director of the VA's Epilepsy Centers of Excellence, which is a network of sixteen different sites across the United States.[1] Its main office is here at Fort Miley. When I met her, Parko had been coming to these supervision sessions for six months because she was, in fact, one of the trainees being supervised as she learned to practice cognitive behavioral therapy.

Several weeks after we first met in Building Eight, I visited her in her office to learn why she has ventured into territory that is, she confessed, quite alien to neurologists and epileptologists. Parko is tall and lean, with long, straight hair that cascades down her back almost to her waist. Her attire displays her twenty-four-year history as a captain in the United States Public Health Service, where she worked in Indian Health Services: her wrists are adorned with Hopi and Navajo turquoise jewelry, and her VA ID card hangs from an intricately beaded lanyard that a Navajo nurse wove for her.

The San Francisco VHA recruited Parko in 2004 to run its epilepsy program, so she returned from the Hopi and Navajo reservations in New Mexico and the Four Corners area of the Southwest. In 2005 she joined other VHA epileptologists across the United States to form the National VA Epilepsy Centers of Excellence. When she first came to Fort Miley, she had not left active duty, and her husband, as a nonmilitary dependent, was eligible for VHA care, which he got in the form of ear surgery. He could have had the surgery, Parko says, from the same surgeon at UCSF, all paid for by the VHA. He chose to have it on-site at Fort Miley, because she quickly discovered while working there that the VHA's commitment to teamwork and coordination of care was second to none.

Parko is an ardent supporter of the VHA, not only because of such personal experiences, but because of the professional opportunities presented to her: notably, the fact that not only can she teach medical trainees, but she can also learn and train with psychologists who have mastered cognitive behavioral therapy. This, she says, is critical to helping certain kinds of patient who often land on the doorstep of neurologists and epileptologists ill equipped to handle their problems.

What brought Parko to Building Eight is known as psychogenic nonepileptic seizures (PNES), and it is a big headache—no pun intended—for epileptologists. "Epilepsy," Parko explains, "is an electrical disorder of the brain that causes seizures. The cardinal symptom or feature is the seizure where people shake and pass out. The seizures PNES patients have look, to all the world, like a classic epileptic seizure"—except they are not caused by an electrical discharge in the brain. Parko says that factors that influence development of PNES are thought to be rooted in trauma—not head trauma of the TBI variety, but mental trauma produced by rape, sexual abuse, combat, or childhood deprivation, among others.

"The only way we know the PNES seizure is different from a regular seizure," Parko says, "is by watching what happens while patients are hooked up to an electroencephalogram [EEG]. An EEG measures brain electrical activity, and in epileptic seizures, abnormalities in brain electrical activity are easily identifiable, while with PNES there is no abnormality in the brain electrical activity during the event."

To show me what seizures actually look like and how PNES is distinguished from regular epilepsy, Parko walks me down to the epilepsy monitoring unit at Fort Miley. The unit has two rooms, each with two beds, where patients are hooked up to dozens of leads that are, in turn, hooked up to monitors. At the nurses' station, two registered nurses sit watching the tangle of gyrating, leaping, and swooping zags and zigs that measure the patient's brain electrical activity. The goal of this monitoring is to identify focal points in the brain where electrical activity is going radically wrong, so that patients whose epilepsy is not well managed by medication can perhaps be candidates for some sort of surgical fix. Standard treatment for epileptic seizures is a class of drugs called anticonvulsants that help to diffuse electrical activity in the brain. If PNES patients are erroneously given medications that change the chemical and electrical balance of their brain when there is no chemical or electrical imbalance, the medications do no good and can do harm.

Many PNES patients do, however, get treated with such medications, because in a normal clinic setting outside of an epilepsy monitoring unit, patients who appear to have epilepsy will be treated with anticonvulsants. When those medications don't work, the gold standard is to classify the spells using epilepsy monitoring (video electroencephalography telemetry, or VET).

When neurologists finally figure out that the patient has PNES, the patient is then sent to a psychiatrist or psychologist for some sort of therapy. But things don't necessarily get better in a mental health professional's office, Parko warns. When the patient is in the psychologist's or psychiatrist's office, the seizures may get even worse as the patient delves more deeply into traumatic memories. So the psychiatrist or psychologist, who may have no training in dealing with seizures, is sitting by helplessly with a patient who has fallen to the floor, shaking uncontrollably. As I watch some patients seizing in their beds, it becomes clear just how scary this can be to a clinician who is not familiar with seizures and PNES. Patients don't just shake; they groan and emit frightening cries and practically foam at the mouth.

Parko role-plays the psychiatrist or psychologist's normal response. "'I can't do CPR,' they say when they call us on the phone to tell us what happened. 'I can't do therapy with this person if I have to call a code blue every time they are in my office.' We put the psychiatrist in a really strange position because they're the only fix the patient really has, but they can't deal with it because how can they possibly treat a patient who is seizing?"

So the patient is sent back to the neurologist. But although the therapists often can't handle the neurological symptoms, the neurologists often can't handle the psychological ones. "Neurologists find it all scary and uncomfortable as well. 'I don't know anything about mental health,' they say. We are not trained to look at unconscious, unresolved issues or the unconscious and somatic disorders. Epileptologists are trained to see people with electrical problems and fix them. If we can't do it with meds, we do it with surgery. The last thing most of us want to do is see someone who doesn't have an electrical problem because we don't want to waste our time with these people." Because these patients need help, they often occupy up to 30 percent of the beds in epilepsy monitoring units, both in and outside the VHA.

In the time she spent managing people with PNES, Parko discovered that one approach that works with them is cognitive behavioral therapy, a treatment whose effectiveness has been documented in clinical trials. It just so happens that one of the two national experts in cognitive behavioral therapy for PNES is William Curt Lafrance Jr. of Brown University and the Providence VA. The VA Epilepsy Centers of Excellence recognized PNES as a priority treatment issue and engaged with Lafrance to develop and implement a training program for VHA Epilepsy Center providers. The original studies done by Lafrance showed that patients would benefit from a twelve-week program of therapy. Parko and her colleagues worked to disseminate this treatment through the national epilepsy center network and encouraged providers to learn it. Lafrance currently trains three to four providers a year.

At Fort Miley, Parko tried to encourage psychiatrists and neurologists to sign up for the Lafrance training. She got no comers and decided if she wanted to get it done, she would have to learn the method and practice it herself. In any other setting, this would have been mission impossible. She would have had to quit her job, at least temporarily, and become a psychologist. Or she could have taken a course, gotten a not-very-robust certificate, and hung out her shingle. She would have received little or no supervision, or she would have had to pay for that supervision. At the VHA she discovered that McQuaid and his colleagues both taught and practiced cognitive behavioral therapy. When she approached them as a prospective learner, they were delighted to welcome her.

She also asked Lafrance to include her in the network he was developing. He became her teacher and supervisor. Once she had her training network in place, Parko began to recruit "beta patients"—those who know that their therapist is in training and getting supervision and agree to sign a consent form and have all the sessions recorded. For a year Parko sent tapes of her sessions, via secure snail mail, to Lafrance, who reviewed them, and every Tuesday at 7 a.m. Pacific Time, the two would go over them on the phone. Once a week, she met with McQuaid, learning more about the overall principles of cognitive behavioral therapy. She also apprenticed with Kristi Chambers, who is a psychiatric nurse-practitioner and expert in cognitive behavioral therapy for anxiety, depression, and PTSD. Chambers invited Parko to colead a cognitive behavioral therapy for depression group.

As I follow Parko, I meet some of her patients. One is Mr. Jones,* a veteran who was a Navy minesweeper in Vietnam but never in combat. Jones has driven hours to get help at the VHA. Like most VHA patients, he has a lot going on. He has PTSD. He was a serious alcohol and drug user—although, as he tells us proudly, he has been sober for twenty-three years. He gives us a semi-toothless smile and greets Parko with enthusiasm. She has been treating him via telehealth from a CBOC about six hours away. He has told her about his spells, but she has never seen them, and she has been unable to assess his brain activity.

He lies in his bed, tethered to a leash that allows him to move only about fifteen feet around his bed—to the bathroom, to the window, and that's pretty much it. His head, which has some sixty-four electrodes pasted to his skull an inch apart, is covered by a gauze turban that keeps them in place. His long gray hair peeks out from underneath the turban, at the nape of his neck. The electrodes are bound into an input channel, which is hardwired into the wall. On his bed table are several AA books, which he keeps close to him, his bibles of sobriety.

He greets me warmly as well and then suddenly jackknifes forward, head to knees, hand clutched to his chest as if he cannot breathe. Parko moves in. A nurse who has watched this on the monitor also comes in the room, as does another epileptologist, Nina Garga.

Parko, who has never seen one of his spells, asks him if that is what they are like. He nods. Then he jackknifes over again, like a ballet dancer executing a precise and difficult choreographic move, and sits up. With tears in his eyes, he sighs and says, "I think it's going away."

But it hasn't, and it doesn't, at least not over the next fifteen minutes. Parko asks him what he is feeling. "Heavy emotions," he stammers, "emotions, hysteria, crying. I don't know—it's never happened twice in a row like this." Out of deep embarrassment, he tries to contain his emotion. "I'm a dude," he whispers. "Epilepsy is one thing," he says, "but this, this is something else. I'm afraid to leave the house, afraid to go to the store. Sometimes a word or expression on someone's face just sets me off. I can never tell when it's going to happen. I am so ashamed," he says, trying to turn away and hide.

Parko tries to reassure him. "This is exactly why you are here," she tells him, her concern bathing him in empathy. "We need to know what's happening, and then we can figure out what to do about it. I have different things I would recommend when you are ready to talk about it more. It's a process you could begin with me on V-Tel so that you don't have to come down here. I can't make any promises about this, but it has worked well with patients."

Jones smiles wanly and says, "Well, it's better than brain surgery."

When I catch up with Parko several months later, she tells me she has completed her didactic training and supervision and is now seeing patients on her own. "It's a brave new world," she quips. "It's hard to have practiced medicine for so long and be so green at something, so I'm pretty uncomfortable. After practicing as a neurologist for twenty-two years and getting really good at it, I haven't been in a place where I haven't been a master for a long time. I'm in a perfect environment to continue to grow my skills." Parko still attends Tuesday group supervision sessions with McQuaid and, in addition, twice a month joins other VA providers who specifically treat patients with PNES on a phone call to discuss any patient care issues.

Parko is not only interested in cognitive behavioral therapy because it can help patients in the VHA. "The VA has the ability to change practice not only in our system but to disseminate best practices throughout the country and even the world. As we grow this program, we will train providers who will leave the VA and take the skills they have learned here along with them wherever they practice."

Parko believes that cognitive behavioral therapy will become the standard of care for every comprehensive epilepsy center because proven therapies are available for PNES. "When the VA does something like this, other people follow suit," Parko says. She adds ironically, "This is even more true today when the VHA has become everybody's whipping boy.

It reflects poorly on outside institutions when they don't offer treatments the VA offers."

Sitting on top of Parko's desk is a stack of papers, research intake forms for a recently approved trial she and Chambers are undertaking at Fort Miley. The study is testing whether this therapy for PNES, which has been shown to be effective in individual sessions, can be effective in group sessions. It's important to scientifically determine that fact because, as it currently stands, the ratio of people who need this therapy to the specialists able to provide it is way too high. As part of the therapy trial, Parko and Chambers plan to enroll any patient, including nonveterans, with PNES in San Francisco. There are two other epilepsy centers in San Francisco, one at UCSF and the other at the California Pacific Medical Center, and both will be sending patients for enrollment in this research trial. Neither offers cognitive behavioral therapy for PNES, which means that the only way any nonveteran in the city can access this trial is through the VHA.

Returning to Civilian Life

Veterans on Campus

In March 2016 I talked with Norissa McLorin, the president of the student veterans' club at City College of San Francisco. McLorin, a tall, slim, twenty-eight-year-old African American soon to be completely separated from the Marines, joined up when she was twenty-two to get a change of scene. After boot camp in San Diego, she worked in battalion administration in South Carolina. When I ask what particular things brought her to the VHA, she rattles off a list of problems: bad right knee, tinnitus, migraines, sinusitis, and then PTSD and military sexual trauma.

Like too many women in the military, McLorin was sexually harassed by a Marine who was higher in rank than she was. They both worked in administration, and at first the two dated. When she found out he had a pregnant girlfriend off base, she called it off. That was when the trouble started, she says. He began a campaign of belittling her, calling her out for every little thing. He would make humiliating comments that were, she understands now, fishhooks dangled in front of her so she would take the bait. When she fought back, she says, he told other people that "I didn't know how to take orders, that I was a shitbag."

Finally, he went too far and began to touch her inappropriately. She filed a complaint, which led to an investigation. McLorin was irate that the investigation resulted only in a slap on her harasser's wrist and that he was easily approved for his reenlistment package. And she got angrier still when the investigators accused her of being immature, not understanding the nature of sexual harassment, and trying to get back at the guy. When she learned she was not the only woman he had harassed, she tried to warn higher-ups that the man could move from touching a knee or shoulder to full-scale rape. No one paid attention. She had to continue working on the same base, living in the same barracks, until she finally left active duty and returned to California.

She says she thought she had got away from the guy. She did not realize he had taken up permanent residence in her brain until she walked into the City College lounge and the back of another student's head reminded her of her harasser.

"I thought it was him," she tells me, "and went into a full-scale panic attack."

Like so many other members of the service, particularly Marines, acknowledging the need for help and actually getting it were not easy. "In the Marines the mind-set is that you're fine," she says. "Even if you need help, you don't need help. You do what you're told and stick to the plan. And unless something is broken, like your arm, you get back up to par and continue. Emotional things are frowned upon." McLorin would not admit to needing emotional help when she was in the service, and she certainly wouldn't as she was about to leave it.

Marines who are in the service and about to be discharged have to fill out medical forms that ask about things like trouble sleeping, irritability, and depression. They may not check the relevant boxes and risk revealing emotional problems because this will lead to a medical hold that can delay discharge for several months.

"They want to get out," she says. "They don't want to hang around for another two months, so we basically lie. Everyone knows that." The fact that this could seriously complicate efforts to get a service-connected disability rating seems to be something people either don't know or ignore.

When McLorin finally walked next door to seek counseling, it took a great deal of effort. It still does, she says, even though she is in therapy. There's the time it takes to get to the VHA at Fort Miley, but more important, there's the problem of delving deeper into painful memories with a therapist. "Sometimes I just scratch the surface," she confesses.

McLorin, who transferred to San Francisco State in fall 2016 to pursue a degree in hospitality, does not view the veterans' club as a bubble that should never be penetrated by the civilian world. Everyone is welcome, she emphasizes. But it is, for her and other veterans, a place where she can be with people with whom she feels a special kinship, which is why she wants to re-create it at San Francisco State.

Between 2000 and 2012, more than nine hundred thousand veterans and military service members received education benefits from the VA. Because of the post-9/11 GI Bill, the largest increase in the number of veterans pursuing higher education was fueled by those who served in the wars in Iraq and Afghanistan.[1] Because many veterans don't have a lot of money and may have delayed or interrupted their academic studies to serve in the military, about 47 percent of veterans who first use their GI Bill after leaving the service enroll in community college. If you want to help student veterans, community colleges are the place to go.

Over the course of the last four decades, the VHA has learned from the experiences of veterans reentering the civilian world and is doing a lot more to help them better navigate the passage from soldier, airman, sailor, or corpsman to civilian—student, worker, father, mother, husband, wife, partner, son, daughter, friend, citizen.

Increasingly, the VHA is providing both outreach and mental health services in nontraditional settings like community and four-year colleges as well as at universities. The San Francisco VA was one of the first medical centers to pilot an on-site mental health center at a community college, establishing a successful local model that has been used as the VA launched a broader national outreach effort. The Walter S. Newman Veterans Resource Center at City College of San Francisco—the largest community college in the state—began when administrators responded to complaints from student veterans by contacting Keith Armstrong, the director of Social Work Services at the San Francisco VA Health Care System.

The lanky, sandy-haired clinical social worker has worked at Fort Miley for more than thirty years and directed its Family Therapy Program since 1991. An expert in PTSD and other veteran readjustment problems, Armstrong eagerly scheduled a meeting to discuss veterans' issues with City College's football coach, who was an adjutant general. At the meeting, college officials asked Armstrong if the San Francisco VA could set up a mental health clinic on the college's main Ocean Avenue campus.

He laughs when he recalls that he had no hesitation saying yes, despite the fact that he did not ask permission from Fort Miley's administration.

"When this medical center gave us permission after I committed us to doing it at the college," he says, "we proceeded to get an office, hire some staff, and then create services that would be friendly to our student veterans."

To be student friendly, he emphasizes, meant finding out not just which services clinicians considered essential but which services student veterans considered useful. To do this, Armstrong and his staff talked to the student veterans to "ask them what the hell they want."

What veterans wanted was a safe place where they could gather before, after, or in between classes, plus they wanted counseling, academic advice, and coordination with the health care they were receiving at the VHA itself.

City College refurbished two old classrooms in Cloud Hall. One has been turned into a student lounge. Right next door is a suite of offices where two full-time mental health providers can meet with veterans for on-site counseling and veterans can also receive academic advice from an academic adviser and credentialing officer. Veterans can also enroll in the VA or VHA on-site.

The veterans' lounge is equipped with a refrigerator that is filled with water, juice, and snacks. There are two flat-screen TVs, a couple of tables where people can eat or study, and ten computer cubbies that line two sides of the room. One of the walls is covered with five flags: one for each of the four branches of the service, plus a large black flag with the silhouette of a man whose head is bowed down forlornly as he stands in front of a prison guard tower. A white banner headline promises POW-MIAs "You are not forgotten." Whenever I visit, the lounge is filled with student veterans—male and female—who peer into the computer screens or sprawl across two comfortable, dark brown sofas.

The VA has assigned a licensed clinical social worker as CCSF's student veteran health program coordinator. A psychiatrist works there part time. Because the program has been so successful, in 2013 marriage and family therapist Brandina Jersky was hired to become the full-time Bay Area student veteran outreach coordinator.

As part of his duties at the San Francisco VA, Armstrong spends four hours a week at CCSF counseling students, as does a psychologist who also works for the San Francisco VA and the VA's National Center for PTSD.

"Veterans will come to us and ask us to help them figure out the best way to handle a problem with a professor or student when something comes up in class," says Armstrong. "It's a balancing act for the therapist. You have to assess the capacity of the professor to be sensitive to certain issues and the capacity of the veteran to handle pushback from a professor who won't accept your perspective, given that you were there."

To avoid as many problems as possible, the center offers primers in military culture to faculty and staff. At the most basic level, Armstrong and other counselors try to help professors be aware that when they talk about a particular war or military engagement, "they may have people in the room who were on the ground in that conflict. The professor can phrase things in ways that are respectful of the veteran experience. Without being overly politically correct, the leadership of the center tries to help educational institutions navigate some tricky territory."

Some professors are more sensitive than others. Jersky cites the example of a professor at another Bay Area school who had assigned a particular reading for his class. "One of the student veterans found the assignment very triggering and asked for a different option. The professor wouldn't budge."

"It's like in family therapy," Armstrong says. "Sometimes you can bring things up, and people are ready to hear them. Sometimes there are things you just need to leave alone. It's important for people to learn nuanced thinking, but sometimes some veterans may just need to avoid certain professors or situations. The last thing we want is for the veteran to explode and get thrown out of class—or worse, out of school."

When I spoke to Armstrong and Jersky in 2015 and 2016, Skyline Community College in San Bruno and the College of the Redwoods in Eureka were setting up similar programs. Jersky is also doing outreach to other Northern California schools. Some are enthusiastic, whereas others express tepid interest or none at all. One of her jobs is, therefore, to evaluate where a school stands on this spectrum.

"Some schools," she says, "have a lounge, some a veteran coordinator, some have academic advisers specifically hired to work with student veterans. Some, like University of San Francisco, want nothing to do with the program because they see student veterans as no different from anyone else on campus. Sometimes it takes a few meetings, and what we end up doing might be just encouraging them to have an event for veterans. We come to it, bring materials about VA health care, and leave it at that. It's better than nothing."

If schools want to go further and give faculty and staff an introduction to military culture, veterans' problems, and their many strengths, the program will also do that. Veterans don't only have problems, the two VA therapists highlight. "They are very serious about their education," Armstrong says. "They respect their professors and go nuts when they see students distracted by their cell phones or laptops in class. They are very disciplined and have a lot of skills."

Plus, it is important for institutions of higher education to understand that treating veterans well is not only, in their view, a moral imperative, but good business practice. The more veterans who choose a particular school for their GI Bill–funded education, the more money a school makes.

"With leadership in our front office," Armstrong says, "we began something very important. And VA central office was smart enough to learn from it and turn it into a national program."

He is referring to Veterans Integration to Academic Leadership (VITAL), which helps "facilitate the transition from Soldier to student."[2] The goal is to foster "positive cohesion between Veterans and the entire learning community through campus and community clinical education and training, seamless access to VA healthcare services and on-campus clinical counseling as well as to provide efficient care coordination of all available services."[3]

In 2013 the VITAL program hired Khamkay Chitaphong to direct the national effort. Chitaphong entered the Army National Reserve as a social worker, where he served on two deployments in central Iraq. He is raising a family of four, and, after nearly eleven years of stop-and-start school-work, he has almost completed his PhD.

Throughout his work on the VITAL program, Chitaphong says he has integrated the principles of combat stress control he learned working in Iraq, where he and his team brought services to soldiers rather than waiting for the soldiers to come to them with their problems. As a counselor he would show up in guard towers, at the gym, or in the chow hall. If he and his colleagues knew a convoy or Humvee had been hit by an IED, they would come and meet soldiers returning to base, even if it was at two or three in the morning. They would be there not only to ask how things had gone but to provide critical information. "If you were hit by an IED," Chitaphong would explain to soldiers, "it's normal to have trouble sleeping, or ringing in your ears, or you may have problems with your appetite or find your mind racing. All of this is normal and might persist for a couple of days. 'If it lasts longer,' we'd tell them, 'then please come to us.'"

He recognizes that students are more likely to persist in their education if they feel committed to an institution. And it's not surprising that they are more likely to feel committed to an educational institution if that institution is committed to them. So Chitaphong began to standardize VITAL's offerings. Programs now include a set of four core components:

- Mental health services are provided by licensed practitioners who can do everything from helping with time management to providing evidence-based therapies.
- Coordinators help student veterans navigate both the VA system and the administration or bureaucracy of the school in which they are enrolled.
- Outreach helps to reach out to veterans who are not enrolled in the VA so they can connect with the VBA. Programs also help veterans make service connection claims, access educational benefits, and get into vocational rehabilitation programs.
- Finally, the VITAL program provides training on military culture for administrators, staff, and faculty at educational institutions that serve veterans.

Just as Armstrong began to educate faculty at CCSF, Chitaphong and his colleagues, who meet on biweekly national teleconferences, have prepared two PowerPoint presentations: Military Culture 101 and the Student Veteran Experience.

The primer on military culture helps staff and faculty get it right. It informs you not to refer to every veteran as a soldier; that's just for the Army. Then there's the importance of military rank and identifying the meaning of the "salad," or insignia, that service members wear on their uniforms. Basic training, or boot camp, the primer tells you, involves "being stripped of individuality" and embracing "camaraderie and teamwork." You have a better chance of helping to create a veteran-friendly campus by setting up facilities like a veterans' lounge, where student veterans can feel safe as well as part of a community that is part of, not apart from, the larger student community. Finally, being veteran friendly also means shattering the myths that all veterans have PTSD or other mental problems and are male, which is why the presentations also convey much-needed information on the expanding number of female veterans.

Chitaphong also spends time reaching out to or answering questions from academic institutions that have a high concentration of veterans. "Oftentimes we talk with senior leadership at schools," he says. "Sometimes there is resistance. They may feel they are doing all they can, and then it's 'kudos to you.' If there are barriers, most of the time, we can negotiate through them."

Chitaphong's end goal is to find institutions willing to provide some sort of dedicated space where VHA mental health providers can set up shop and provide services to any veteran enrolled in that particular school.

As of 2017, twenty-three medical centers had a VITAL program, serving 115 college and university campuses like City College of San Francisco. Obviously, this is only a tiny percentage of institutions in which student veterans are enrolled. But it's a start, and one that veterans as well as school staff have told me not only helps with academic success but may even have saved some lives.

One VITAL program counselor told me about a thirty-four-year-old Marine gunner who had had two tours in Iraq and Afghanistan. He had received a 100 percent service-connected disability for PTSD. After he enrolled in a community college outside Boston, his PTSD became so severe that he sought help from the VITAL program, got some housing and financial support, connected to Vocational Rehabilitation, and entered therapy. In May 2016 he graduated North Shore Community College and in the fall continued his studies in business management at Northeastern University in Boston.

Erica Shelly, a Colorado State University veteran success coach, e-mailed me about three student veterans at serious risk for suicide who were then connected to therapists through the VITAL program. "In my opinion," she says, "this likely saved their lives."

10

Suicide Prevention

VHA Programs That Save Lives

At first glance, the Canandaigua VA Medical Center, located in the Finger Lakes district of upstate New York, about half an hour from Rochester, looks more like a small Ivy League college than a medical facility. Built as a VA neuropsychiatric hospital back in 1932, in Tudor and Jacobean revival style, the main buildings are brick with half-timbered facades, steeply gabled roofs, and medieval arches. The facility has been designated a historic hospital and is located in a national historic district next to the Sonnenberg Gardens and Mansion State Historic Park. Over time the rural location saw fewer patients, and so, to avoid facility closure, the VA decided to house the National Homeless Veterans Line, the Women's Health Line, the Caregiver Support Line, and the Veterans Crisis Line on the campus.

I have come to spend the day at the Veterans Crisis Line. In 2015 it was the subject of an HBO documentary, *Crisis Hotline: Veterans Press 1*, that won an Academy Award.[1] The film depicted the difficult daily work of mental health workers responding to suicidal veterans. Like the VA itself, the crisis line has also had its share of bad press. A few days before my arrival, the *New York Times* published an editorial entitled "For Suicidal Veterans, a Frayed Lifeline," calling attention to an inspector general's report stating that Veterans Crisis Line calls weren't being expeditiously answered, or were being sent to voice mail, and that the center was in "disarray," lacking sound leadership and sufficient staff.

The *Times* editorial also noted that studies show veterans who do receive VHA care are less likely to kill themselves and that the veterans who are in trouble are those over fifty who aren't signed up for VA care. The editorial quoted Donald Trump, who called the VA a "horrible, horrible and very unfair system."

The editorial agreed, but with an important caveat: "The VA is horrible, horrible and very unfair. And it's saving people from suicide. Both those statements happen to be true." It went on: "The only real solution is to sign up more veterans, and to serve them better, with greater access to mental health care and a well-run crisis center that has the staffing, oversight, and attention needed for its critical mission."[2]

So how well is the VHA doing on its "critical mission"? Why are veterans killing themselves, and what is the VHA doing about it? Let's start with some of the facts about suicide in the United States in general and among veterans in particular. In August 2016, the VA released a comprehensive report on veteran suicide. It examined fifty-five million records of veterans in every state. Twenty veterans—not twenty-two, as some media reports suggest—die of suicide every day. Only six of those veterans used VA services. Fourteen had not made use of VA services. "Since 2001, U.S. adult civilian suicides increased 23 percent, while veteran suicides increased 32 percent in the same time period."

But, as the *Times* said in its backhanded compliment, veterans who used the VA reduced the increase in the rate of suicide dramatically—by a factor of four, in fact: "Since 2001, the rate of suicide among U.S. Veterans who use VA services increased by 8.8 percent, while the rate of suicide among veterans who do not use VA services increased by 38.6 percent," the report found.

And in 2014, the most recent year studied, the report noted that "veterans accounted for 18 percent of all deaths from suicide among U.S. adults. This is a decrease from 22 percent in 2010."

The report also noted that most veterans who commit suicide are not fresh from the battlefield, as you might imagine if you're reading the media accounts. "Approximately 65 percent of all veterans who died from suicide in 2014 were 50 years of age or older," the report said.[3] Two-thirds of veteran suicides are by firearm (68 percent for males, 40 percent for females).[4]

Between 1979 and 2014, the VHA examined the health records of fifty million veterans from every state in the nation to analyze trends and problems. It has tried to figure out what factors influence veteran suicide and create models that will predict and, hopefully, prevent it. Once veterans with the highest risk for suicide—the 0.1 percent who are forty-three times more likely to attempt suicide in a month—are identified, they are targeted for special outreach. This includes calls if they missed an appointment, along with follow-up visits and offering plans for safety and care. The VHA also offers mobile apps that deal with depression and coach mindfulness, and it provides one called Moving Forward, which is designed to help veterans develop problem-solving skills. Another VHA program is called Coaching into Care, which offers individual telephone advice to families that are trying to encourage a veteran to seek help.

Each VHA medical center has dedicated suicide prevention coordinators, who reach out to veterans in trouble to connect them with needed services and help VHA staff recognize the problem of suicide. As we shall see, all new VHA employees are introduced to the basics of suicide prevention as part of their required staff orientation.

The Veterans Crisis Line is an integral part of this prevention effort. When I visited, it had 253 crisis responders and other staff working on the crisis line 24/7, 365 days a year. Several months after my visit, the VA opened another crisis line in Atlanta, Georgia, adding two hundred more suicide prevention staff. Since 2007, the Veterans Crisis Line has answered 3.3 million calls and dispatched emergency services ninety-three thousand times—saving thousands of lives.

Veterans Crisis Line staff have to respond to calls within thirty seconds—not just from every veteran or veteran's family member who calls in from anywhere in the world, but also from every active-duty service member across the globe. They must also respond to ordinary civilians who have no connection to an active-duty service member or veteran. If a suicidal man or woman dials 1-800-273-TALK, the number for the National Suicide Prevention Lifeline, and hears a voice telling them, "If you are a current US military veteran or current service member or are calling about one, please press 1," they may be too upset to register the information and punch in "1" by mistake. Responders who get the calls must talk with the distraught individual and get them help.

Plus, if any veteran or veteran's family member sends a letter to the White House or to a political representative, or even to the president's or vice president's spouse, and it contains key words or phrases that hint of suicide, this will trigger outreach to the Veterans Crisis Line. A responder will then be assigned to follow up, find the person involved, and offer assistance.

In a meeting with the staff of the Veterans Crisis Line, including interim director Randy Johnson and deputy director Betty Johnson (the two are not related), I learn that not all veterans or family members call because the veteran or a loved one is about to commit suicide. Sometimes veterans are lonely during the day and need someone to talk to. In the evening, after holding it together all day, some begin drinking and may pick up the phone. In the middle of the night, many call because they've woken up from a horrible nightmare or had a flashback. And some call because they are angry at the VHA, the government, or life in general.

Of course, some do call because they are a genuine threat to themselves, their loved ones, or the community. "The goal is to work through the crisis, de-escalate the situation, create safety for now, and outline steps and actions that the veteran can take while working toward a long-term solution," Julianne Mullane, the team operation manager, explains.

If the veteran is in real danger, then the responder does a number of things to ascertain the immediate risk of an actual suicide attempt. "We have impressive investigative skills," says Randy Johnson. Responders are trained to find any hint of ambivalence the caller may express. "If someone is calling with a gun to their head, we need to keep them talking, to find out what brought them to this point," he says. While they talk to the veteran, others on the team will be calling the emergency services and police where the veteran is.

Emergency service personnel cannot enter the home of a suicidal veteran or approach that veteran alone, because veterans may be armed and thus a danger not only to themselves or family or friends but to rescuers. Sending out an ambulance and police to engage in a dramatic, Hollywood-style rescue is the last, rather than first, resort. As Mullane explains, the first thing responders do is ascertain the urgency of the situation.

"For veterans, it's very invasive to have police show up at your door, with the neighbors wondering what's going on," says Tracy Wilt, who was a crisis line responder for seven years and has now worked for several years as a supervisor at the call center. "Once we make the phone call to dispatch, it's out of our hands. We work with dispatchers all over the country; some are trained, some are not and have little familiarity with mental health issues. We're always trying to avoid an unfortunate situation." She is referring to the danger of what is known as suicide by cop, where a veteran brandishes a weapon in an effort to get the police to pull the trigger first.

As I sit with one of the crisis line responders—Maureen Henry, who was featured in the HBO documentary—I learn even more about what it's like to do this kind of crisis intervention. Forty-four years old, Henry has worked at the Veterans Crisis Line for six years. A trim woman with jet-black hair and tattoos on her arms, Henry got a BA in psychology and worked in mental health care for twenty-four years. Five days a week, from eight-thirty to five, she sits in a small cubicle adorned with pictures of her four sons, who range in age from nine to seventeen. As soon as she enters her cubicle, Henry logs on to two computers that track and record all her calls. She has a list of every suicide prevention coordinator in the country, as well as another list of local mental health resources.

Henry then puts on her headset and begins to take calls. She can immediately identify her first caller. That's because he calls at least seventy times a month, every month, and he's not the only one.

"He talks to us about news articles, things in the paper," she says. "We have a protocol to deal with him. We ask him if he's had thoughts of suicide, and if he hasn't, then we just end the call so we can talk to the next veteran in line. We have four or five who call a lot. It's hard because he calls and complains about how we're not helping veterans on the phone, but he's tying up the phone lines so we can't help other veterans. You want to say, 'Do you understand the irony here?' But you can't say that."

When she answers the next caller, all frustration has been erased from her voice. The man tells Henry his name, and she asks, "Are you a veteran? Well, thank you for your service. What's going on today?"

He stammers something I am not privy to on the other end of the line, and she tells him that she is happy to listen to him if he would like to talk. He wants to enroll in a substance abuse program. No one from the program has called him, and even though it's been only twenty-four hours, he is frustrated with the delay. She tries to reassure him and give him a bit of comfort, but she cannot spend time dealing with veteran loneliness or frustrations about life. After ascertaining that he is not in crisis and has no thoughts of suicide, she hangs up, sighs, and takes off her headphones. She explains that this is the fourth time he has called since yesterday. "It's very hard because you want to help veterans like this," she says, "but this is not a chat service; it's a crisis line. You can give them a little bit of time, but you can't chat and chat."

The next caller is a veteran's sister, who is very concerned for his safety.

"What's going on with your brother?" Henry asks politely.

The woman tells Henry that her brother is a Gulf War veteran who is drinking and depressed.

"Does he realize he needs help?" Henry asks.

No, the woman replies, he thinks he's fine.

"That must be very stressful for you," Henry says. "Do you have any thoughts of suicide?"

"No," the woman replies.

"Does your brother talk about suicide himself?" Henry asks.

"Yes," the sister says.

"Would he talk with me?" Henry asks.

The phone is silent for a moment as the woman asks her brother, who says no, he will not.

Henry realizes the veteran may be right next to his sister. "Is he sitting there? Answer yes or no," Henry asks.

"Yes," the woman says.

So carefully, Henry asks more yes-or-no questions.

"Has he exhibited dangerous behavior?"

"Yes, sometimes."

"Does he go to the VA now?"

"No."

"Well," she says, "the VA has all kinds of different services." She then explains how he can get into treatment and asks, "Do you think you can encourage him to get help?"

"Yes, maybe. I hope so."

Henry tells the woman she can put in a referral to his local VA. The brother, she then learns, is homeless.

"We have all kinds of resources for homeless vets," she informs the woman. "We have all kinds of help available. All you have to do is pick up the phone and call." She then suggests the woman call Coaching into Care and tells her it is for family members whose loved ones are reluctant to seek care. She gives the woman the number.

"We're here twenty-four hours a day, seven days a week," Henry tells the woman, who is worried that she might put in a referral against her brother's wishes.

After ten minutes Henry hangs up, takes a very deep breath, and says, "These calls are very hard, because the family is really suffering."

Henry tells me that one of the hardest calls she had was from a veteran who was angry and abusive while on the phone. This is not unusual. "We try to redirect them, to help them, but also encourage them to call when they are not so angry. If they are too abusive," she adds, "we can hang up on them."

This particular man had called several times during her shift, and she tried to deflect the veteran's anger and figure out what was really going on. "He was swearing at me, but I gave him time," she recalls. "I listened to him. It turned out he was a really young Marine and was calling from a naval hospital. He had just gotten back from Iraq. An IED exploded, and he lost his arm. Because of his injury, he wasn't able to pull his friend to safety, and his friend died. He got to cover, but he feels tremendous guilt. He was crying at the end of the conversation and apologized for swearing at me."

Henry explains what he was going through. "He had wanted to be a Marine, and now his purpose was gone, his self-image was gone, everything about him had changed after five seconds on the battlefield," she says. "No wonder he's angry. Sometimes those calls from angry veterans are my favorite calls, because if you can get past that anger and find out what is going on underneath, there's usually such pain and such hurt, and if you can tap into that, you can really help."

She is also often a help to people who are not veterans and call the hotline by mistake. She tells me the story of a teenage girl who punched 1 and told Henry that she had skipped science class and was in the school bathroom cutting herself. She wasn't a suicide risk, but she was deeply troubled. "I asked her if we could call the school while she was on the line, but she hung up on me. But she'd told me the name of her school while we were talking." Henry talked to her supervisor, and they called the school and informed the principal about what had happened.

Henry feels lucky—"blessed, really"—that she has never had a veteran "complete" on the phone. Nonetheless, it is hard to imagine the toll of this work, of listening to story after story day after day. Henry tells me that she has had people call and tell her stories about horrific abuse. "You have to tread very carefully," she says, about how deeply you probe and how much you encourage people to reveal. "If you unpack all their luggage and they're sitting at home with all this stuff, all alone, and you have to move on to the next call . . ." She pauses to reflect on the possible consequences. "You have to be careful and talk about today—'How can I help you today?'"

After spending time with Henry, I talk with Jon Geller, a crisis line responder, and Melanie Haw, a social services assistant. In her late fifties, Haw wears neat khaki pants and a T-shirt and has cropped, graying hair. Between 1981 and 1995, she served in the Navy on the USS *Yellowstone*. She tells me that, as a veteran herself, she understands how difficult it is for veterans to ask for help.

She took a medical retirement and spent the next ten years of her life living out of her car behind a grocery store in upstate New York, smoking marijuana and drinking. She did enroll in the VHA, but only used its services for a variety of physical problems.

She would not tell her providers about her mental health problems. "No way in hell. Not in a million years," she repeats emphatically. "I would see my doctor once a year or whenever. He'd ask if I was fine, and I'd say, 'Yes, doing great.' Finally, I called a homeless hotline, and they gave me a HUD-VASH voucher. [The US Department of Housing and Urban Development and the Veterans Affairs Supportive Housing program—HUD-VASH—provides rental assistant to homeless veterans as well as extensive case management and clinical services to those veterans.] The next day I got a call from the head of Behavioral Health. She said, 'You need a job.' And I said, 'No, I have a HUD-VASH voucher and my $1,000 retirement check, and I have gas in the car and money for weed, and that's all I need."

The woman persisted, and Haw finally relented, "kicking and screaming," and got some help. Now she's working for the crisis line herself. "I have been here six years," she says. "I am clean, sober, and own my own home."

Haw says she is content to work in the background as a social services assistant. She does not want to be a responder. "I am not qualified," she says, "and besides, I would be too mouthy. I call a spade a spade. I would say, 'Hey, you called us fifteen times today! What are you doing?'"

As a social services assistant and a vet, she feels she is able to make a significant contribution by offering her perspective to responders and supervisors. They might come to her with a problem locating a homeless veteran who called in, and she will pinpoint where they are. Or she tells them, "They are blowing smoke up your butt. There is no way they are doing that."

Or maybe responders won't think the situation is dangerous enough to warrant a rescue, and she will disagree and encourage them to do just that. "If someone expresses frustration about a frequent caller, I say, 'Hey, dude, that could be me.' Having been where I've been," she says, "gives me an edge."

And having experienced the support the hotline has given her has changed her attitude toward asking for help. Now she feels completely comfortable going to her supervisor after a difficult call and saying, "Look, I'm about to have a meltdown, and here's why."

"Working here is a challenge, and it keeps me stable," she says. "It's part of my program, and that's a huge reward for me."

Jon Geller is a former Marine. At the crisis line, he tells me, his job is to sell hope. "We offer support when others may not be around," he says. "We let people know that they matter. Whatever they are going through, they don't have to go through this alone. If I'm able to get that across and connect on that level, it's really powerful."

Geller stresses how important it is to respond in a nonjudgmental way to the men and women who call the crisis line. "I am a veteran myself. I served in the Marine Corps and got out in 1992 on a medical discharge. It is not easy for people to make that call, and the whole thing is having a 'brother or sister's six'" (translation: having their back).

To give me an example, he tells me about the Iraq War veteran who called the other day. "The call actually came through the White House," Geller says. "We got it and reached out to him." The caller's monthly benefit for PTSD had been cut because someone had discovered that the twenty-six-year-old was enrolled in a graduate program. If he was well enough to go to school, it was assumed that he no longer needed a 100 percent service connection.

The veteran told Geller that he was not in a traditional classroom in a community college or university. Instead, he remained, as he had been for years, isolated in his apartment, taking classes online. He confided that he hadn't showered in two weeks. "I haven't been with a woman in years," he told Geller. He also told Geller that suicide was definitely an option for him. "I don't want to die, but I am not afraid to die, because this is worse," he told Geller.

"By the end of the phone call," Geller adds, "you know what he agreed to do? Shower. This may not seem huge, but in the short term, it means a lot."

After telling the veteran to reach out any time, Geller contacted the veteran's local suicide prevention coordinator and began to work on the issues that, in his view and the veteran's, led to an inappropriate cut in benefits.

Handling call after call—dealing with frightened, anxious, suicidal people hour after hour, day after day—takes its toll. "When I'm training new people, I tell them it's like walking down a dark alley, and there's rats and piss and garbage strewn all over the place," says Henry. "As a responder, you have to walk down that alley with the veteran and see what's going on. Hopefully, you walk with them to the other end, where there's light. That's the referral and the help. But as a responder, you have to brush that all off of you and go down the next alley with the next veteran."

Mullane agrees. "The type of exhaustion you feel after you've done this work all day is very hard to explain to someone who hasn't done it," she says. "My husband recently worked on a grand jury and had to look at all kinds of horrible pictures with graphic details of motor vehicle accidents, crime scenes, and child abuse. He came home and complained, and I said, 'Now you understand what I do every day.' For us, when we come home and show our battle scars, people don't know how to react. This work is not something you can talk about at a neighborhood barbecue or cocktail party."

A Focus on Wellness

One way the Veterans Crisis Line is trying to address the problems of burnout and other side effects of this work is by focusing on the wellness of staff as well as the safety of veterans. Part of ensuring wellness involves making sure staff are well trained. A lot of civilian crisis lines are staffed by volunteers who don't have much training. At the Veterans Crisis Line, responders and other staff receive three weeks of training.

The Veterans Crisis Line has also started a formal wellness program and hired as its acting coordinator Emily Dumee, who worked for four years as a responder on the night shift. Dumee explains that the program was devised with the help of experts in the field and a heavy dose of input from responders and social service assistants. It focuses not just on physical fitness and nutrition but on emotional, spiritual, financial, social, intellectual, environmental, and occupational wellness.

It's especially needed when tragedy strikes and one of the callers does end up committing suicide within two weeks of a conversation with a responder. In those instances, first responders and social service assistants must be notified and offered counseling themselves. Responders are not put back on active phone duty for several days and are assigned other duties. Any responder who has a difficult call can talk to a supervisor for support. There are biweekly team meetings and monthly individual meetings where responders and social service assistants can get coaching and further support.

The program has also set up a peer-process group, where frontline staff can come together—with no supervisors or others present—to talk about problems they have with callers or conflicts they may have with supervisors or other employees. They also help one another with personal issues. Fifty percent of frontline staff members participate in these groups.

The Veterans Crisis Line is only one part of the VHA's national effort to prevent veteran suicide. That effort is coordinated in Washington, DC, by psychologists Caitlin Thompson and Megan McCarthy, who was the director of Suicide Prevention at the San Francisco VA Health Care Service.

"Suicide risk is very complex, and the science is not well advanced," McCarthy says. "We know what factors indicate a risk of suicide, but many people exhibit those problems. We're bad at predicting who, among all the people who share these common behaviors or attitudes, will actually commit suicide."

A veteran might tell someone that he is having a really hard time and his family would be better off without him. Or he may exclaim that he can't bear it anymore and, by the way, last week he went out and bought a gun. The provider he is talking to may then ask if the veteran is thinking of killing himself. The veteran says no, and he may very well be telling the truth at that moment.

"Some suicide attempts are very impulsive," McCarthy says. "A person might not be thinking of killing themselves today. Then tomorrow things get really bad, and suddenly suicide becomes an option." In fact, surveys have found that 24 to 74 percent of people who attempted suicide began their attempt within ten minutes of making the decision.[5]

To make sure that those who might make these decisions get real help, outreach about the Veterans Crisis Line and veteran suicide goes on at every VHA facility and in local communities throughout the nation. When I was recently at Fort Miley, the suicide prevention team had set up a table near the cafeteria in an effort to inform veterans, staff, and family members about the crisis line. They gave out brochures, gun locks, and cards and answered questions about the hotline and other suicide prevention efforts.

Every VHA medical center has a suicide prevention coordinator and team. They respond to any calls from the Veterans Crisis Line. "If a veteran tells a responder that they are not enrolled in VHA care, or haven't seen a doctor in a year, they are referred to the suicide prevention/crisis team at the local level," McCarthy says. "A member of that team will reach out to the veteran to see if they want to come in to receive care. If they are not signed up for VHA care and are eligible, a sign-up can be initiated within hours. If the veteran isn't eligible for care, they will be referred to outside resources. No one who is actively suicidal will be refused services. They will be treated in a VHA emergency room or sent to one in the community. It is the policy of every VHA hospital to provide emergency and humanitarian care for everyone."

If the veteran already has a VHA provider, the suicide team will contact that provider, who will, in turn, reach out to the veteran. "It's much better if someone the veteran knows is in contact rather than a complete stranger," says McCarthy. If veterans do come in for help, they will not only get psychological and behavioral counseling and care but also can get help with their finances, housing, and employment.

Suicide prevention coordinators educate VHA staff at every level. Brian Tate Guelzow, a clinical psychologist, is the suicide prevention coordinator at Fort Miley. Every two weeks, he gives an orientation session on the problem of veteran suicide to all new employees. The people in the room may be physicians, clerks, social workers, transport workers, or engineers. No matter where they are in the health care hierarchy, they can come into contact with veterans and need to understand the facts, myths, and realities about suicide. They also need to recognize the signs so they can understand what to do if they hear a stray comment, encounter a despondent patient, or even overhear a worrisome discussion in the hallway.

The tall psychologist with salt-and-pepper hair and a neatly trimmed mustache stands in front of the room and packs facts, figures, and critical advice into his thirty-minute presentation. Although it seems a short time to go over such a vast amount of critical material, this is a presentation you will rarely see in a private-sector hospital.

Guelzow begins his presentation by reassuring the audience that he does not expect them to be experts on suicide in just thirty minutes. What he does hope is that they will be able to identify risks of suicide and feel more comfortable intervening when necessary. He begins to outline some of the general facts and then debunks some of the most prevalent myths about veteran suicide.

Perhaps the most common myth is the idea that merely mentioning the issue will lead someone to taking his life. Asking people whether they are contemplating suicide, he reassures them, will not lead them to kill themselves.

"I have never known anyone who said, 'Oh, now that you mention it, what a good idea,'" he tells the group. Asking people about suicide does, however, give them permission to talk about their problems, which in turn allows you to give them hope and reassurance and get them the help that will be lifesaving, he says.

He also cautions them: don't for a moment think that people are divided into two camps—the talkers and the doers—and don't believe that even if you're dealing with a very determined doer, there's nothing you can do to stop them. The acute risk for suicide is often time limited, and the conditions or circumstances that lead to it are treatable. Most important, he reiterates, helping someone find a safe environment for treatment can save a life.

Guelzow's goal is to encourage all employees to take part in what the VHA calls Operation SAVE, which is an acronym for

- Signs of suicidal thinking should be recognized.
- Ask the most important question of all.
- Validate the veteran's experience.
- Encourage treatment and expedite getting help.

What the VHA is trying to do is identify people who are thinking about hurting or killing themselves; looking for ways to die; talking about death, dying, or suicide; or engaging in self-destructive or risk-taking behavior, especially when it involves alcohol, drugs, or weapons.

Any or all of this should trigger the staff member to ask what Guelzow calls the most critical question: "Are you thinking about killing yourself?"

"It's easy to ask this question in a way that's mumbled or jumbled," Guelzow acknowledges. "You don't want to ask the question as the veteran is about to leave the room or in a way that suggests you really don't want to know. Saying something like, 'You're not thinking of killing yourself, are you?' communicates that you really don't want to know the truth," he warns.

A hand goes up in the audience, and a young woman, newly hired as a clerk, asks, "So what do you do if the answer is yes?"

The first thing Guelzow tells them is what not to do. "Don't keep the veteran's suicidal behavior a secret," he says. "Do not leave him or her alone. Inform appropriate staff immediately, but stay with the veteran till help arrives. Or walk the veteran to the emergency room to get that help ASAP."

Finally, Guelzow warns, no one should ever negotiate with someone who has a gun. If that happens, he says, "Get to safety and call 911, VA Police (extension 2222). If the veteran has taken pills, cut himself or herself, or done harm to himself or herself in some way, again: call 911, VA Police (extension 2222)."

Later, when I interview Guelzow in his office in Building Eight, he says that this orientation is only a small part of what the suicide team does at Fort Miley. Guelzow and his team provide more intensive educational sessions for mental health providers, psychology interns, and residents. Most important, they work with other providers to identify patients who are at high risk for committing suicide, immediately implementing a series of mandated protocols once someone is flagged as a suicide risk or has attempted suicide and survived.

Guelzow gives me the example, all too common in San Francisco, of a veteran—let's call him Joe Smith—whom the police found about to jump off the Golden Gate Bridge. Smith is hospitalized in the inpatient psychiatry ICU at Fort Miley and, after he has been treated and stabilized, is discharged.

A high-risk flag is activated in the medical record, which is shared by all Smith's providers, and a carefully monitored protocol is followed. This includes post-discharge follow-up visits at which the veteran's continued risk for suicide is evaluated. If Smith doesn't show up for any of these appointments, that is a signal that triggers outreach efforts. Three attempts are made to contact the veteran. If he does not respond, this may then lead to a "welfare check."

If Smith does come to his follow-up appointments, he may be offered a variety of different therapies. If the veteran declines, there is no way to force him to get further help. Throughout this follow-up period, the suicide alert stays on the veteran's electronic medical record. At the end of ninety days, providers once again assess the veteran's suicide risk and may remove the flag on his record.

The suicide team also functions as on-call consultants throughout the hospital. Consider, McCarthy says, the case of an audiologist who has gone through an initial suicide training. One of her patients says he's feeling depressed. When he leaves the office, the audiologist says, "See you for your next appointment," to which he responds that he isn't sure he'll make it. Given her introduction to suicide risk and her concern about the veteran's state of mind, she may call the suicide prevention team for a consult.

"This is a very delicate process for providers," McCarthy says. "Many veterans are very concerned about their privacy, and providers don't want to violate confidentiality. But they are equally concerned about patient safety." She continues, "We constantly tell people to please pick up the phone and call us, even if it's outside our normal business hours. If people are showing any warning signs or displaying worrisome behavior or saying things that concern you, please don't hesitate."

The VHA doesn't just wait for veterans in crisis to reach out via the Veterans Crisis Line or suicide prevention coordinators. It has used its vast data bank of information on veterans to develop a program called REACH VET. I first learned about REACH VET from clinical psychologist Spencer Beck, whom I met at the newly opened Southwest Community Based Outpatient Clinic, which is part of the VA Phoenix Medical Center. Beck explained that REACH VET, which was launched in December 2016, identifies the top 0.1 percent of veterans who are at the highest statistical risk for suicide and other adverse outcomes. These veterans are thirty times as likely to complete a suicide.

"The program," Beck says, "is a joint effort between the National Institute of Mental Health and the VA. The project looked at sixty variables that contributed to statistical risk based on veterans who are using the VA health care system. One of the variables," he says, "is veterans who are on multiple psychotropic medications. We also know there is a higher risk of suicide for older white males, so we're also looking at veterans' race, age, and relationship status—whether they are divorced, married, separated, or widowed."

Beck stresses the importance of this data. "It allows us to more effectively target our outreach efforts and see if we can engage the veteran to enhance their care in some way," he says. It also serves as a warning or caution to providers that particular veterans are at a higher statistical risk and to keep that in mind when thinking about their patients' needs for care and attention.

Russell Lemle, psychology director at the San Francisco VA Health Care System, emphasizes how important and unique this program is. "We can look at all the records of all the veterans in the system, medical center by medical center. This includes not only veterans who are seeking mental health services or have talked about suicide, but those who have not but are at high risk. This is critical because we know that many people who complete a suicide have never talked to anyone about this or may not be seeking mental health treatment. Nobody but the VA is doing this kind of sophisticated targeting. Kaiser is trying to identify people at risk for suicide, but they are only dealing with people who are in mental health treatment."

Each VA major facility has a REACH VET coordinator (there are now over one hundred) who can reach out to veterans in the facility's area. Once a veteran is identified, a mental health or primary care provider reaches out to the veteran to check on how he or she is doing. They also review charts and treatment plans and make recommendations for further treatment. In the area of suicide prevention, Thompson, one of the coordinators of the VA's national suicide prevention program, calls REACH VET a "game changer."

The Gun Conundrum

One of the toughest problems VHA caregivers face when it comes to preventing and reducing veteran suicide is navigating the contentious issue of gun ownership. Although there are many murky and little-understood factors that determine whether and why a person chooses to kill himself, one thing is not at all ambiguous. When veterans try to kill themselves, many of them pick up a firearm. This is a significant problem because, as the statistics underline, at least 85 percent of suicide attempts with a firearm are fatal.[6] That's because, unlike many other methods, when someone initiates a suicide attempt with a gun, it can almost never be reversed. People with guns at home are more than twice as likely to die by suicide as people who don't have guns at home. The risk is even higher if the guns are stored loaded and unlocked.[7]

Separating veterans with serious depression, problems with substance abuse, or suicidal ideas from their firearms is thus one of the best ways to prevent them from succeeding in killing themselves. Although this makes total sense, any whiff of gun-control talk or of relinquishing firearms, even on a voluntary and temporary basis, raises deep concern in the veteran community. To deal with this significant problem, VHA suicide prevention experts have had to walk on proverbial eggshells, crafting solutions to a major problem without invoking a firestorm of suspicion or protest.

The way VHA suicide prevention experts have dealt with this problem that has divided the entire nation is to partner with suicide prevention groups outside the VHA, as well as veteran gun owners and civilian gun dealers. "If we are going to forge effective approaches in the broader veteran community, we need the voices of gun advocates, veterans, and their families," says Lemle. The San Francisco VA, adapting work from the Means Matter Project at the Harvard School of Public Health's Injury Control Research Center, was given a three-year grant from the VA central office to develop a pilot training to teach staff how to talk with and counsel veterans about safe storage of their weapons when they are at risk for suicide.

On March 4, 2016, I attended a conference that Lemle helped organize where all these groups came together. The conference, "Counseling Veterans at Risk for Suicide: Safe Storage of Firearms and Other Lethal Means," was sponsored by the San Francisco VA Health Care System and the American Foundation for Suicide Prevention's Greater San Francisco Bay Area chapter. Presenters and participants included veterans (many of whom had contemplated or even attempted suicide), the mother and father of a veteran who had actually committed suicide, mental health care professionals, suicide prevention researchers, and three firearm dealers. All of them agreed with Christine Moutier, MD, chief medical officer for the American Foundation for Suicide Prevention, who said in her presentation that one way to reduce the suicides that are ending the lives of twenty veterans a day is to encourage veterans in crisis to safely store their weapons.

This is not easy, said Jason Zimmerman, a former Army medic who has PTSD and is now a peer specialist at the James H. Quillen VA Medical Center in Mountain Home, Tennessee, as he explored the central dilemmas the conference addressed. Many veterans come from regions where gun ownership is part of the culture, and when you're in the military, you get further attached to guns.

"In the military service," Zimmerman explained, "we learned that our weapons are our friends." Once out of the service, Zimmerman continued, veterans may be reluctant to go into counseling or report a mental health problem or suicidal thoughts because they erroneously believe their weapons will be taken away from them. They and their families will then be unprotected from threatening strangers, which many report to be the primary reason they own firearms.

To reduce the threat of suicide in a population committed to gun ownership is therefore a challenge. Catherine Barber, director of the Means Matter Project at the Harvard School of Public Health's Injury Control Research Center, explained that many people erroneously believe that people who try to kill themselves will eventually find a way to succeed. According to the scientific evidence, she said, only 10 percent of those who attempt to kill themselves will go on to die by suicide at a later date. Reducing access to lethal means thus reduces the overall suicide rate. For instance, in 2006 the Israeli Defense Forces required service members to leave their weapons on base when they left for weekend leave; the suicide rate dropped by 40 percent.

Suicide prevention advocates and researchers thus want veterans in crisis to leave their guns with friends or store them at shooting ranges or in safes in their own homes. To encourage veterans to do this, of course, involves asking them the right questions in the right way and at the right time. To make sure this happens, the VHA asked McCarthy to create a pilot project, in collaboration with Means Matter, that developed a veteran-specific program to train mental health providers in lethal means safety counseling.

McCarthy told the audience that providers need to "engage in a collaborative conversation with an at-risk veteran that explores options for temporarily storing lethal means more safely." Even seasoned mental health professionals need to understand that directly telling a veteran he or she shouldn't have access to a firearm during a crisis will not work as well as guiding the veteran to think about how to keep himself safe when things look unremittingly bleak.

Since the conference, the San Francisco VA has turned over its pilot project on safe storage of firearms to the Rocky Mountain VA VISN's Mental Illness Research Education and Clinical Center. At a national meeting held in 2017, this clinical center trained all suicide prevention coordinators in dealing with lethal means. It has also held four national webinars to provide further education around the issue. As in suicide prevention training, Lemle explains that education involves dealing with things like the common myth that you can never stop someone from committing suicide. What is perhaps most important about this ongoing work, he says, is how much support it has received from veterans and their families. "Most veterans and their families support inquiries about the availability of lethal means and also support the development of safety plans that temporarily and voluntarily encourage safe storage of firearms if a veteran is in crisis."

As is typical with public–private partnerships in the VHA, all the information, research, treatments, and training the VHA develops about suicide prevention is available to private-sector researchers and practitioners, which is one reason why researchers like Barber are so impressed with the VHA. "I don't understand the image the media is painting of the VHA," Barber told me candidly. "It bears no relationship to what I see happening and what I experience when working with VHA providers and researchers."

How We Understand Veteran Suicide

Over the past decade, the topic of veteran suicide has received more heated attention than perhaps any other. The media and members of Congress blame the VHA often for not fully understanding the issue and certainly for not solving it. The rain of accusations seems unrelenting. Observing this debate, I am constantly struck by the rancorous and often superficial nature of the blame game. Suicide is a horrible, tragic problem—one that is unique not to veterans but to the human condition. Although we often expect the medical system to analyze, understand, and remedy every aspect of the human condition, this is beyond the power of science. When it comes to suicides that are a product of war, things become even more heated and complicated. As McCarthy succinctly states, "What so much of this discussion about veteran suicide overlooks is the state of the science when it comes to many persistent and truly awful mental disorders."

Many VHA patients enter the military with a host of psychological and behavioral problems. Going to war—even preparing to go to war—does not improve their state of mind or psyche. In many instances it creates other problems that the veteran never experienced before. Yet VHA caregivers are being asked to do what we would never ask of caregivers in the private sector. (Imagine, for example, blaming an oncologist for not fully parsing the mystery of cancer or railing against a pulmonologist who was unable to cure a miner with black lung disease.)

"When people come back from war with terrible mental problems, not all of them can be fixed if we just applied ourselves better," McCarthy says. "The problem is not that we are not trying hard enough."

"It's very frustrating when people constantly ask why the VA isn't solving this problem [of veteran suicide] or doing more," says Craig Bryan, executive director of the National Center for Veterans Studies at the University of Utah. A psychologist and veteran himself, Bryan points out how much the VA is actually doing. "When I'm asked that question by journalists, I always say, 'What are you talking about? The VA is doing more than anyone else. Yes, there is room for improvement, and yes, mistakes are made, but we have to contextualize the issue.'"

To understand the context, Bryan says, you have to recognize several critical facts. One is that the increased rate of suicide nationwide is a serious problem with complex social roots that no single organization has been able to fully understand or solve. We also have to understand, he says, that the VA is not the only organization about which veterans complain. Many veterans leave the military feeling misunderstood and alienated from much of society. At least at the VA, he points out, there are specialists who are trained in dealing with the unique traumas that veterans face.

"When a Marine's buddy commits suicide, the Marine veteran will often say, 'I didn't do enough,' and will blame himself," Bryan says. "He will get frustrated when private-sector providers don't seem to understand what he's going through. Private-sector providers will tell them that their problem is they are too perfectionist and that they just have to get rid of that sense of perfectionism and honor," says Bryan. "And they stop going. These providers don't understand that for many years of their lives, these guys were taught that you have to give 100 percent; you can't make mistakes, because if you do, someone dies. And so then, when someone like one of their buddies does die, they blame themselves. It's very hard to help someone deconstruct the difference between their value system and exaggerated self-blaming."

And it's even harder, Bryan says, to encourage people to seek help when they've been socialized to believe that mental problems are a sign of weakness and they should be able to tough it out on their own. When they do seek help from the VHA, Bryan says, they do better.

"It's tragic," Bryan says, "that I never get calls from journalists asking me about veterans who are treated appropriately and effectively at the VA. I only get calls when there is trouble."

11

OVERCOMING DISABILITY

VA Rehabilitation Services

Chris York, a tall, gaunt former Marine in his early thirties, is staring intently at the large, black Dynavision machine in front of him. Small plastic squares are scattered across its surface and blink, apparently randomly, in the center, top, bottom, or around the periphery. York tries to hit each one as it flickers for what seems like only a nanosecond. Numbers also periodically flit across the screen. And York shouts out each one that he sees: "Twenty-four, fifteen, forty-six."

By his side a smaller, trim woman, occupational therapist Cate Dorr, cheerleads every strike he makes and every number he repeats by exclaiming, "Great, Chris!" or "That's super!" or "Go, Chris!" or "Wonderful!"

The Dynavision machine is used in neurological rehabilitation for patients trying to improve reaction time, balance, visual scanning, peripheral vision, gross motor skills, and many more cognitive neurological functions that have been impacted by strokes, TBIs, and other conditions. It's one of the many tools used in the VA's nationwide Polytrauma System of Care to help veterans and active-duty service members recover from complex traumatic injuries. York has spent time in the acute brain injury inpatient unit and has now progressed to the residential Polytrauma Transitional Rehabilitation Program (PTRP), which will help him get back to the community.

After leaving the Marines, York worked in roofing and construction in Salt Lake City. Then he got into a car crash. After spending a month in a coma in intensive care, he came to Palo Alto. His head is a road map to his injury. Lines of scarred skin bisect his buzz cut where his skull was opened and a section removed so surgeons could repair the damage to his brain. He now talks with the slow, almost affectless speech of those who have suffered from a severe TBI, and he walks slowly, with pronounced attention to every step.

He is frank about his ordeal and his current disabilities. He spent weeks, he tells me, relearning everything. "I could get out of bed, but I looked real bad and couldn't make it to the chair," he says. "I wasn't strong enough to walk, and they made me go everywhere in a wheelchair. The injury affected my ability to talk. My tongue isn't very strong, so I don't have enough muscle to push the food back anymore. I have to work to strengthen my tongue. I still do my exercises every meal. I have a tongue depressor and push it out over and over and over."

"One of his cranial nerves that controls his tongue was impacted," Dorr explains. "The nerve that controls facial muscles on the left side was affected. He couldn't blink, and his eye was sewn shut. It still isn't working properly, and he has double vision, which is a huge piece of balance."

York is working on the Dynavision machine because he wants to drive again. Dorr is optimistic that he will. "We are targeting the left side of the brain that controls Chris's dominant right arm," Dorr says. "We're using it partially for motor control, muscle strengthening, muscle movement, and accuracy. We're practicing dividing attention between multiple stimuli, scanning all of your peripheral visual fields as well. Chris," she says, turning to him as she talks to me, to include him in the conversation, "is definitely making progress. The first time we did this, he got about four out of ten on the numbers in the middle. Now it's nine out of ten."

York is also determined to return to marathon running. Before he got into the car crash that changed his life, his goal was to run half marathons. "I do not want to let this injury get in the way of that," he insists.

With the help of physical therapist Pat Wager, he has, in fact, gone from barely being able to move from the bed to the chair to running. Wager recounts the beginning of York's journey as we sit talking in the physical therapy room in Palo Alto. "I didn't know if he could do it because of his vision. But he asked if he could try, and I said, 'Sure.'"

When he saw York try to run, he noted that one of his biggest problems was his right leg. He couldn't bring his toes through a stride, and they would catch. His balance was entirely off. But York, whom Wager describes as going a hundred miles on everything, would not give up. So when Wager finished his day's work with a full caseload of patients and York finished his full day of therapy, the two headed out to run the 2.25-mile loop around the Palo Alto VA campus.

"It was very scary in the beginning," Wager recalls. "I ran really close to him. I had my hand out ready to grab his T-shirt." A couple of problems cropped up right away: York would run to the left side of the trail in the lane of runners coming the other way. Another problem would occur every time York cleared his throat and spat. "He'd lose balance and take a dive into the bushes," says Wager.

York continued. In fact, he had the idea of starting a running team, which is now called Team Trauma and includes staff, military liaisons, and patients. Their first race was a fund-raiser for the Stanford Pulmonary Hypertension Program.

Team Trauma is now a fixture at the Palo Alto VA Medical Center's Polytrauma Transitional Rehabilitation Program, which is one of five VHA Polytrauma Rehabilitation Centers around the country. They are part of the VHA's extensive Polytrauma System of Care, which spans the spectrum of rehabilitative services for patients, with sites that are strategically located across the many regions of the VHA.

Rehab programs at the VHA don't only serve veterans. Because the DoD's hospitals do not deliver extensive rehabilitation services, it has a memorandum of understanding with the VHA, whose rehab programs also serve active-duty service members. When active-duty service members have sustained complex injuries on the battlefield—TBIs and resulting PTSD, burns, amputations, and more—they are treated in the field and then sent to a military hospital, where they are cared for in the most acute and intense phase. Once they are stabilized, they are sent to polytrauma rehab. Rehab programs also serve active-duty service members who have complex injuries that were sustained outside of combat. Most of the active-duty service members I met when I was at Palo Alto had been in motor vehicle—mostly motorcycle—accidents while they were on duty in the continental United States. Some had previously been in combat.

The VHA works in such close collaboration with the DoD in this area that each branch of the service has a special liaison officer with a Wounded Warrior program assigned to major rehab facilities. At Palo Alto, members of the different branches of the military serve as nonmedical case managers to patients in various programs. They have their own dedicated offices on-site so they can maintain constant contact with patients who are active-duty service members. As Lieutenant Peter Reichenbach, nonmedical care manager with the Navy Wounded Warrior Safe Harbor, and Debra Bruton, the Marine Corps liaison, explained to me, their role is to help people who have been socialized not to ask for help.

"You can't just march into someone's room and ask if they need help." Reichenbach recounts what he has learned the hard way. "From watching Deb, who's been my mentor, you have to go in and establish rapport. You have to ask permission for them to let you use the knowledge you have to help them out."

Nonmedical liaisons like Reichenbach and Bruton assist families in many ways. They help them obtain financial resources to travel to visit a loved one and make sure they can stay in a local hotel or one of a national network of Fisher Houses—lodgings built to house military or veteran families when a loved one is hospitalized. Perhaps most important, they help active-duty service members deal with medical boards that will decide if they are fit to return to service, get compensation for their injuries, and access VA health care.

These military liaisons serve an important function, says Odette Harris, the neurosurgeon who directs the Polytrauma Rehabilitation Center. They are there so that "active-duty service members who have sustained significant injuries do not feel isolated and abandoned by the military."

I expected to see mostly younger veterans in rehab programs at the VHA, but many of the patients are older. Some had fallen off a ladder, had a stroke, had a knee or hip replacement, or been in a car crash.

For veterans, stays in the Polytrauma Rehabilitation Centers are not time limited as they are by private-sector insurance, Harris says. In the private sector and under Medicare rules, patients are given a limited number of days of inpatient rehab accompanied by varied levels of co-payments. Then the meter runs out. In the VHA, by contrast, discharge is determined by the patient's progress in recovering function and rehabilitation, Harris notes. In their acute phase, rehab patients focus, Wager tells me, on recovering basic motor and cognitive skills: getting from the bed to a chair, going to the toilet, walking. The goal of the program is "to return each individual to the least restrictive environment possible. This may include return to active duty, work, school, or independent living in the community with engagement in meaningful daily living activities."[1]

Patients in these programs have a vast array of services. The PTRP includes the Return to Work Tech Shop as well as the Warrior Canine Connection, which uses service dogs to help veterans learn how to relate, control their emotions, communicate, and navigate. It also helps them return to their families and communities—and to school and work.

Finally, the Polytrauma System of Care includes seven Regional Amputation Clinics and eighteen Polytrauma Amputation Network sites that provide the latest in prosthetics and methods to increase mobility after an amputation. Then there are nineteen Polytrauma Network Sites, which provide outpatient rehabilitation for brain injury and polytrauma patients. One of the Polytrauma Network Site programs, School Workshops for Academic Success, works in collaboration with the Army Wounded Warrior Program, the Assistive Technology Center, and the Polytrauma Medicine Initiative to help veterans who have had brain injuries go to or finish school and move back into the civilian world. The VA also provides a network of outpatient polytrauma rehabilitation services for people who need longer-term cognitive therapy, physical and occupational therapy, and speech therapy, among other things.

In each of these areas, teams of clinicians and other caregivers work together. These include neurologists; orthopedists; physiatrists who specialize in rehabilitation medicine; prosthetists; psychologists; psychiatrists; social workers; nurses; physical, occupational, recreation, and art therapists; speech language pathologists; and chaplains. Freda Dreher, a physiatrist who works at the White River Junction VA, one of the spokes attached to the hubs of both the Spinal Cord and Polytrauma Systems of Care, says that one of the reasons she left the Dartmouth–Hitchcock Medical Center to work at the VHA in White River Junction was the VHA's focus on teamwork.

"I made a deliberate choice to come here," she says, as her colleagues in speech language pathology and nursing nod in agreement, "because I have a team to work with." Social workers, nurses, occupational therapists—you name it, she says, all work together and talk together. In the private sector, Dreher tells me, all those different professionals were there; they existed, but their work was not coordinated and integrated, as it is in the VHA.

Dreher says the care she and her colleagues provide is "like a dance." As a member of that dance troupe, Dreher evaluates and treats and writes out traditional medical orders. But, she says, she depends on her colleagues, who are constantly conveying their own responses and ideas. "We are interdependent on each other's knowledge, skill, and scope of practice," she insists.

In the choreography of this dance, as Dreher has explained, the patient's family plays a central role. To facilitate their participation on the patient care team, the VA helps to assure that service members' or veterans' families who may live far away from a center of care can stay closer to their loved ones who are in treatment. If families do not have the money to pay for a stay in a hotel, the VA works in conjunction with a special network of Fisher Houses to provide shelter for family members, and it provides travel money. The Fisher House in Palo Alto is a calm, well-equipped residence with kitchen facilities. The Defenders Lodge is also available for shorter stays.

Scott Skiles, the polytrauma social work supervisor, says that the VA also pays stipends for family members to care for patients when they return home through its caregiver support program.

"We will rent the family member a car if they need it, paid for out of funds we have raised in the community," says Skiles. "We have even worked out a deal with National Car Rental to get extra insurance if a veteran's partner or family member is too young to rent one."

Assuring family involvement in a patient's rehabilitation is critical, psychologist Elizabeth McKenna tells me as we sit in her comfortable office in Palo Alto. The head of family therapy for the Polytrauma System of Care, she says the VA understands serious injuries affect not just patients but their families as well. If family members get sufficient initial and ongoing support, this will help them in caring for patients who may need care for years, perhaps decades.

"We are talking," McKenna says emphatically, "about everything from doing a loved one's intimate hygiene [e.g., helping with bathing, going to the toilet, dressing, eating] to assisting the patient in transferring from a bed to a wheelchair or with basic communication." Family members may have to make sure a bed-bound patient doesn't develop a bedsore, or they may have to deliver and monitor complicated therapies for patients who have multiple injuries.

Most difficult, perhaps, McKenna tells me, is helping children adjust to a parent's injuries. To demonstrate precisely how, she pulls out a red plastic doctor's kit with toy syringes and stethoscopes. She shows me dolls with walkers and one young man in a wheelchair holding a basketball. McKenna uses these toys to help children who have trouble understanding that "my dad or mom is different now."

"Their parents may be using profanity they never used before, or they're increasingly irritable," McKenna continues. "These kids have gotten used to fathers—or mothers—who are away on long deployments, and now they're home all the time, but they are injured. Kids and spouses have to reconnect with someone who is not only physically injured but often has PTSD."

Dealing with an injured loved one is a process, McKenna says. "The husband may have lost both legs and has a brain injury. The wife is only concerned with whether he will survive. When they discover that their loved one will, in fact, survive, they are incredibly relieved. And then suddenly they discover that the spouse can't walk, or has trouble forming or understanding words, that they have speech impediments. They may be impulsive or lack inhibitions." The catalog of disability—and possible disaffection on the part of the caregiver—is almost endless.

And then, McKenna adds, there is sex. Spouses naturally have concerns about whether their loved one will ever be able to have sex with them again. Complicating matters further, sometimes a neuropsychiatrist may actually have to determine whether the injured patient can even consent to sexual activity.

"When someone suffers a devastating injury, family dynamics are just turned topsy-turvy," McKenna adds. "Family relationships change completely. They change again as a person gets better; you have to reestablish a marital relationship, as opposed to a caregiving relationship."

Family counseling has been invaluable, says Becky Johnson,* the twenty-two-year-old wife of twenty-four-year-old Marine Errol Johnson.* The three of us talked during one of the dinners that the Polytrauma Residential Rehabilitation Program, with the help of different community groups, puts on each week for veterans and their families. While on active duty stateside, Errol had a motorcycle accident and ended up at the Palo Alto VA after a monthlong stint at a private-sector rehab hospital. Becky has been able to accompany her husband through this part of his recovery only because of generous VA programs and benefits. She has stayed for over a month at the Fisher House and received help with transportation to and from her home in Southern California. If her husband needs ongoing care, she will be able to take advantage of a program that pays and supports caregivers of post-9/11 veterans.

"They've explained a lot of things about brain injury and what to expect in his recovery," Becky says. "They're very quick to respond to any issue. For me, it's a total role change from wife to caretaker." Looking over at her husband sitting at her side, she adds, "Talking with a therapist has also helped me deal with his anger."

"I'm the kind of guy that likes to scare the locals," Errol interjects. His brain injury, both agree, has made this worse.

"He was very angry," Becky says. "There were all these older people in the convalescent facility. There were patients roaming around, yelling and screaming. He was really angry being around all these older people, and I couldn't take care of him. Coming to this hospital, I've noticed a drastic change. He's around people his age that he can talk to; they're in the military. They give dinners like this here. He isn't just stuck in a room."

Another patient, an older veteran, underlines the importance of being treated in a community of active or former service members. Colonel David Rabb, an African American retired career military officer, served in the Army and Marine Corps for thirty-three years. From 2004 to 2005, Rabb was in Iraq as commander of the 785th Medical Company. Then, between 2007 and 2009, he was the US Army Western Region Medical Command care and transition coordinator and worked at the Palo Alto VA as a VA–DoD military liaison. Rabb served on active duty as the director of psychological health for the Sixty-Third Regional Support Command in Mountain View, California, from 2009 to 2011, where he managed the psychological health of forty thousand reserve soldiers who were deployed to or returned from war. In 2013, after he retired, Rabb returned to the VA as director of the VHA Diversity and Inclusion Office, where he served from San Diego as a virtual employee whose scope was the whole country.

Rabb, who is wearing a black Army T-shirt and shorts, is back at the VHA as a patient. He suffered a stroke, which has been complicated by PTSD, with which he was diagnosed in 2003. He has loss of vision in one eye and many other physical and cognitive problems. As we talk, he rides on a Vasper machine, a recumbent exercise bike that is hooked up to a compressor with a tangle of electrical leads. Blood pressure–style cuffs circle his arms and thighs, returning messages to the machine's command center. These messages trigger a response in the brain that stimulates the growth of anabolic hormones that repair muscle. The cooling mechanism is designed to keep the user's core temperature lower and maximize blood oxygen exchange. When he has finished his twenty minutes of intensive workout, he will lie on a cooling pad for ten minutes, which he says he finds very calming.

When he first had his stroke, Rabb says, he went to a Sharp Rehabilitation Hospital in San Diego for two months. After a monthlong stint at Fort Bliss, Texas, he came to Palo Alto. "The VA," he says, "is heads and shoulders above the private sector. People here are mission driven; that's what they do here. They also have military cultural competency. They know me here. They know where I came from. They speak my language and understand concepts near and dear to me. At Sharp I felt like I was a fish out of water. They provided good quality care, but they couldn't treat my soul. They could treat what was visible, but a lot of what was wrong was invisible. For me the physical problems are about 20 percent of it. The rest is about the psychosocial environment where you feel you can grow."

Polytrauma care at the VA includes a long-term outpatient program. In the physical therapy room, I met a stocky, bearded vet in his fifties who was working out. Kai Azada, who lives in Santa Cruz, takes the shuttle every week and stays at the Defenders Lodge while he engages in long-term rehab. Azada was in the Army between 1982 and 1988. While he was on active duty, his weapon blew up in his face. It was, he says, like a shock wave from an IED. When he was examined after the accident, "They told me," he recalls, "that there was no bleeding from my eardrums, no physical damage, so I went right back to duty. They never like to have to report training accidents, especially when things blow up." Bleeding or no bleeding, Azada knew something was wrong with him. "I was slower, in a fog," he recalls. "They thought I was being lazy."

When he left the Army, things got worse. "I couldn't hold down a job, had trouble working with people. I was twenty-four when I got out of the Army in 1988. I'm fifty-one now. For me it was a long, slow decline. I was obviously depressed. I had PTSD and became worse."

Azada said he lived like a hermit for years. He didn't leave the house and gained almost a hundred pounds. Finally, he went to the Vet Center and spent three years in counseling. The Vet Center also helped him prove his claim for benefits, which took eight and a half years to wend its way through the VBA.

When he finally got benefits for PTSD and depression, he was sent for neuropsychological testing. Asked if he had ever been in an explosion, Azada said, "I had to think for a minute. I said, 'Yeah, a weapon exploded. An M-16 rifle split clear in half.'" He was then diagnosed with a TBI. "It made a huge difference," he says. "I started having cognitive behavioral therapy, learning how to work with deficits in executive function, decision making, planning, prioritizing, and memory."

He is proud of the progress he has made. "Oh my gosh!" he beams. "We really maximized my time here. I had gotten up to 245 pounds and had zero fitness. I was completely deconditioned: riding a tricycle was a challenge. I had balance problems and was afraid to do anything. Then I started working on a recumbent bike, and I got hooked." Suddenly Azada found a "sense of freedom and began planning bigger, longer rides." He also did a seven-week kayaking course and routinely uses the elliptical machine. "The VA," he concludes, has been a lifeline. "I don't know how I would have dug myself out of the hole I was in."

One of the things that helped Azada and so many veterans is recreational therapy. Jocelyn Reyes-Pagsolingan, who is the supervisor of recreational therapy for the Polytrauma System of Care, is a petite Filipina with short, dark hair. She has been a recreational therapist for twenty years and has worked at the VA for ten. She explains a persistent misconception about the rehabilitation of people with a variety of injuries—that it includes only physical or perhaps occupational therapy, minimizing the role that sports, art, or other activities play in regaining a sense of hope and normalcy.

"We work with other therapists and members of the interdisciplinary team," says Reyes-Pagsolingan, "to find out what a person is interested in and what activities they enjoy. Then we figure out how they can do it. If a person can only walk thirty or forty feet and they liked to play golf before they were injured, then we can help them return to playing golf."

She tells me about a veteran who had a TBI with weakness on one side of his body—the side, as luck would have it—with his dominant hand. He was becoming increasingly depressed because of his disability, so a recreational therapist worked with his physical and occupational therapist to help with his balance. He was able to use a four-point cane, and—with someone standing by to assist him in case he fell—he went to the driving range and began relearning how to play rounds of golf. Because he had a brain injury, one of his problems was attention to detail. The veteran became frustrated because he wasn't as good at golf as he used to be. So part of the job of the therapist, Reyes-Pagsolingan says, was to give constant encouragement.

"Sometimes recreation therapy involves going to a restaurant as a form of community practice," she says. This is something that seems simple if you are not disabled, but which can be like climbing Everest to someone with a brain injury, PTSD, amputation, or all three. In the real world, as opposed to the world of the hospital, there are uneven surfaces, which people have trouble scanning, architectural barriers, and environmental cues about which they need to be reminded. Plus, there are organizational skills and social etiquette—all of which may have been lost.

An outing to a restaurant is a perfect occasion to assess whether a patient can ask for a table, understand or communicate wishes to a waiter, pay a check, or add on a tip. "These are little skills that become big barriers that can be overcome," she observes. "We can also help someone figure out which environment may be too overstimulating or overwhelming, where they might sit, and how that will affect their experience." She cites as examples Outback versus Chipotle. The first has such an extensive menu that a patient may find it overwhelming, whereas at Chipotle the menu is more limited. Some restaurants are so noisy they would be unbearable for someone with PTSD. In others it's easier to find a quiet place to sit.

Taking patients on an outing can be quite complicated, she says. For example, her patients were recently invited to an exhibition of vintage airplanes at the Livermore airport. On the face of it, what could be simpler and more engaging? Get in a car or van, drive to Livermore, and see the exhibit. Not so fast, she warns. In order to execute this particular mission, a therapist has to first go and do some reconnaissance. Is it safe for patients? Where can they park? It's outdoors—is there shade? Where are the bathrooms, and how easily accessible are they?

"We have to pay attention to the overall experience," she says. Something as simple and appealing as this could turn into a real problem if attention is not paid to the smallest details.

Some of the details to which attention must be paid include a therapist's knowledge of, and sensitivity to, military culture, recreation therapist Andrew Duprey explains. Duprey is an expert in that culture from professional and personal experience. His father was a master sergeant with a severe case of PTSD. The younger Duprey did not want to join the military to serve his country. ("Been there, done that," he says, referring to his childhood.) But he did choose to serve: providing care to veterans. And he admires the care the vets receive at the VA.

"If you're going to have a psychiatric diagnosis, pray you're a vet," he says. "If you have a brain injury, you couldn't ask for better."

He has seen a lot of change in the VA and veterans since he began working at the VA in 1989, he says. "Vietnam vets didn't trust us because we were too government," he recounts, laughing at the contradictions. "Today's vets don't trust us because we are too civilian."

Which is why Duprey conducts a short course for his students and new therapists on military culture. "It's important to these patients to be addressed by rank and last name. To do otherwise alienates them," he warns. "People have to know basic military culture. They have to know a person's MOS, or if someone is [an] infantryman in Eleven Bravo or Eleven Charlie, or that a Navy corpsman attached to a Marine platoon is often called Doc. You want to know the history of the different services and the rivalries between them."

A sports clinic that the VA offers is popular with the vets, Duprey says. "One of the coolest things we do is our adaptive sports clinic." The whole team of providers—from sports medicine doctors to orthopedists to physical, occupational, and recreational therapists—all meet together in the same room. "We watch the veteran as they are training, cycling, whatever they may be doing," he says. "We talk through whatever problems they are having and adapt equipment so they can do it better." The goal of all these services, Duprey says with both passion and compassion, is "to try to put a warm blanket [on] and create a developing sense of comfort for our veterans."

This warm blanket can be furry and walk on four legs. Dogs are one of the most effective tools used in the rehabilitation and recovery of many veterans. For instance, as Dorr was working with York on the Dynavision machine, Errol Johnson came in the room with his personal canine connection, Ford, a service dog that is helping him work on problems with attention. I watch a smile flash across his face as he commands the dog to turn the lights on and off, and then he drops a pen on the floor and orders Ford to fetch it, patting him and saying, "Good boy, good boy," as the dog obeys his commands.

While he is working with Ford, Dorr explains why service dogs are so effective. "Here, we're working on fine motor control skills, visual scanning, leg strength, dropping and picking up things, as well as practicing the reinforcement of a positive affect," she says. "We know repetition builds skill, but it's really boring. So if you can do it in context of training and handling, it has more meaning."

At the Welcome Center in the Menlo Park VA, Ellen Fisher, a canine therapeutic instructor at Paws for Purple Hearts, and Sandra Carson of Warrior Canine Connection outline the programs they have for veterans. As we speak, several dogs being trained by veterans to be service dogs are scampering on the lawn outside. Fisher explains that the group, which also works with the Homeless Veterans Rehabilitation Program, has dogs that interact with twenty to thirty veterans every week. The Paws for Purple Hearts program has three service dogs in training that stay and live on the campus and work with two trainers each.

These dogs help veterans with mobility problems open a fridge or undress. Kevin Brady, a former Marine who had two deployments to Iraq and suffers from PTSD and a TBI, explains that service dogs were an important part of his therapy. He now works with the Paws for Purple Hearts program and accompanies Fisher to the polytrauma and spinal cord injury programs.

"You get to play with dogs and see their effect on patients," says Brady. "Being in the Marine Corps, you're trained to be a certain way, speak a certain way. You can't do that with dogs. In my mind, it's a kind of trick. They think they're training dogs, but really the dogs are retraining them.

When they're holding a puppy, playing with a puppy, their affect changes. People with PTSD are uncomfortable in public, but the dog acts as a social buffer. Sometimes dogs even wake them from nightmares."

After visiting the canine therapy program, I pass by a large room decorated with paintings, drawings, and watercolors. It's the art therapy room. José Rodriguez,* a Vietnam veteran who sports a ponytail and a bushy beard, is sitting at a long table working on an art project. Rodriguez served as a Navy cryptographer and electronics technician between 1967 and 1970. Fifteen years ago, he had a major stroke and was paralyzed for nine years. "They pronounced me dead five times," he recounts, proud that he defeated such high odds. With the help of rehab, he started walking six years ago. "I can't feel anything on my right side, but I'm gaining back muscle," he says.

Rodriguez says art therapy "is good for motion, concentration." It has also helped with his irritability, as have anger management classes. He has used different forms of therapy to deal with his anxiety and depression. "I would have killed myself without all this," he states matter-of-factly. "I was thinking about it."

Spinal Cord Rehab

Another critical rehabilitation service is the Spinal Cord Injuries and Disorder System of Care. The VA has the largest system of care in the country serving those with spinal cord injuries and disorders, with twenty-four centers located around the country.[2] Veterans who were injured while in the service aren't the only ones who use the centers. Younger and middle-aged patients who have been discharged from the military and are eligible for care use these services after they sustain a spinal cord injury in a motor vehicle accident, for example. Older adults might have arthritis of the neck or spine deterioration, which then injures the spinal cord. The centers serve as hubs connected to the spokes of other specifically designated facilities where primary and specialty care providers who are familiar with spinal cord injuries and disorders can follow patients over their lifetime.[3]

In Palo Alto, physical medicine and rehabilitation specialist Doug Ota directs the program's Spinal Cord Injuries and Disorders Center. Ota has a spinal cord injury himself and greets me in his office in a wheelchair. In his third year of medical school, Ota was in a diving accident and sustained a C6 spinal cord injury. He has thus personally experienced all the stages of treatment, recovery, and follow-up care through which he now guides his patients. As he describes it, the first stage of treatment is acute medical stabilization, which also frequently includes some sort of surgical intervention. After surgery, patients move to inpatient acute rehabilitation units, "learning," he says, "to do everything—eating, toileting, bathing, dressing—all over again."

"After the basics," like learning wheelchair propulsion, he continues, "there come higher-level skills: discharge from the hospital and reintegrating back into the community, figuring out transportation, using a wheelchair on uneven surfaces, follow-up visits to address issues and spinal cord injury–related conditions you have over a lifetime."

One of these problems is pain. "A lot of people don't think pain is a problem for patients who are paralyzed," Ota says, "but 78 percent of our patients suffer from shoulder pain during the first year from transferring from their wheelchairs. Plus, there is neuropathic pain: Nerves may become hypersensitive above or at the level of the injury or below, and patients may experience burning or electrical pain, which requires a very specific treatment approach."

What he and his patients then have to deal with are the lifetime consequences of their condition. "People think that walking is the most important thing that affects people with a spinal cord injury," Ota says. "But the main problems voiced by individuals with a spinal cord injury are bowel and bladder and sexuality problems. When your bowel and bladder don't function," he explains, "you are at risk for all sorts of infections. When your mobility is limited, there is the risk of obesity and pressure ulcers. Fortunately, we can develop strategies to trigger the bowel and manage many other problems."

People with spinal cord injuries are very reliant on medical equipment. They need the right kind of wheelchairs, chairs for bathing, and myriad other devices to help them gain function. They are also dependent on follow-up care. "Every year, we see our patients for an annual assessment," Ota says. "Within the VA system, we recognize the importance of providing transportation for patients to come and get those assessments."

Most important, Ota says, patients who have spinal cord injuries must be cared for in an integrated system that can follow them when they leave the acute and rehabilitation phases of their treatment. "This means," he says, "working with primary care providers and specialists who understand their specific problems and are willing to coordinate care with us to prevent a host of complications."

From both his own experience and that of his patients, Ota has learned that private-sector facilities and providers simply can't provide the level and duration of services available in the VHA. When it comes to surgery and acute stabilization, patients may do well in private-sector hospitals. When it comes to inpatient rehabilitation and obtaining the lifetime services they need, the private-sector system is severely constrained. Private-sector primary care providers do not have the expertise or even facilities to help spinal cord injury patients. Nor do they tend to have available the teams of physicians, nurse-practitioners, physical therapists, occupational therapists, social workers, and psychologists that see the patient in an organized, collaborative appointment as they do at a Spinal Cord Injuries and Disorders Center in the VHA.

Sunil Sabharwal is the neurologist in charge of the Spinal Cord Injuries and Disorders program in West Roxbury. When I met him, Sabharwal introduced me to the new rehab gym, as well as many other programs and the patients it has helped. One of those patients is Samuel Jay Keyser, an emeritus professor of linguistics at the Massachusetts Institute of Technology. Keyser discovered the importance of the VHA on the morning of his seventy-ninth birthday on July 7, 2014. That was the day an ambulance drove him from the Spaulding Rehabilitation Hospital in Charlestown, Massachusetts, to the West Roxbury VA Medical Center's Spinal Cord Injury and Disorders Center. Ordinarily, you wouldn't want to spend your birthday in an ambulance. But, as Keyser puts it, "It was a blessing."

On April 26, Keyser was doing his daily stretches in his home in Cambridge. His right leg collapsed, and he fell flat on his back and suddenly found that he couldn't move. Raced by ambulance to Massachusetts General Hospital, Keyser was rushed into surgery, where a neurosurgeon said he found the "crappiest spinal column" he had ever seen. Keyser had serious damage to his spine, of which he had been totally unaware. "The forest of bone spurs that sprouted along my spine bruised the nerves between the third and sixth cervical vertebrae," he explains. "After hours of surgery, a doctor at MGH told me I would never walk again."

Before his fall Keyser had played trombone in the oldest continuous jazz ensemble, the Aardvark Orchestra, in the country. Then, "in a nanosecond," as he puts it, "I was transported from the bipedal world into the world of tetraplegia. My arms and legs were paralyzed. I had no control over my bowels. I was, for all intents and purposes, an infant."

During his thirty-three days at Massachusetts General—twenty-two in the intensive care unit—Keyser suffered a series of postsurgical infections and almost died. He was then transferred to Spaulding Rehabilitation Hospital in Charlestown. "It was one of the best in the country," he says. "Nonetheless, they had to discharge me after seven and a half weeks because of the 'length of stay' problem. My Medicare insurance was running out. The hospital planned to send me to an assisted-living complex with little or no rehabilitation capability because I couldn't afford to pay out of pocket the $3,170.75 a day it cost to stay there. The next facility would house me for three weeks. Then what I thought was good health care insurance would again run out. After that, I was on my own."

Just before he was about to be discharged, a Spaulding case manager discovered that Keyser was an Air Force veteran and might be eligible for care in the VA's spinal cord injury program. After leaving the military, where he served for three years forty-nine years earlier, Keyser couldn't have imagined that the VA would be a possible source of assistance. He'd had a good job, and, he thought, good health insurance came with it. "In my own mind, the Air Force had receded like an object in a rearview mirror." (Even if he had applied for VA care, his income and lack of service-connected problems would have made him ineligible.) But because he had a catastrophic injury, the case manager found that he could go to the spinal cord injury program and then receive care for the rest of his life.

Keyser spent July 7 to November 3 in inpatient rehab in West Roxbury. He was discharged home with a hospital bed and a hover mat, a device that would make it easy for his wife to move him in bed. He was also furnished with an overhead freedom bridge that could help lift him out of bed. "A $30 remote switch saved the government a lot of money a year for nurses who would have had to stay and turn me," Keyser recounts. "They also gave me two walkers, a Rollator, and a superb motorized wheelchair that enabled me to stand up. It has a built-in mechanism that allowed me to be pushed upright, to stand in the wheelchair and get the weight of my upper body on my legs. This allowed me to do the exercises prescribed. They told me to do the exercises once a day, but I did them twice a day. The VA also provided a wheelchair-accessible package to make the van we purchased on our own wheelchair accessible."

After his discharge as an inpatient, he waited the requisite two weeks and became an outpatient, which he has been ever since. "While an outpatient I went to VA hospital three times a week for physical therapy," he recalls. "That lasted a year. Now I see them once a month. I can go anytime and make an appointment and go swimming. I also see them for ears, eyes, my nose." Keyser chuckles as he prepares to enumerate the obvious ways everything in the body is, in fact, connected.

Now, with the help of a walker, the man who was told he would never take another step can walk a mile a day. He is back to playing jazz trombone and has played six concerts and one half-hour TV program.

He has nothing but praise for the VA, noting the little things that made a big difference to him. "One day," he explains, "I wheeled myself into an elevator. Hospital workers I didn't know were already there. As I was about to exit at my floor, they said, 'Thank you for your service.' Shortly after that, Eddie, a painter in the hospital, invited me to listen to the jazz he was playing while he worked in the corridor outside the gym. A week later, a CD player and a stack of jazz CDs showed up in my room next to my bed. Eddie had put them there."

He credits a unique attitude at the VA for the success of its programs. "That I am able to walk now and to live a relatively normal life is evidence that the staff at the West Roxbury VA are superb at what they do, from my primary care provider, to the nurses in my ward, to the extraordinary physical and occupational therapists who showed me how to use my body again," he says. "But on top of this expertise, they bring something else. Helping me was their way of thanking the thousands of veterans who had sacrificed so much on behalf of our country. The VA hospital people have a unique perspective. They see what they do as a way of giving back. No wonder they are so good at it. If they hadn't been, my wife would be taking care of a man who would be as good as dead. We would also be destitute. My wife would be a widow of a husband who wasn't dead."

Blind Rehabilitation

They say that seeing is believing, and this is certainly the case when it comes to the VHA's programs for veterans with impaired vision. Although these veterans are all legally blind, 90 percent of them have some vision.

Most patients' vision problems are not a result of combat but of a host of eye conditions related to age, genetics, ill health, and poor health habits. Every major VA medical center has a full-time visual impairment service team coordinator who functions as a case manager for veterans and active-duty service members with serious vision problems. Blind rehabilitation outpatient specialists help veterans in their homes and at VA medical centers. The VHA also has Intermediate and Advanced Low Vision Clinics, Vision Impairment Services in Outpatient Rehabilitation Programs, and Visual Impairment Centers to Optimize Remaining Sight programs.

Thirteen Blind Rehabilitation Centers strategically located throughout the country also serve veterans who have severely impaired vision or are totally blind. Over the course of a year, more than two hundred veterans stay in each center in residential units with private rooms and shared bathrooms for between four to eight weeks (or longer if necessary). Nurses are on staff 24/7 to manage any medications or medical problems.

Mark Matthiessen is a specialist in low vision at the VA's Eastern Blind Rehabilitation Center located at the VA Connecticut Health Care System, which I visited in 2015. He asked me if I would like to learn what it's like to suffer from low vision or total blindness. Of course, I reply, assuming he would sit me down, give me a brief lecture on various ocular conditions, and hand me some articles and brochures to read. Instead, Matthiessen reaches over and pulls out a bunch of heavy-duty eye gear that look like my swimming goggles on steroids. They are called occluder kits. The devices, he tells me, simulate the way people see when their vision is impaired by conditions like diabetic retinopathy, retinitis pigmentosa, macular degeneration, glaucoma, or total blindness, among others. Everyone—nurses, ophthalmologists, optometrists, vision specialists of various sorts, psychologists, social workers—who works in the Blind Rehab system trains extensively with these goggles, Matthiessen says.

So one after another, I don different goggles designed to simulate a particular condition. The first set produces the kind of vision characteristic of the inherited disease retinitis pigmentosa. Suddenly I can see nothing directly in front of me, but, as through a constricted tunnel, I can spy a dime that Matthiessen has placed on the floor ten feet away. Donning another pair of goggles with lenses punctured by tiny holes, I experience the fractured world produced by diabetic retinopathy. High blood sugar levels produce tiny particles that speckle and occlude the visual field. Then there is macular degeneration, the most common cause of low vision, which severely restricts your central vision even if you can discern things in the periphery. The biggest challenge is the goggles that entirely black out the world, simulating total blindness.

Handing me a long, white cane, Matthiessen invites me to take a walk outside. Standing by my side, he encourages me as I try to navigate along a corridor, through an exit door, and down a ramp at the side of the building. It takes only a second to experience the terror and dislocation of this temporary sightlessness. It's clear to me that these goggles produce not only understanding but a profound sense of empathy that can help erase the clinical distance and detachment in which so many health care providers are assiduously schooled—or any skepticism family members or friends may have about a patient's condition.

Over the course of the day, I listen as providers and patients amplify my understanding of how the VA deals with problems that afflict so many veterans. Fourteen million Americans suffer from visual impairment. Most can be helped with corrective lenses. More than three million, however, have problems that are not correctable with such lenses.[4]

In a recent report titled *Improving the Nation's Vision Health: A Coordinated Public Health Approach*, the Centers for Disease Control and Prevention describe the national burden of vision loss, which, because of an aging population, is expected to double by 2030 and fall hardest on African Americans and people with low incomes. It argues that the only way to deal with this growing problem is through a public health approach. This would include better evaluation and preventive services and more comprehensive, integrated assistance when people suffer from vision loss. This approach, the report points out, is generally lacking in the provision of private-sector health care.[5] Indeed, in most cases, optometrists and ophthalmologists are not skilled in helping people who suffer severe vision loss or total blindness live independent lives or cope effectively with their disabilities. As in the delivery of primary care, in geriatrics, mental health, and end-of-life care, the VHA is once again a notable exception.

Jonathan Hamilton, an optometrist, is director of the Low Vision Optometry Externship and Inpatient Low Vision Optometry at the West Haven VA. Tall, lanky, and bespectacled—although with no severe vision problems—he says when he was in training, he saw optometrists and ophthalmologists who were skilled at diagnosing and treating eye diseases but who were untutored—or uninterested—in the long-term management of patients whose conditions impair their daily function. An emphasis on function rather than cure, Hamilton says, does not fit the fee-for-service model of medical care in the United States. "Working with these patients," Hamilton says, "just takes too much time, and it is difficult and challenging to make a living doing that in private-sector health care." So patients are given reading glasses, told to stop driving, and basically dismissed with a standard, "I am sorry, there is nothing further we can do to help you."

Hamilton recounts a typical example. "I was observing an opthalmologist who was with a patient who was legally blind. Her best corrected vision with glasses was 20/400. She asked him what she could do to read. That was all she wanted to do. He said, 'There's nothing more I can do; everything is stable, and there's nothing anyone can do to make you read.' As someone who is passionate about low vision, and who was doing a residency program in low vision at the VA, I was sitting there thinking, 'Give me five minutes with her, and I will get her reading newspaper print.'"

Hamilton evaluates patients who are candidates for the VA's Blind Rehab Center and works on a team, with whom he meets weekly, to devise and monitor plans of care that are constructed around the needs and goals of each individual patient. To discover what patients need, he and his colleagues take a long functional history.

"We are trying to live a day in the life of the patient," he says. "We ask them what they have been living with, what they have difficulty with, what they enjoy doing. We ask about their hobbies and goals. When they first come into the program, we see patients twice, back to back. At the end of their first exam, I give them some homework to do before they come in again. Their homework is to think of anything and everything they want to be able to do—from rebuilding a car or computer, to playing an instrument, or to something as simple as reading. You name it, and our goal is to help you do it."

As an optometrist, he helps them fulfill these goals in a variety of ways. He will give a person with retinitis pigmentosa a reverse telescope to help them see. He will stick prisms, which act like rearview mirrors on a car, on the back of glasses to expand their field or teach patients how to move their eyes to similarly expand their visual field.

"We do a lot of blue-blocking tints that reduce glare and enhance patients' contrast," Hamilton says. "This won't get them seeing farther on an eye chart, but it will get them functioning better on a contrast sensitivity chart. It's another way of measuring function. We'll do a pair of everyday glasses that they'll use indoors with a tint in them for reading. We'll do sunglasses as well. Bright sunlight is more functionally disabling for a vision-impaired person whose eyes can't adjust. They experience much more glare, which throws off contrast and causes more discomfort and photosensitivity."

Hamilton says they also can tailor-make devices for particular patients. Hamilton cites one example. "I had a guy who was in a wheelchair who told me that every time he maneuvered his wheelchair outside he couldn't tell if it was a shadow or wet pavement or a pothole he was seeing. Sometimes he would hit a pothole, and he would fall over in his wheelchair. We made a special bifocal so when he looked down, he could tell what was a shadow and what was a pothole. Between the tint and the prescription, we could get him functioning better."

In the Blind Rehabilitation Centers, veterans spend their days relearning orientation and mobility and acquiring low-vision and daily living skills: everything from walking with a cane and listening for traffic sounds to cooking, cleaning, doing laundry, and going shopping. Manual Skills programs help veterans acquire confidence and mastery through wood shop or arts-and-crafts activities.

In West Haven, for instance, Matthiessen has constructed a planting garden. Veterans choose what to plant and where to plant it, and Matthiessen helps them both sow and harvest. And at all Blind Rehab programs, veterans can take advantage of a Computer Access Skills Training program that lasts another two to six weeks.

In Menlo Park, John Kingston, supervisor of the Western Blind Rehabilitation Center, gave me a tour of the large, well-equipped shop. The hallway in front of the entrance has displays of the stunning wooden pens veterans have made. Inside, what might seem daunting and dangerous equipment is specially designed to protect veterans from harm. I watch them peering at large-print tape measures, listening to talking tape measures, or—for someone totally blind—using click rulers that employ touch and hearing to measure accuracy within one-sixteenth of an inch. A twenty-four-inch SmartTool is a precisely calibrated digital level. I watch as a veteran does copper plating and another creates an iPad-like image of a poem he has written.

The Menlo Park Western Blind Rehabilitation Center has a program for patients whose vision has been impaired by TBI. (Optometrists throughout the VA are trained to discern between the headache caused by eyestrain and that caused by a TBI.) The center has also launched a program that works on helping veterans with balance. Anyone who has tried to do the yoga tree pose knows that sight and balance are intimately connected. When you begin to lose vision, your balance is significantly impaired, and you are at a greater risk for falls.

When veterans leave the program, they are also given many devices that help them function in daily life. "When a veteran comes in, we give them a full technology assessment," says Elizabeth Bottner, a computer access technology specialist in West Haven. "We find out what their goals are and how technology can help. They will learn how to use and leave the program with special computers, iPads, cell phones adapted to help the veteran, for example, access a contact list on his iPhone through voice-over. Apple devices have special zoom features. Adapted color contrast provides ways to access a computer keyboard and voice-overs, and verbal feedback is also available."

There are special knobs and voice adjustments for kitchen equipment, the bathroom, and for reading and television. As Bottner explains, for those who are totally blind, technology may entirely replace vision. For someone who still has vision, the goal is not to replace but to support the use of that vision as much as possible.

Veterans may also be involved in group or individual therapy sessions with psychologists or social workers to help them better cope with their disabilities and navigate the stages of grief they may experience because of the loss of their vision. What plays an equally important role, explains Joan Cummings, a social worker in West Haven, is what happens at night and on the weekend, when veterans with similar problems and a shared background live and socialize together. Veterans also gain greater confidence because, in many Blind Rehab centers, staff who have low or no vision may be their teachers or instructors. The fact that they work and function, and even flourish, is an example to patients of the distance they can travel from despondency and social isolation to better function and community.

Family Relations

One of the most important aspects of the VA's Blind Rehabilitation programs is its emphasis on educating family members in not only how to take care of their loved ones once they leave, but how to allow those family members to use the skills they have mastered in the program to understand their veteran's problems. The goggles I donned when I first observed caregivers in New Haven are designed to help family members gain more understanding of, and thus empathy for, their loved one's disabilities. As Matthiessen explains, it's imperative to teach family members what their loved ones are experiencing, because sometimes they may think they are faking it. They'll say, "What do you mean, he can't see me? He can see that speck on the floor way over there." Or, "He can't have low vision. He just stopped me from getting run over by a bus that I didn't even see out of the corner of my eye." When family members don the occluder kits and see what their loved ones see—or can't see—those reactions dissolve.

So, hopefully, do family members' fears and objections to a loved one playing a larger role in daily life and achieving greater independence. The program teaches veterans to overcome the kind of learned helplessness that often occurs when illness leads a family member or friend to take over in many areas of life. In the program, veterans don't only learn how to do things they thought were once impossible; they also learn to advocate for themselves, to tell a loved one, "This is how you can help me, and this is how you cannot help me."

Helping family members learn how to help—and not help—is critical. With the best of intentions, families and friends want to protect a loved one. Some family members have spent months, perhaps even years, caring for someone with deteriorating vision. They may be convinced that allowing a husband or wife more independence will do far more harm than good. A wife may be convinced that if she lets her husband into the kitchen, he'll burn down the house. A husband may worry that if his wife goes out by herself, she'll get run over by a bus.

To help family members or friends understand a veteran's newfound ability to function, they are invited to visit during a veteran's stay and, at graduation, Matthiessen explains, to spend three days with veterans. "We bring in family members multiple times to show them what people can do," Matthiessen says. "It's not mandatory, but we really push it. Family members stay at a local hotel, and the VA pays 50 percent and, if necessary, helps with travel. If, because of work or other obligations, a family member can't stay, this kind of training is done via telehealth."

I attend one of these weekly graduations at Menlo Park. Early in the morning, the room is packed with patients, staff, and family members. The average age of the group is late sixties to early seventies. One World War II veteran is ninety-one. They come in with walkers and canes and take their seats. Veterans are then invited up to a podium, given a graduation certificate, and asked to make some comments about the program and their progress. One man seems to have a bit of trouble negotiating his way up to the podium, and his fellow patients shout out, "Use your cane." He does and reaches the podium, where he proudly tells the group that he has loaded all his music and comedy albums onto his new iPhone and has begun texting his daughter. He thanks everyone who has helped him, including the janitor. Another veteran says that three is supposed to be a magic number. This is, he says, his third time in the program, and he is now applying newfound skills to his business.

In a moving speech, another veteran, who is in his seventies, chokes up as he tells the group, "I've never graduated from anything before. This is the first time I have graduated from somewhere, and it's been a pleasure and a wonderful experience to be in a place with this wonderful team where everyone works together." Embarrassed by his display of emotion, he then jokes that the only thing he has to complain about is the food, reflecting that "We didn't come here to eat." Tearing up again, he concludes: "This place is like a second home. It feels like family when I come here."

Watching the men and women who come to and work in this program also reminded me of my own family. I am, in fact, the daughter of a world-famous ophthalmologist who developed the use of cortisone and adrenocorticotropic hormone for inflammatory eye diseases. Growing up, my famous father used me as a guinea pig when child patients were afraid to let my father turn their eyelid. He would call me over, and dutifully I would demonstrate that having your doctor stick a finger under the lid and flip it wasn't bad at all.

I visited my father's office at New York Hospital hundreds of times, saw the books he wrote about eye diseases, and listened to his stories of the surgeries he performed and the people for whom there was nothing further to be done. Not once, in all the years I spent with my father, did I ever hear him talk about how to help patients live with their diseases. And I know for a fact that my father never donned a pair of goggles simulating those diseases. Did they exist before he died in 1970? I have no idea. But even if they did, I don't think the nature of his training in fixing things, "failing" to do so, and then forgoing any long-term involvement in helping patients manage daily life would have encouraged him to participate in or value such an experience. Once again, I was learning from this VHA program what health care could and should be, if one is devoted to more than fixing but also helping patients function in a world in which the imperfect is the very definition of the good.

Prosthetics

One of the things that make it possible for patients like the ones we have just met to return to more independent life is the VHA's extensive state-of-the-art prosthetics. In the VA, prosthetics include everything and anything that replaces, augments, or supports bodily function damaged by disease or traumatic injury. This can include everything from an artificial limb, to a wheelchair or cane, to supplemental oxygen, eyeglasses, a knee or ankle brace, all the way to a computer or cell phone. The VA's provision of prosthetics is not only far more advanced but relatively hassle-free when compared to the obstacles patients must navigate in the private sector. The VHA is far more generous in its provision of prosthetic devices than private-sector insurers or government programs like Medicare or Medicaid.

The first visit I made to a prosthetics department was at the San Diego VA Health Care System in 2014, where I talked with Tristan Wyatt, who was then the chief of prosthetic services. Wyatt has a very intimate understanding of the difficulties of fitting a prosthetic and getting it right. After 9/11, when he was eighteen and fresh out of high school, Wyatt signed up with the Army. In 2003 he was sent to Iraq. "I was shot in a firefight with insurgents and lost a leg," Wyatt recounts. He also had multiple other injuries. He was stabilized and then shipped out to Walter Reed Hospital in Washington, DC, where he spent almost a year. Wyatt had fourteen surgeries to repair his leg and other injuries before he could even be fitted for a prosthesis.

"At Walter Reed a VA case manager came to meet me and helped me file for benefits: VHA health care, compensation for injuries, a pension, the GI Bill." Once he was able to leave Walter Reed, he went to work at the VA central office in Washington in a program designed for combat veterans. A Vietnam veteran then introduced him to the Technical Career Field program, where he had an internship in prosthetics at the VA in New York City. "It was a natural fit," Wyatt says, adding, "no pun intended."

From his dealings with suppliers of the precision artificial limbs that are routinely provided to veterans, Wyatt has come to understand what would have happened to him if he had had similar injuries (say from a construction or a motorcycle accident or being shot in one of America's increasingly common mass shootings) and had to depend on private health insurance. His prosthetic options would have been much more limited and the limbs he received much less advanced. The VHA will care for these veterans for their entire lives, and it makes sense to promote wellness in any way possible. If patients with serious disabilities are just stabilized, given a wheelchair, and wheeled out the door, Wyatt explains, they may start drinking, do drugs, gain weight, and amass a whole host of problems.

At the VHA a veteran whose limb has been amputated will not only get one designed for everyday use, but also get another for athletic purposes. "We have a lab that does artificial limbs and custom bracing for athletic rehab." Wyatt outlines the kinds of services the VHA provides. "We have recreational equipment and athletic wheelchairs. We provide various limbs. We just made a prosthetic arm for someone who does rock climbing. Patients tell us what activity level they are at and what they hope to achieve." Multidisciplinary teams evaluate patients for prosthetic items and then put in requests for different equipment. "When requests come in from veterans who want to play tennis or do wheelchair basketball," Wyatt continues, the VHA acts to help the veterans realize their goals. He concludes proudly, "We provide the latest and greatest. In the private sector, you would have a hard time getting these things approved—or a heck of a co-pay."

One of the most fascinating hours I spent was with Francisco Pinedo, chief of prosthetics and sensory aids services, and Dan Ramsey, who is a prosthetist and orthotist who actually makes the limbs on-site that many veterans use at the VA Clinic in Las Vegas. Also present was Miguel Miralles, who is a technician who assists with the fabrication process. The clinic opened in August 2012. The hallways are decorated with beautiful art and greenery. Several waiting rooms have glorious water sculptures whose cascading bubbles gently sway aquatic grasses in a mesmerizing, almost hypnotically calming rhythm that makes waiting for an appointment a meditative exercise.

In their well-equipped prosthetics department, Pinedo and Ramsey and their colleagues fit veterans with limbs, orthotics, braces, diabetic shoes and socks, and many other mechanisms that are used to prevent further damage and help veterans adapt to daily life. They make prosthetics from scratch and repair and replace them as needed. Other people within the department help modify veterans' homes to make it easier for them to navigate with their disabilities. The prosthetics unit purchases power wheelchairs and scooters and repairs them when needed. When it comes to artificial limbs, their goal, they tell me, is not only to make sure prosthetics are comfortable to wear in a variety of situations but also to minimize the exertion and exhaustion that can be involved in using them. As Pinedo explains it, "You have two veterans, one's in his mid-twenties and one is in his mid-sixties. They have the same amputation, but the younger is stronger and may be able to handle higher-end technology and heavier components, while the older one may need something that is lighter in weight."

When Pinedo and Ramsey talk about comfort and exertion, they, like Wyatt, do so from personal experience. Thirty-nine-year-old Pinedo lost his arm in Iraq. Ramsey, a Marine Corps veteran, lost his leg in the Vietnam War when a land mine exploded. "I've been through four generations of different artificial limbs," Ramsey says with a chuckle. "Each one is smarter than the previous one."

When it comes to designing artificial legs, the trick, they tell me, is to figure out what kind of activity a patient wants to do and then design, for example, a prosthetic leg—and foot to go with it—that will be light and smart enough to accomplish the tasks of getting through daily life without leaving the patient totally wiped out at the end of the day.

"There are so many things, like microprocessors, that are attached to artificial limbs today that can help with the articulation of a knee or foot, but they might be so heavy they will exhaust the veteran wearing them," Pinedo explains. "If veterans are older, it takes more energy for them to walk because their joints are wearing out. We also have to make sure that any prosthetic doesn't negatively impact how a veteran walks or moves, thus creating pains in a hip, or back, or knee, or other unaffected part of the body."

There is no "one size fits all," they tell me. Nor is there one limb that fits all possible uses. If someone wants to walk and run in a full-on sprint, that person will need two different prosthetic limbs. If someone wants to go scuba diving, then a limb has to accommodate a fin. Locking mechanisms also have to be carefully chosen and adjusted. Plus, limbs with microsensors can fail without notice. Veterans are given not only one leg but also a second replacement limb that can be used in case the primary one suddenly gives out and needs repair.

"It's an honor and privilege to serve my fellow veterans who are amputees," Pinedo tells me. "I know what it's like to need help and get that help from the VA. I know how important it is to make sure veterans have the equipment or prosthesis they need."

Using the kind of limbs that veterans receive is more than a matter of assuring the right technical fit. Managing life with a prosthetic device requires physical mastery and continuous follow-up care. In San Diego, fifty-nine-year-old Navy veteran Susi Black, a tall woman with dark hair falling around her shoulders, explains the need for constant readjustment to new prosthetic devices. Black is wearing sweatpants and a T-shirt and working with physical therapist Leslie Straukas when I meet her. She is adjusting to a new prosthetic for a below-the-knee amputation on her left leg. While Straukas observes her gait, Black moves along a walking frame. The physical therapist notices that she is shifting her center of gravity and slapping down as she walks. In this kind of gait training, Straukas is trying to help Black build not only strength but also awareness of how she is moving her body.

After her exercises are over, Black sits down and recounts her history. She served in Guam between 1978 and 1982 as a Navy cryptographer. She didn't enroll in the VHA when she separated from the military because she was married to a career service member who was enrolled in Tricare. In 2000 her marriage failed, and Black was divorced. In 2003 a hit-and-run driver crashed into her, shattering her left leg. Both bones were broken, and she endured numerous operations with bone, skin, and muscle grafts in an attempt to save the leg. But over the years, it became infected, and in October 2007, it was amputated. Black is now totally disabled but manages to function. With help from her caregivers, she lost over a hundred pounds and now weighs about 157. The VHA monitors her type 2 diabetes, carefully checking her good leg and foot for any signs of problems.

As far as her prosthetic limb goes, she quips that she is now on "Henry the Eighth." This is the latest limb she has been given, and, she says, it's the best so far. Black says she doesn't know where she would be were it not for the VA. "I didn't have any insurance," she says. "I have just enough money to pay the rent, which they're raising by ninety dollars, which I don't know if I can afford."

When she hears politicians talk about privatizing the VA or limiting eligibility to only combat veterans, she is simply aghast. "It's a bunch of poppycock," she says. "This place is amazing. They should come here and sit in our shoes, see what it's like. It keeps changing for the better. I've seen differences just in this past year with the beautification project they're doing. It used to be so dark and dingy. Now it's great. Why don't they come and talk to people like me to find out how we're doing? I have never had better care anywhere."

She especially appreciates the caring attitude of the staff members. "Sure, there are some people you meet who must have gotten up on the wrong side of the bed sometimes," she says. "But mostly, over the many years I've been coming here, I see people who know me and care about me and are familiar. Sometimes I will come in for a couple of appointments, and they'll realize I need something else and arrange for me to go to those appointments. For someone who has trouble getting around, that really means a lot. The VA pays for cabs and shuttles. I don't have money for buses and taxis."

Black pauses and looks at her therapist, who is helping another veteran. She inhales and then, slowly, lets out her breath. "If it weren't for the VA," she says matter-of-factly, "I would probably be dead."

Home Care

Part of the long-term rehabilitation process at the VHA also includes home care follow-up from nurses, nurse-practitioners, therapists, and psychologists. On the morning before Thanksgiving 2016, I visit one of the patients who receive these home-based services. Thirty-nine-year-old Demond Wilson, who lost the use of his arms and legs, lives with his family in the house in which he grew up.

The family's long rectangular living and dining area has been converted into Wilson's permanent living space. It's filled with an array of state-of-the-art equipment—all furnished gratis by the VHA—that is critical to his survival. There's a folded-up ramp that permits Wilson's wheelchair to descend the small step that separates the dining area from what used to be the living room. A standing chair allows Wilson, with the assistance of a caregiver, to hold himself upright, thus helping to maintain his muscle tone. A portable shower allows Felicia, Wilson's sister, to shower him three times a week. His manual wheelchair sits next to the hospital bed that occupies the space that would have held a dining room table.

Wilson's injury is not the result of battlefield trauma acquired during his eighteen-year stint as a mortarman in the Second Battalion, Fifth Marines, where he served in Kuwait, although not during the first Gulf War. When he left the service in 2004, he got a job as a union carpenter at the Conoco–Phillips oil refinery near Vallejo, California, got married, and had four children. Then, in 2014, after leaving work, he was in a motor vehicle accident that broke his neck with a C1 fracture and ruptured his C4, C5, and C6 vertebrae. He woke up in a hospital after a week in an induced coma to find his life had been upended.

After two months at a Kaiser rehabilitation facility, he was about to be sent home because his insurance had run out. "They would have sent me home with the city or county social worker," he says, "and I would have had to pretty much do everything else on my own from there. It would have been GFL [good fucking luck]."

Fortunately, he was a veteran, so his catastrophic injury gave him VA eligibility. He went to the Palo Alto VHA's spinal cord injury program. That was when things changed for him both medically and psychologically. "In Kaiser you felt like they kind of rushed you through it," he says. "You had the feeling that as long as you could get out of your bed, then you were okay. When the insurance stops, it stops, and that's it."

His experience at the VHA Spinal Cord Unit in Palo Alto was entirely different. "They did a total reassessment of my body and injury," he says. They found out, for example, that his wrist had been broken in the accident, which was one reason he had trouble gaining strength and function. Every day, he did physical therapy, met with a social worker, did occupational and recreational therapy, and attended computer classes. When he left Kaiser, he had no use of his hands. When he left the VHA, he could open and close his hands to grab things and now has learned how to use a computer, with the help of a special mouse and a voice recognition program.

He candidly broaches another subject. "There was no discussion of sexuality at Kaiser," Wilson says. "I mean, you could go to a class with a bunch of other people, but sexuality is kind of personal. It's something you want to talk about one on one." He also found it helpful to be around other veterans, who created an informal peer support network. "There were just so many resources available at the VHA," he says.

Those resources have followed him as he returned home, first to his wife and four children, then, when the marriage snapped under the strain of his care, back to the home he grew up in that he now shares with his two sisters, one nephew, and his mother, who is aging and increasingly infirm. Now the VA pays his sister to provide his nighttime care, which involves a complex bowel regimen.

Wilson also values the assistance he has received from psychologist Bill Collins, who works out of the Home-Based Primary Care Program at the VA Clinic in Martinez, California. Wilson met Collins when he was at a very low point in his life. Before the accident he had been an athletic, muscular guy used to fixing things, taking his kids out to play sports, and, in his words, "holding his own." Suddenly, he was reduced to the status of a newborn, dependent on everyone, looking forward only to being an endless burden on those he loves. "I just didn't want to be here," he says. "I felt I would be better off dead. I couldn't do anything for anybody. How can I talk to my son when I can't take him to basketball practice or play ball with him?" he tells me, his eyes tearing up.

In sessions in his home with Collins, he learned to contend with his disability. As I visit with Collins and Wilson together, Collins explains how he helped Wilson change his perspective. "We're all interdependent," Collins says. "We're all able-bodied until we're not." Then he turns to Wilson. "What you had to do is learn about what's really important," he tells him. "Yes, there are losses, but you can adapt, you can still do things with and for the people you love, just differently."

With the help of people like Collins, Wilson began to recognize that he had value and could overcome obstacles and be a functioning part of his family and society. He now uses his manual wheelchair every day, can open and close doors, uses the computer, and plans eventually to go back to work helping other veterans.

More than this, with the VHA's financial and emotional support, he has participated in both winter and summer Paralympics and has done kayaking, snowboarding, hockey, scuba diving in a pool, and archery. He even found himself dancing, which is definitely something he never expected to do. Engaging in the kind of sports that would have been second nature to him before his accident involved overcoming his shame at exposing his body; he didn't want people to see the catheter bag hanging down his leg (permanently attached to his lower torso). After a few hours, he realized that no one cared about it.

Through all his experiences, the most important lesson he says he has learned is that he can be a father to his children and a functioning member of his family and society. "I feel I am a good dad now," he says. "I can watch my son play basketball and be around him and feel he loves me. It took a while, but I have learned to advocate for what I need."

He has also learned how to accept and even ask for help from his sister and other family members and friends. His sister showers and dresses him, changes his catheter, and makes sure it functions efficiently. She has learned to recognize the signs of any obstruction, which could be lethal. As twenty-eight-year-old Felicia explains, her ability to care for her brother is a direct result of the help she has gotten from the VHA.

"They have helped with physical therapy and supplies," she says, "and they have taught me how to take him on airplanes and trips. When my brother first came home, I did feel overwhelmed to see him like this. But I got my strength from how much I love my brother. I learned how to cook his meals, how to help him bathe, stretch his legs, and give him night bowel care. All of this takes a lot of time—hours and hours—but," she pauses, pushing back the tears herself, "this has been really rewarding."

"I went to school and wanted to do nursing," she continues. "I got a degree as a medical assistant. Nurse Laurie [the nurse-practitioner who is part of the VA's spinal cord injury program] taught me how to care for my brother. They taught me how to give him his meds and change his catheter.

He can get bad urinary tract infections, or AD—autonomic dysreflexia—which is a potentially fatal problem for people with spinal cord injuries."

Felicia inspects her brother's skin every night for the tiniest hint of an irritation that could indicate a bedsore. "The VHA has been very supportive," she says. "They give me real practical help. The recreational therapist and nurse come out here all the time." She herself has, in fact, become a skilled nurse for at least one patient.

After two years of rehabilitation, Wilson wants to go back to work. He feels that, with the help of the VHA, he will be able to do just that. "Without the VHA I would be lost," he says. "If you don't have support, if you don't have help getting through this situation," he points with his eyes at all the paraphernalia of recovery and survival that surround him and at his sister, who stands by his side, "well, you are just totally lost."

Mark Smith

No Ordinary Bike Shop

When I met Mark Smith, a slim, sandy-haired twenty-nine-year-old occupational therapist with a trim beard and Mohawk-like buzz cut, he was an occupational therapy fellow at the Errera Community Care Center in West Haven, Connecticut. I caught up with Smith again a year and a half later, after he had finished his training and gotten a job at the San Francisco VA Medical Center working with the Psychosocial Rehabilitation and Recovery Center.

Smith is a dual Canadian and American citizen. His father was Canadian and his mother American. His maternal grandfather was an infantryman in the US Army and served in World War II, and the VA took good care of him in his later years, Smith says.

Smith spent most of his life in Canada and did his graduate training at the University of Alberta. He was first introduced to the health consequences of military service when his youngest brother decided to join the US Marines, drove down to Montana, enlisted, and saw combat in Afghanistan.

As an intern Smith also worked with Canadian veterans who had been peacekeepers. "I got a chance to facilitate a therapy group with veterans. I heard their stories and interacted with them, and I had this—" Smith pauses, and an embarrassed smile flashes across his face. He flushes as he continues. "Well, all I can say is, and I know it sounds cheesy, but I felt like I had this sense of calling to the work I was going to."

"I was doing rehabilitation, which is what OTs do," he continues. "We help people do what they want to do on a daily basis. I realized that I could help, that this was work where I could make a difference."

Smith began looking for opportunities to do rehabilitation with veterans in the United States, through the VHA, because it was far more like the Canadian health care system that he grew up with and values highly.

"I did a couple of internships in American private health care systems. I couldn't ethically do that work. No way," he says adamantly. "I saw the difference between doing rehab for brain-injured patients in the US and in Canada. In Canada you would do rehab till the patient stopped making progress. In the US you would do rehab until insurance stopped paying, even if the patient was still making progress. In the US I'd also encountered patients with serious brain injuries who had basically lost everything, even though they had health insurance. They just used up their benefits." He shakes his head in disbelief. "That was very distressing to me," he says. By contrast, he adds, "The VA is a public health care system. The clients I am seeing are not worried about who's going to pay for it or whether they should come in for care."

Smith applied for training programs at the VA. He was accepted as a fellow in the Interprofessional Fellowship in Psychosocial and Recovery Oriented Services at the Errera Center, where he helped veterans with serious and persistent mental illness. "They were veterans experiencing psychosis, extreme mood disorders, severe PTSD—really folks who are struggling," Smith says. "They were also dealing with homelessness or substance use disorders, and I was helping them to learn how to manage and live fulfilling and meaningful lives despite those challenges."

In trying to help veterans integrate into the community, he and his colleagues taught classes on managing extreme anxiety, distressing voices, and disturbing thoughts and beliefs. They helped veterans who had disorganized thinking, problems with concentration, and those who were harming themselves. "One of the ways occupational therapists do rehab,"

Smith says, "is by using an activity that is meaningful to the person as therapy. This way, it's intrinsically motivating and rewarding and helps build skills they might need."

Smith had heard about programs that taught low-income young people how to build bicycles. They built the bike and kept it afterward. This not only gave them confidence but taught them marketable skills. Some even got work in bicycle shops. So, Smith thought, why not develop a similar program for the veterans he was working with?

He reached out to Joel LaChance, who ran a nonprofit program in New Haven called Bicycle Education, Entrepreneurship, and Enrichment Programs (BEEEP), and asked if he could work with him developing a program for veterans. "He was really excited about the opportunity to teach veterans. If it weren't for him, there would be no program," Smith happily acknowledges.

In one fortuitous instance, the head of the Transportation and Parking Department for the City of New Haven was on Smith's kickball team. He told Smith that the department had space in the basement near City Hall that served as a bicycle workstation for employees the city was trying to encourage to bike to work. He made the space available to veterans.

Smith recruited five or six veterans who would come to the bike workshop once a week for two or three hours. The police department of New Haven contributed broken bikes, and LaChance taught the veterans how to refurbish them. Once the bike was up and running, the veteran could keep it. What happened next was an unexpected surprise. Veterans liked the program so much that they wanted to continue repairing bikes that they could give to other veterans in need.

"It was great," Smith says, "to see a group of people who tend to be quite marginalized socially and economically have this opportunity to not only build a mastery of skills working with their hands and completing a project, but also to have this meaningful role to providing something useful to another veteran. We had one veteran who was working at Ikea from 6 a.m. to 10 a.m. He had no transportation and a bad knee. But he got up at 2 a.m. to walk to work. He was given a bike and wrote us a letter to tell us that now he thinks about how happy he is with his bike instead of all the ways he had wanted to kill himself."

Like so many innovations that occur at one VA facility, this one has inspired activities in others. After his fellowship finished, Smith came to

San Francisco to work with more veterans with serious mental illness. The bicycle program he had launched was ongoing in New Haven, and he wanted to continue helping veterans in San Francisco through similar activities. As he wandered the grounds of Fort Miley, which is located in Lands End National Park, with its fabulous views of the Pacific Ocean and Marin coastline, Smith thought that the best way to do this would be to bring veterans into nature.

"We know from research studies," Smith says, "that getting people out into the wilderness and nature has healing benefits both for physical and mental health." He was aware that the Park Service had piloted a program to encourage low-income city residents to use the city's parks. Shuttle buses would pick people up at neighborhood libraries and take them to various parks. Suddenly, urban residents who thought of nature as the inaccessible playgrounds of the rich or tourists began to realize that these were their parks as well.

Just as he had found allies in New Haven, Smith found others in San Francisco. Jen Green at the Golden Gate Parks Conservancy was enthusiastic about Smith's idea and worked with him to create a public–public partnership. Smith and his colleagues reached out to health care providers in the San Francisco VA system, asking them to suggest veterans who might benefit from the monthly walks that he, with Green's help, now leads. So far, the response has been heartening, he says. About thirty-five people signed up for an outing to Alcatraz. In May, when I met him at Fort Miley, Smith handed me a flyer advertising a visit to Muir Beach, located just across the Golden Gate Bridge in Marin County.

Wheelchair-accessible shuttle buses pick veterans up at Fort Miley at 10 a.m. and return them at 3 p.m. Veterans can go on these trips no matter what their level of activity. "At Muir Beach," Smith says, "if you want to go for a hike, you can. If you just want to sit on the beach and have a picnic and gaze at the ocean, that's okay too." The Muir Beach outing includes a "savoring walk," which is part of mindfulness practice. "We will walk past gardens near the Green Gulch Zen Center farm, paying attention to all the senses. The idea is to notice the colors of plants, the smells, the temperature, the feel of the wind on your skin." While not a substitute for traditional therapy, these programs are important supplements that really heal.

12

TRANSCENDING TRAUMA

The Martinez Cognitive
Rehabilitation Program

It's Wednesday morning and time for the weekly process meeting at the Martinez VA's Post Deployment Assessment and Treatment program. PDAT is an inpatient cognitive rehabilitation program that helps veterans from Iraq and Afghanistan who have mild TBI and PTSD, as well as other post-deployment issues (insomnia, chronic pain, depression, and substance overuse). Most were discharged from the military years ago but are still struggling with divorces and failed relationships, unemployment, and the resulting financial problems. They have tried to start or to return to school and have dropped out. Some are enmeshed in troubles with the police and the legal system.

The PDAT program serves both male and female veterans who spend between four and six months on an inpatient neurorehabilitation unit. At the Martinez, California, VA facility, veterans may also make use of an innovative post-hospitalization community-based transitional program of eight VA-subsidized apartments. While they live in these apartments, an interdisciplinary treatment team supports these veterans. The team helps veterans cope with returning to school, finding employment, reconnecting with their families. It also helps them learn to tolerate the stresses of life outside of a structured hospital setting or even their own homes, where they tend to isolate themselves to avoid the complex business of everyday life after the military.

Today seven of the eight veterans in the program meet with its director, neuropsychologist Jeff Kixmiller, in the clubhouse in the basement of the Center for Integrated Brain Health and Wellness. Although there is a more formal conference room upstairs with high-tech telehealth equipment, the veterans prefer the informal clubhouse with its comfortable leather couches and chairs, pool table, and wide windows that look out onto a patio furnished with picnic tables and a full-service outdoor stove and barbecue.

Because I'm an invited guest, the meeting doesn't begin with the usual conversation about current problems and progress on realizing a variety of goals. It begins instead with an interrogation of the journalist—me—who is asking the veterans permission to observe them in their therapy sessions. Kixmiller and one of the veterans—we'll call him Ty—are vouching for my trustworthiness. I interviewed Ty several days earlier as he described his journey from high school to the Marine Corps, then to Iraq, and finally to this program. He seems to like me, or at least is prepared to accord some trust in my good intentions. But I haven't met the other six guys, and they have to vet me—no pun intended—as well.

This is not an easy group to win over. Since they entered the military, they have been taught not to trust, to be vigilant to attacks that can come from anywhere and everywhere. They see enmity and menace in the most innocent appearances: a garbage bag thrown carelessly on the side of the road or a seventy-year-old journalist, armed only with a reporter's notebook.

The first thing they demand is that I swear that I will not use their names and identifying details unless they specifically request it. I agree. We decide that they will choose their own pseudonyms: Stud, Ranchero, Buford, Giovanni, Pedro, Ty, and Kyle.

Buford is a slim, handsome twenty-eight-year-old with a classic buzz cut. He is not at all comfortable with me, even though Ty has told him I'm cool and that he talked to me because "if my story can save one guy from blowing his brains out, it's worth it." Buford, all edges, jitters, and indirect glances (as if direct gaze would actually hurt) is nonetheless one of the most vocal of all the veterans in the room. What am I writing? he wants to know. Why am I writing it? What's my take on the VA? If it's to trash it, we're not interested.

When I tell them I'm actually a big fan of the VA, the veterans shift gears and begin their own attack. Why couldn't they get hearing aids right away? Why did it take weeks? What about their records? A slew of complaints follow. Like family, they can say whatever they want about the VA. But I am not family, and I can nod, and maybe ask the odd question, but mostly I have to let them vent. This is, I figure out, what they want from me. And then, grudgingly, I'm in, and their session begins.

These men have been through the overlapping circles of hell. Stud talks openly about how long it took him to come out of his room and participate in group meetings. He was in charge of cleaning vehicles that had been bombed, which means picking body parts off windshields. Stud talks about learning how to "conduct ourselves in the community. How I conducted myself in the community was what got me in here."

Under his breath Ranchero says that he "feels like a frigging freight train is running through my head most of the time. I feel like I always have to do something to feel I'm okay. I have to be running in circles, chasing my tail or someone else's. Face it, I'm never going to be like a civilian. Maybe, just maybe, I'll be civilianized," he concludes. He stares at his friends, gets up, and walks out of the meeting.

Because veterans are free to come and go as they like, the group continues talking without him. Kyle talks about his kids and the guilt he feels because their father has so dramatically changed.

Ty offers that "It would be easier if I got my legs shot off, then people wouldn't look at me and go, 'Shit, like, you look fine.' Fine—I'm not fucking fine, lady. I'm a fucking mess."

Giovanni boasts that yesterday another veteran, not one of the group, was making too much noise, bothering both patients and staff, and so he shouted out, "Hey, heads up, veterans are healing."

Kixmiller, a tall, stocky man who exudes empathy and kindness, laughs, turns to me, and says, "They get protective of our staff and each other. If people are acting out, they try to help, even if we don't need their help." Turning to the group, he smiles broadly and adds, "You guys have our backs; we've joined the club."

"Yeah," Giovanni agrees. "I have little brothers I can beat the shit out of that no one else can. You're our little brothers, whether you like it or not."

As we've seen in an earlier chapter, veterans who come back from Iraq and Afghanistan and go to the VA are routinely screened for TBI and other post-deployment conditions. Those with positive screens may be referred to the Polytrauma System of Care. The Martinez VA is a Level Three Polytrauma/TBI Support Clinic and one of five national Polytrauma Network Sites. Kixmiller and a group of Martinez clinicians developed the PDAT program to serve the needs of veterans who have a set of complex problems that restrict their treatment options. Most of PDAT's patients have mild or occasionally moderate TBIs. The Polytrauma System of Care will take veterans with mild TBI and provide some mental health support, but the system is not designed to take the kind of patients who have many serious mental and behavioral health problems, like severe PTSD, active substance abuse, behavioral impulsiveness, and intense anger, among others. "Many of our veterans," Kixmiller says, "would also be ineligible for PTSD inpatient programs because they are too behaviorally impulsive and still actively drinking or using drugs. They would need to go to detox and residential substance abuse treatment to be eligible for PTSD treatment. The problem is they won't—or can't—make it through a detox or PTSD program without relapsing. Another complicating factor is that their traumatic brain injuries have produced attention and memory problems that make it hard for them to make it through PTSD and substance abuse programs. These rely on verbal therapies based on learning abstract psychological concerns and associated coping tools and strategies. Our patients are the outliers, the extremes." The PDAT program is designed specifically to deal with these outliers and extremes.

From 1997 to 2007, when the PDAT program was developed, Kixmiller spent his time in Martinez in a neurorehabilitation program working with inpatient veterans who had had strokes or other neurological illnesses. The goal was to help veterans attain as high a level of independence and community functioning as possible.

Many of his patients were Vietnam veterans who educated him about the gaps in services they encountered when they returned from the war. With the entry of Iraq and Afghanistan veterans into the system, Kixmiller and his colleagues started seeing a new kind of patient. He began to recognize the same kinds of gaps in care that emerged in the Vietnam era. "These new veterans are young, complex, live in rural areas, are years post-discharge, and experiencing a multitude of community and family conflicts or stressors. They are divorced, bankrupt, can't get or hold a job. They have pain problems, and because the military gave out painkillers like candy, they're abusing or overusing opioids."

Kixmiller, who was at the time helping to set up Polytrauma at the Martinez VA, knew that that system of care did an excellent job dealing with patients who had brain injuries, and burns, and amputations as well as mental health problems. It just wasn't set up to accommodate a subset of veterans that were high users of emergency care services or refused to go to—or dropped out of—mental health and substance abuse programs. These veterans were ending up in acute psychiatric wards or even jail. Many of these veterans also lived in rural areas, hours away from a major hospital or large clinic. To be comprehensively evaluated, they would have to drive hours back and forth from Chico or Redding or Yreka to the Sacramento VA. They had PTSD, road rage, and insomnia. Because they couldn't work, they may also have had child care responsibilities. It was therefore difficult, if not impossible, for them to make it to the multiple appointments with myriad specialists needed to even begin to evaluate, much less treat, their complex conditions.

Kixmiller was working with a treatment team made up of neurologists, nurses, speech language pathologists, physical and occupational therapists, physiatrists, chaplains, social workers, and mental health providers. He went to his team to talk about the need to serve this subset of veterans. They were, he said, more than happy to create a service that would welcome veterans on an inpatient unit for one to two weeks to do a comprehensive evaluation of their problems and develop an outpatient treatment plan for each of them. In 2007 the group set aside a few beds in the Center for Rehabilitation and Extended Care (CREC) at Martinez and started seeing post-9/11 veterans.

Even though their injuries did not show up on brain scans, many veterans riding in Humvees and in other settings were subject to dozens, if not hundreds, of blast exposures. "Because of these blast exposures," Kixmiller says, "their brains were knocking against and squishing around their skulls. Even in a rollover, there might be a brief loss of consciousness, and then boom—they were back to fighting. Then there were the EODs," he continues, "people on explosive ordinance details, who were experiencing lots of blasts as they were trying to defuse the IEDs.

"The veterans told us about all their problems. They also told us stories about PTSD leaking out all over the place." Kixmiller summarizes a long list of behaviors. "They were angry, raw, ready to fight. They were having nightmares. They would sleep all day but not at night, couldn't handle stress, new people, or unfamiliar contexts. They were beyond irritable. Irritable was their baseline, and they would flare up from there. They told us about their man caves"—and, he adds, you didn't have to be a man to have one—"the places they holed up in, where they could go so everyone would leave them alone."

The problem was what happened when they left those caves. These veterans were also having serious pain problems and using alcohol and drugs to self-medicate.

Kixmiller goes on to describe a pattern with which we have become all too familiar. These veterans were also unwilling to admit to mental health problems. "They don't want to be called crazy. They would rather be diagnosed with a TBI than PTSD, because then there's no mental health stigma."

By 2009 the group had developed a way to systematically evaluate them. The veterans who had come to the fledgling program were overwhelmingly enthusiastic about the process, Kixmiller reports. "They finally felt they were being understood and heard. They also appreciated the fact that their problems were viewed as interconnected and treatable."

Through the feedback it received, however, the group learned that the veterans were unhappy with one thing. The outpatient treatment plans the team developed required the veterans to return to their homes and then drive miles to multiple appointments, in multiple locations, where providers with great expertise and the best of intentions were, nonetheless, treating one problem at a time. "What we realized was that veterans this complex, with intense interconnected issues, needed the kind of inpatient treatment that could deal with all of their problems over an extended period of time. We needed to do more than hand them a great treatment plan as they were going out the door. We needed to provide them with an intensive, comprehensive inpatient treatment program that would ready them to enter and benefit from other VA treatment programs, like inpatient residential or outpatient PTSD, substance abuse, pain, or other programs."

This recognition gave birth to PDAT, which is, Kixmiller says, deliberately defined as a cognitive rehabilitation readiness program. By 2010 PDAT had developed its basic model. By 2017 the program had ten dedicated beds and hoped to expand to sixteen. Most veterans are male (of the two hundred people who have gone through the program, fewer than 10 percent are women). The men share a room and bathroom. If there is a single female, she has her own room and bathroom.

Although PDAT is a unique, stand-alone program, it is, like all the local VHA innovations we have visited, embedded in a web of integrated care and a community of interdependent caregivers. Its inpatient beds are located in the CREC, and it benefits from nursing staff who deal with other patients. Staff from other areas of the Martinez VA—from the interdisciplinary pain team to primary care providers and specialists—work with its patients. Its therapy sessions, classes, and meetings take place in the Center for Integrated Brain Health and Wellness, which is lodged in a building specially designed and constructed to attract younger veterans who have been through the conflicts in Iraq and Afghanistan.

Neuropsychologist Jim Muir and polytrauma and TBI social worker Katherine Miller explain that the building's design was meant to overcome the resistance of Iraq and Afghanistan veterans to seeking care at the VHA. Younger veterans who suffer from a variety of problems, they tell me, often either fail to sign up with the VA or repeatedly are no-shows for the appointments they do make.

"You're dead in the water if you can't get them to come in for help. They didn't want to be sitting in a waiting room with a bunch of older veterans," Miller says.

"They don't want to acknowledge mental health problems, like PTSD," Muir adds.

Recognizing the needs of these veterans, Muir says, "we spent years in meetings with architects to design this building." Instead of a traditional medical waiting room, we walk into a brightly lit, atrium-like entrance looking over a well-equipped gym. There is, of course, a check-in desk and waiting room area. But the first thing that attracts your eye as you walk through the front door is a giant climbing wall that extends from the gym downstairs to the building's roof.

Veterans, Muir tells me, selected the colors of the walls and floors. "We wanted it to be serene and calming. When we showed veterans samples of flooring and paint that was burgundy and maroon, they immediately thought 'dried blood.'" Needless to say, those ideas were instantly jettisoned. The pale sand walls and vinyl flooring convey the serenity veterans so desperately need. There's an outdoor picnic area with a barbecue, a clubhouse with couches and flat-screen TVs, and a kitchen.

Therapy rooms are designed without windows. Windows can freak people out if they have PTSD. Bullets, after all, can fly through windows. Each therapy room also has multiple options for seating. "Some people," Miller says, "want to sit facing a door so they can see what's coming through. Some want to be facing a wall."

All the therapists in the various programs on offer—chiropractors, neuropsychologists, speech language pathologists, pain specialists, social workers, nurses—dress in casual attire. No suits and ties here. Muir sports a buzz cut with ponytail. "You have to make the veterans feel comfortable," he informs me. He says he was trained to look authoritative, with the requisite distance-affirming attire. No way will that work here. "The veterans also use a lot of profanity. So I've allowed myself to use profanity; it makes them feel more comfortable."

Kixmiller, who uses the occasional swear words himself and always dresses in casual shirts and pants, tells me the PDAT program focuses on a number of what he calls "domains." They are cognition, mood, PTSD symptom management, chronic pain, communication, and sleep disorders like insomnia and sleep apnea. "We use a harm reduction approach to substance abuse," he says. "This means that veterans can be admitted to the program with existing substance abuse problems as long as they are actively engaged in reducing or eliminating their overuse of substances. Substances," he adds, "can include overuse of caffeine, as well as the usual retinue of other drugs."

Veterans will attend two groups or more a day. These include anger management, PTSD, stress management classes, social communication strategies, techniques to improve attention and memory, and compensation for problems veterans have with thinking efficiently and effectively. In addition, veterans also go to a multitude of weekly treatment sessions that can include physical therapy, chiropractic, acupuncture, exercise with a dedicated trainer, mental health support, and cognitive rehabilitation, as well as any needed primary care and other medical services.

A critical part of the program is cognitive rehabilitation, which involves teaching and helping the brain to relearn ways to pay attention to, and remember, important information. It teaches veterans to problem solve, to reflect on how they are behaving and how their actions impact others, and to make appropriate changes in their behavior. "Psychotherapy and cognitive therapy," Kixmiller says, are "literally helping the brain learn new ways of thinking about and problem-solving real-life situations."

To cite an example, veterans may complain about hating one of the nurses or not being able to tolerate going to the grocery store because of a rude clerk. "We teach them to recognize the way they escalate emotionally and to intervene with new coping strategies and thinking," Kixmiller says. "Instead of focusing on the clerk's behavior or how much you really hate the nurse, think about your next responsibilities or a self-soothing activity that you can do when you leave the grocery store. Just taking three deep breaths, or getting up and getting a glass of water, or texting a friend about the frustration without verbalizing it to the clerk are strategies these veterans would never have thought of—or at least never used." He pauses and adds, "Sometimes it's the simple stuff that's hard to get them to use. They think it's hokey and scoff at it."

Planning and preparing a meal, which the group does once a week, along with learning to shop and cook, is another way to retrain the brain. It's an exercise in learning how to cooperate. Veterans take turns planning the meal and shopping for ingredients, subbing out tasks to different participants. They also go to restaurants, Starbucks, the bowling alley. "They go out as a group so they can protect each other in settings they find stressful," Kixmiller says.

Cognitive rehabilitation also helps veterans unlearn typical military thinking. "In the military," Kixmiller echoes what other therapists have said earlier, "you don't ask questions. You act on first impressions because everything is, after all, a threat. Plus, you do not admit weakness or vulnerability. In the military there are no gray areas; there is just black-and-white thinking. That's the shoulds, ifs, have-tos. You have to stand at attention. You should always have an exit plan. We teach that while those had survival value to get you through the military and combat situations, they have less application and relevance to civilian living."

Kixmiller attributes the program's success to the fact that staff pay a great deal of attention to developing trust, rapport, and collaborative relationships with veterans. Winning the trust of patients who have trust issues—and this is a massive understatement of the term—involves, Kixmiller candidly states, "huge and constant understanding and negotiation. When veterans come at us with frustration and anger, we have to understand that that is just another symptom of their hurt, their confusion, their sense of being lost, as opposed to reacting to their anger and frustration with our own. Some veterans come into the program insisting they will not ever, no way, take medications. We tell them, 'Okay, that's fine. We'll take you where you're at.'"

Deborah Chesnut, the registered nurse who was the PDAT care coordinator when I visited the program in 2016, told me, "Some veterans insist they will never, ever, go to a group therapy session. 'I hate groups,' they tell me. So I ask if they would be willing to go for just fifteen minutes just to check it out. If they say yes, then I encourage them, because even getting there for a short time is a big milestone."

Some veterans will spend the first few weeks in their room before they come out to a group meeting or individual therapy session. In those cases individual therapy is brought to them in their rooms, and they are not required to go to group sessions. When I attend the morning session, one of the veterans in the program has been in his room for two weeks.

When the group is coed, negotiations can become even more complicated. "All the women who have gone through our program have military sexual trauma, with rape the most common. This is a major added factor," Kixmiller emphasizes. "This means that the negotiations with these women is around men. If they were gang-raped by buddies, commanding officers—well, clearly being in a program with men is a significant challenge. We try to provide ample access to female nurses and providers, and we carefully negotiate the work with staff and how staff approach patients. We don't let male nurses go in at night. The veteran may wake up and see a male in their room, and even though it's a nurse, well . . ." His voice trails off as we imagine the female veteran's response to a man in her room in the middle of the night.

The staff are very careful and respectful of all patients' special needs. "Nurses are used to walking into patients' rooms without knocking. That doesn't work here," Chesnut says.

"You can't walk into their rooms without knocking. They are hyper-vigilant from PTSD. If they are asleep, they may have nightmares," Kix-miller adds. "We talk to them about how to wake them when needed. We let them put up signs to staff to warn them about what their room restrictions are. Some say, 'Do Not Knock or Wake Up Veteran before 10 a.m. for Sleep Hygiene or PTSD Purposes.' Some have written, 'Don't fucking bother me at night for stupid requests!'

"We work with them by asking, 'What will help you at night to get to sleep and stay asleep? What will work with you when you're angry? Can we text you later? Do you want us to follow you so we can talk about it, or do we need to leave you alone until you approach us?'" Kixmiller says. "We are dealing with people who feel they have consistently failed, that nothing has worked. We are trying to set them up for going back to school, living in an apartment, dealing with their kids. We get them ready to do other things. We help them with legal issues—for example, if they haven't paid child support, don't have service eligibility. If things don't work, our attitude is, 'Thank you for telling us.' If one relaxation technique didn't work, we have fifteen alternatives to relaxing, earbuds for visualization, or yoga, mindfulness meditation. The most popular one right now is ceramic painting at a place in Concord called Color Me Mine. They thought it was going to be the hokiest thing, but now we take vets weekly. They love it."

"There is never any criticism for not working," Kixmiller states ada-mantly. "All we ask is that you try."

Although the PDAT program emphasizes flexibility, there are, however, certain nonnegotiables upon which the team insists. Veterans eventually have to engage in individual and group treatments where they disclose vulnerable things about themselves. "I might not like groups," Kixmiller elaborates. "But eventually, I have to start talking about issues in the group. In individual therapy they have to progress to revealing and pro-cessing and reflecting on their habits, patterns of thinking, and problem-atic thinking styles."

They also have to abide by group rules: avoiding politics and religion, talking about their history from their own point of view rather than engaging in group stereotyping—we as veterans all think like this; civil-ians think like that. Similarly, they cannot, under any circumstances, rag on other veterans. When the morning group was meeting, the guys began to vent about a veteran—the one who was still in his room—who had joined the program in spite of the fact that he hadn't been in the shit, meaning in combat. Kixmiller didn't hesitate to stop the trajectory of competitive victimization right in its tracks. This program, he reminded them firmly, is a safe place not just for you, but for everyone in it. You cannot attack—even verbally, even out of his earshot—another veteran resident.

What Kixmiller was interrupting was one of the drawbacks of working with a group of veterans who have had similar experiences. On the one hand, Kixmiller explains, the men and women can really help and support each other. They like to think they have each other's proverbial back. On the other hand, they can easily slip into groupthink that pits them against the world, aggravating a tendency to engage in one-upmanship contests to establish who had the worst experience: noncombat vets can't possibly have PTSD or TBIs or any problem as serious as theirs; officers didn't have a hard time like they did; civilians do not and can never understand what they've been through. Kixmiller says he and his colleagues must constantly remind these veterans that their problems reverberate across generations. Everyone who signed up signed up to serve and possibly die. And you definitely didn't have to be in combat to have had significant problems, either as a child or adult, that can be as crippling to deal with as hundreds of blast exposures.

In helping veterans adjust their thoughts and actions, the PDAT program makes use of many different therapists and many different kinds of therapy. One of these consists of an innovative combination of mental health and physical therapy. Physical therapist Liza Katz and clinical psychologist Sasha Best work together to treat patients who are in physical, mental, and spiritual pain. In Katz's large physical therapy treatment room—or sometimes out walking and talking in a nearby state park—the two therapists help veterans who are reluctant to talk about experiences they would rather repress or drown with alcohol and drugs.

Katz, who is in her seventies, is a trim woman with short gray hair. She originally worked at the VA in Fairfield, California, where she first met Best, a psychologist in her late thirties with curly black hair, who specializes in cognitive behavioral therapy. Best spends most of her days treating patients at Highland Hospital in Oakland and donates one day a week to the VA in Martinez. In treating patients, both therapists have come to understand the deep connection between psychological and physical pain and trauma. "When PTSD is exacerbated, your shoulder injury becomes even more painful. In fact, I have had patients who have begun to have nightmares about how they got their shoulder injury," Best tells me as she sits next to Katz in the physical therapy room in Martinez. "It's all linked together—pain, stress, and anxiety."

"When you treat someone's shoulder in PT," Katz adds, "that can bring up the experiences that happened when someone injured their shoulder. It all comes flooding up."

Despite never having been in the military or combat, I can certainly relate to the connections they are exploring. I have had back pain for years and quickly realized in physical therapy sessions that manipulating my body can unleash fears and anxieties that remind me of both the initial injury and the resulting pain. Seemingly matter-of-fact recommendations for follow-up exercises, rather than being viewed as the road to relief, can easily be construed as an invitation to further injury, disability, and God knows what. In other words, the "cure" can produce the kind of catastrophizing tendencies with which most physical therapists are ill equipped to cope but with which psychologists like Best are all too familiar.

Best and Katz discovered how effective combined therapy can be in addressing these fears and anxieties when Best was treating a veteran who had a lot of pain and was open to talking to a physical therapist. Best knew that Katz had worked with Colin Fernandes, the director of the chronic pain clinic in Martinez. She was told that Katz was a physical therapist who would do more than palpate, massage, apply ice or heat, and prescribe stretches, strengthening, and other traditional remedies. She would not only try to find and relieve the physical source of the pain but also address the veteran's experience of pain. The veteran was willing to go to Fairfield to talk to Katz but wanted Best to be there to sit in on the session. "After that session," Best recounts, "the veteran continued to see me and Liza separately, but we realized there were other patients in our caseloads who could benefit from working together with the two of us at the same time, and we decided to try it out."

Many veterans liked the approach, and Katz eventually came to work at the Martinez VA full time, where she works with Best on Tuesdays. The two have the space and time to listen, as Katz puts it, to the story the body has to tell them. This is a story, Katz elaborates, about more than injured tissues, cells, and muscles. It's a story about fear, anxiety, anger, despair.

"In our work, information that arises from the body has an equal place at the table with all the other information we get through X-rays and MRIs and mental health and behavioral and cognitive therapies. What Sasha and I have now is a rhythm where we can explore bodily sensations, physical feelings, and negative thoughts that emerge together." Katz recognizes that the brain isn't the only part of the body that holds on to memories of trauma. The body has its own muscle memory and reactions to those traumas that can be used for healing.

I met with Katz and Best and two of the patients they have been treating for years. Because the patients wanted to remain anonymous, they, like the veterans in the morning group, chose their own pseudonyms. Mojo, a female Army veteran, chose both her name and that of her friend from the PDAT program, William Wallace. "It's like after William Wallace—you know, Braveheart, the Scottish warrior," she explains eagerly.

The first time I met Mojo, she was walking into the Brain Wellness Center, accompanied by her service dog Jimmy. She was wearing shorts and a short-sleeved shirt, and her arms and legs were covered with tattoos. A hank of straight black hair arced down to her neck, but the sides of her head were buzz cut. You could see the slashes of white scar where surgeons put plates in her skull against her shining dark hair. She also has the look I have come to recognize in so many of the younger veterans from Iraq and Afghanistan who suffer from both PTSD and TBI. Her eyes are wary, on full patrol. So I was surprised when, upon hearing that I am writing a book about VA health care, she immediately exclaimed, "I can't believe they are trying to shut down the VA! Can you believe it? It's like closing a door on all of us who have served!"

The second time we meet, it's with her buddy William Wallace. Both wanted to talk to me about their experiences in PDAT, but only if Katz and Best were present during the interview. "If you're okay with them," Mojo announced, referring to Best and Katz, "you're in."

They also chose not to meet at the VA in some enclosed therapy room but outside in a local park, where they often go to do therapy with Best and Katz. Mojo is also accompanied by not one but two service dogs, who strain against their leashes as we find a quiet place to lay out a blanket and sit. Once comfortably settled on our blanket, surrounded by low hills, grasses, and wildflowers, with the pleasant sound of a lawnmower humming softly in the distance, I begin to ask them about their histories and experiences at the VA.

Mojo enthusiastically jumps in. Wallace is more circumspect, as if he has trouble not only revealing but also processing. It's a problem he readily acknowledges. "I haven't been the same since I left the service," he candidly admits.

Mojo tells me that she joined the Army in 2000 and was eventually sent to Germany and Kosovo. In Germany she was assaulted by a group of Turks. She fought back and proudly informs us that she sent one of them to the hospital. But a year later, she was again assaulted by another group of Turks. Were they friends of the first group of guys? Why did they attack her? What really happened? She doesn't know because she had a bad brain injury, followed by neurosurgery, and can't remember anything prior to the assault.

What she does know is that her brain was badly affected. She was nonetheless sent back to active duty and deployed to Iraq. "I could have fought it," she says, "because it was against medical advice, but hell, why would I? Never in a million years."

When she was on R&R, she went to a doctor because she had forgotten her prescription. "The doctor took one look at me and said, 'What the fuck are you doing here?'"

To which she replied, "'Excuse me, sir, sorry. I forgot my medications.' He went, 'No, that's not it; you should have never deployed. You're going home, blah blah blah.' And I said, 'Sir, I'm not. I'm going to stay.' I got medevaced to Landstuhl, the Army's hospital in Germany.

"After I got back from Iraq, I got really tired of not getting any help and tired of the medications I was taking," she recounts. "So I sort of went the wrong way about it. I started to smoke weed, and I got in trouble for that and got out with a general medical discharge but under honorable circumstances."

Mojo was twenty when she went into the Army and twenty-five when she got out in 2005. "When I got home, my parents didn't know who I was. I didn't know who I was. I'd look in the mirror, and that wasn't me. I was totally soul raped," Mojo states bluntly. Although she resisted getting help for a number of years, a physical therapist at the VA in Sacramento directed her to the PDAT program, which she entered in October 2009. She didn't like one of the psychologists to whom she was assigned and lasted only a week in the program.

"Dr. Kix was awesome enough to give me another chance, and I came back in January of 2010. I got the chance to observe Sasha, and I began going to Liza in Fairfield," she says, turning to Best, who is reclining on the blanket, listening intently to her patient as she recounts her on-again, off-again treatment history.

When I turn to Wallace to ask him about his history with the military and the problems he has coped with ever since, he looks desperately at Mojo for reassurance. "Take a breath," she advises, which he does, and then, slowly and gingerly, pausing occasionally to regroup, he begins.

In 1999, at age thirty-one, Wallace joined the Marines. He had worked in construction and was married. "The marriage was shitty," he recalls, "going downhill, so I thought it's time to change and joined the Marine Corps. How dumb was that? I did boot camp, SOI [infantry school] weapons, security forces, and then did a lateral move to another MOS, EOD [explosive ordnance disposal]. When it's a high-attrition, high-demand job, they'll take anybody. I went to EOD school. That school was no joke."

Wallace was deployed to Iraq for eight months in Fallujah and then careened around other bases and other parts of the world until he was discharged in 2005. His first marriage had ended, and he got married a second time, but things were not going well. He doesn't offer up the kind of details Mojo recounted, and I don't ask for them. What he does say is that getting into the PDAT program in 2010, when Mojo entered, was a lifesaver.

"He was very fragile when he came in," Mojo says, looking at her friend, who nods in agreement.

"Yeah, when we came in, they didn't even have a name for it," Wallace chuckles. "They called it the CREC, and we called it the Crack." Both stayed for months. Mojo left in July, and Wallace in June.

Speaking for herself and Wallace, Mojo says that the program "offered a lot of really great tools: classes in anger and sleep management. The cooking class was great because I don't know how to cook. The whole thing about the program, as much as we were learning from the classes, we were also able to learn from each other. That was huge as well."

Mojo and Wallace also began working with Best and Katz in co-treatment sessions. It's hard for them to articulate why they believe these treatments work so well. "The body–mind thing—William and I call it witchcraft," Mojo says.

"Great stuff happens in there," Wallace concurs. "You have the bones in front of you—you put the flesh on it."

"Mind and body are connected all into one," Mojo jumps in. "I found out I don't like being on my left side. I don't like people on my left side because of the injury and my body. If I hadn't laid down on the table, I wouldn't have known that."

After Mojo and Wallace left the PDAT program, they continued treatment at the VA in Martinez with Best and Katz. "We've been working with Sasha for six years, working with Liza for four." Mojo says. "We also work with Dr. Chan [the chiropractor we met earlier]. When I left the program, I was living in Antioch. I tried to stay close to continue treatment." Then Mojo's mother became ill, and she moved to Redding, three hours away, to be near her. Each week, she drove to Martinez with her two dogs. She would not, she says, have considered going anywhere else for treatment. After her mother died, she faced a "big, big loss," she says. "I was kind of lost a bit, trying to find my place. This all," she turns and incorporates Katz, Best, and Wallace with a grateful gaze, "became lifesaving again after that."

Wallace adds that he has also benefited from years of work with Katz and Best and includes TBI social worker Dan Barrows in his list of therapists who have consistently "been there" for him. "There are some days," Wallace says, "when they've got to drag me in here. Sometimes it just gets too intense. We're all sitting around talking, and my leg is doing its own thing. If I was alone, completely alone, it's too intense. I've had days where I've had to stop."

"We back off," Katz interjects, "but we don't quit."

"It's like putting it on pause," Mojo clarifies.

And then, echoing her friend's comments, she emphasizes that what she has found are relationships she can trust. "When I start going wing nuts, I trust that they can reel me back in." Mojo stops for a moment, lights another cigarette, and continues.

"On the positives of it working, I've been able to get back into the veteran community a little bit. Last year I was junior vice commander at my VFW post. This year, I was senior vice commander. I did honor guard at the VFW. All this has helped me being able to get out, literally out of my door, to do things. Other than that, this is the only place I'll come: the VFW, down here, or to William's house, which is a way bigger circle than

I had before, which was just my house, literally. I'm working on getting that bigger. I'm hoping to be able to walk my dogs. I walk them when I'm here. I don't feel safe, otherwise, I guess. We're working on that, hence doing the VFW."

I ask Mojo and Wallace if they could imagine what it would be like to have private-sector insurance, where they would be limited to a number of therapy sessions a year. She explains that, in that case, her gun would be loaded with two bullets: the first for the insurance company and the second for her. Then she adds, more in sorrow than anger, "The thought of that makes me want to cry. It would be like a sentence. That's crazy; I can't imagine that. It would be a nightmare."

Kixmiller and his colleagues seek out veteran feedback about the program and are thrilled that veterans like Mojo and William Wallace respond positively to it. Because the VHA is a research institution, they have also conducted outcome research showing positive treatment gains in a variety of areas. Veterans who have been depressed or anxious report less anxiety and depression. Those with PTSD say their distress has improved. Kixmiller says veterans who have been in the program report "better cognitive functioning." Translation? They make better decisions, are more reflective, stop before they act, solve problems more successfully, and report greater family and community reintegration than previously.

"We don't promise to fix any of their problems when they come into the program," he says. "What we say is that we'll help you manage better and move on with your life." The statistics confirm that more veterans who leave the program have returned to school, started and completed school, or returned to part- or full-time work.

Kixmiller is proud of the program's success, but he is careful to attribute it to more than colleagues who have developed great expertise in veterans' mental and physical health care conditions, as well as supportive local and regional administration. The program, he says, "is a microcosm of the innovative spirit of the VA in general. We do well at the VA because we listen to vets. Throughout the whole system, we try to put their needs and priorities first and treat them as equal partners in care and collaboration. The PDAT program was developed to treat some of the most complex patients that exist, but we can only continue to do that if the entire system supports us."

Two years after I met them, Mojo and Wallace still depend on that support. Mojo no longer comes to Martinez every week but drives down only monthly because she is doing better. In fact, she has gotten married. Wallace has had, not surprisingly, a harder time. He did very well for a while, then had a significant setback and started drinking. He had a couple of drug overdoses and is now back in treatment. He is struggling and may struggle for the rest of his life. But he is alive and trying.

13

OFF THE STREETS

Reducing Veteran Homelessness

Charlene Phipps is on the prowl. The sixty-year-old social worker is the coordinator of the Homeless Patient Aligned Care Team for the San Francisco VA's downtown clinic. Today she is homing in on a vet we'll call Harold. Phipps has been searching for Harold for almost a year. She finally got closer to finding him when she got a phone call from the agent (known as the payee) who receives Harold's Social Security checks and then doles out a weekly allowance for him. The homeless, who have no fixed address, obviously can't receive any money through the mail or online.

"The payee was trying to find out if anyone in our clinic was working with this particular veteran," Phipps recounted. "I said, 'Are you kidding? I've been looking for this guy for almost a year.' The payee told me that Harold hadn't been picking up his allowance for several weeks and that he was concerned about him. He informed me where the veteran might be staying."

The payee thought Harold was staying in the West Portal neighborhood of San Francisco, sleeping in a parking lot near an unidentified restaurant located in an unidentified shopping mall where he helps out by sweeping up the street and parking area. So Phipps and I drive from downtown San Francisco toward the ocean and begin the search.

The first place we investigate is a small strip mall with a taqueria, a Chinese laundry, and a pizza parlor. We go into the market and ask the two workers who greet us if they have seen any homeless men in the area.

Yes, they say.

When Phipps shows them a picture of Harold (she was careful not to reveal his name), they shake their heads. No, that's not the homeless guy they know. Sorry.

So we move on to the main street in the West Portal neighborhood, with its fancy clothing stores, cafés, and restaurants. Starting our search at Starbucks, we run into a helpful private security guard. Phipps shows him the picture of Harold, whom he instantly recognizes. He's always here between six and seven-thirty in the morning distributing marketing flyers around the neighborhood, the guard tells us. He suggests we talk to a storekeeper nearby who may know how to locate him.

As we walk down the street, Phipps spots another homeless man with wavy white hair, dressed in a blue windbreaker. She calls out to him. "Sir, I'm a social worker working for the VA. Can I ask you a question?" Her polite introduction provokes a hostile response.

"I don't talk to social workers," he shrieks, flapping his arms as if he were about to take flight and attack her.

Unfazed, she tries to explain that she works with the VA and is looking for a homeless veteran to help get him housing.

"I don't give a fuck who you're working for," he retorts. "I make $900 a month, and a studio apartment costs $3,000. How much do you make? You're not a social worker; you're a parasite." He spits and moves along down the block. Phipps merely gives an "all in a day's work" shrug and continues down the block.

Finally, we enter a café where two Asian women tell us that yes, indeed, they know Harold. He comes almost every morning with his marketing flyers. He's really sweet, very friendly. Phipps gives them her card and asks them to tell Harold she is looking for him. Several days later, she calls to tell me she's finally found her man and is getting him set up with housing and other VA services.

On another day Phipps invites me to accompany her as she visits the area around San Francisco's famous tourist attraction, Union Square—also a favorite haunt of the homeless—as she searches for homeless veterans. Before we leave for Union Square, she stops off to pick up a vet who had just gotten out of jail for shoplifting and deliver him to his parole officer. Then we go to a homeless shelter near the Tenderloin to search for another vet. From there we move on to a board-and-care home several blocks away to check on another veteran who had burned bridge after family bridge, abandoning daughters and sons along the way. The only link he has to anyone who cares about him is this middle-aged lady tearing through the city on her mission of connection, scouring the neighborhoods for the men and women most people just want to forget.

On our next stop, we visit Mr. Richards,* a paranoid Vietnam vet who is now lodged at the edge of the Tenderloin and Nob Hill in the Granada Hotel. Phipps tells me that it took her ages to gain his trust and even longer for him to agree to shelter at the hotel. After surgery for colon cancer, Richards had a colostomy bag, which he refused to learn to empty and change. He was always covered in feces. Finally, he was involuntarily admitted to a psychiatric unit at San Francisco General Hospital. Phipps tried desperately to delay his discharge so that she could get him into Fort Miley for surgery that could reverse the colostomy. The surgery failed, but being in the hospital—where Richards had a comfortable bed and three meals a day—apparently convinced him that maybe it might not be so bad to get off the streets. While he was in the hospital, Phipps and her colleagues were able to get him his non-service-connected pension with aid and attendance, which gives him extra money so Richards can pay someone to help him with laundry, shopping, cleaning, and other needs.

He is now living in a small room with a bed, dresser, and a bathroom, where he can stay for at least six months. Phipps has been able to find someone who comes in three days a week to help clean up the room. She bought shower curtains from a secondhand store to lay on the floor because he still refuses to learn how to deal with the bag, and feces are everywhere. Richards objected to the three-day-a-week schedule, so now his aide comes only twice a week. This, Phipps says, makes it harder for the cleaner to do her job; she shrugs again and says, "You do what you have to do."

Phipps is holding a box of colostomy bags for Richards. She knocks on his door, and a tall, thin man with wild, black bushy hair, wearing a down jacket open over a naked torso, opens it. There is no polite greeting or "How are you, Charlene?" All he wants to know is if anyone received his check. Upon learning that the check is not right there, in her hands, he cannot contain his ire and shouts out, "I have no money." She leaves, promising to get him the check.

On her way out, she walks into the sunny dining room where aging men and a few women eat three meals a day served by staff circulating throughout the room. "I just want to check in on a couple of guys," she says, and goes over to one toothless white gentleman named Mr. Johnson,* who is wearing a baseball cap. She tells me that Johnson lived in an SRO (single-room occupancy) facility, where one or two people shared a room and bath. When he was recently hospitalized, he was illegally evicted from his room. Phipps helped Johnson get a lawyer to challenge the eviction and then found him housing in this new residence, where he can stay for up to six months. After that the VA will help find him a new residence.

Every weekday, Phipps drives from her home in the North Bay to Vallejo to take a ferry into San Francisco. She has made this commute, almost two hours each way, for the last seven years. Phipps is one of thousands of VA staff whose work is dedicated to ending veteran homelessness in the United States. Staff members at the highest levels take a hands-on approach to this problem. When I was visiting the Phoenix VA Health Care System, Chief of Staff Maureen McCarthy, Director Rima Nelson, and Nurse Executive Alyshia Smith, along with Kevin Hanrata, assistant secretary of security and preparedness for the entire VA, were up at four in the morning attending an annual point-in-time count of homeless veterans in the Phoenix area.

"Our mission is to engage veterans and wrap them in all the services we can provide," says McCarthy. "In order to engage them in care, we have to find them. So we do all kinds of outreach and participate in different local efforts. The moral of the story from this particular day was that we didn't find very many homeless veterans on the streets because so many of them have been housed, even temporarily. For us that was the real beauty of the day—that so many veterans were in treatment."

It wasn't always so. The problem of veteran homelessness is a large one, and the VA hasn't always been a leader in addressing it. The National

Alliance to End Homelessness estimates that in 2014 there were 49,993 homeless veterans when homelessness groups did what are known as point-in-time counts,[1] and that veterans then represented 8.6 percent of the total homeless population in the United States.[2] According to the National Coalition for Homeless Veterans, these veterans have served in all of America's recent wars or, if not in combat, have suffered from the mental and physical afflictions that affect noncombat service members. Most—over 90 percent—are male. And 45 percent of all homeless veterans are African American or Hispanic, although these two groups make up only 10 percent of the veteran population. Another 1.4 million veterans, although not currently homeless, are deemed to be at serious risk for being without housing "due to poverty, lack of support networks, and dismal living conditions in overcrowded or substandard housing."[3]

For decades, veterans' service organizations like San Francisco's Swords to Plowshares and many other community groups across the nation were pushing the VA to do more, much more, to deal with this problem. But apart from the Grant Per Diem program that provided veterans with temporary housing, according to activists like Swords to Plowshares executive director Michael Blecker, the VA was not adequately addressing veteran homelessness.

Then things changed. In 2009 General Eric Shinseki, secretary of veterans affairs under President Obama, announced that one of the VA's top priorities would be to end veteran homelessness in five years. Shinseki approached Secretary of Housing and Urban Development Shaun Donovan, and the two formed a partnership and created the Housing and Urban Development–VA Supportive Housing (HUD-VASH) program for the most vulnerable, chronically homeless veterans. The program recognized what groups like Swords to Plowshares had long been advocating. "You cannot treat the kinds of mental and physical health needs of homeless veterans if you don't get them off the street. Period," Michael Blecker says.

The HUD-VASH program, which is available only to veterans who are eligible for VHA care and excludes those with other than honorable discharges, is grounded in this "Housing First" approach to chronic homelessness. Initially developed in 1988 in Los Angeles and then applied in New York in 1992, Housing First (also known as Harm Reduction) has become the accepted way of dealing with chronic homelessness in programs throughout the nation.

"Whereas other programs require people to engage in psychiatric or substance use treatment and attain stability and sobriety before they can receive housing, Housing First offers permanent supportive housing without these prerequisites," an article in the *New England Journal of Medicine* explains. "This approach bundles financial support for housing with offers of psychiatric, medical, and social rehabilitative support."[4]

As a HUD-VASH guide states, "The VA Housing First approach combines rental assistance with ongoing case management and other services."[5] Case managers and other VA staff make sure they target the most vulnerable and most chronically homeless veterans, offering them the support they need to master the skills necessary to remain in the housing the VA finds for them. VA case managers also link homeless veterans to health care, mental health, substance abuse, and employment services.[6] Along with HUD-VASH, the Supportive Services for Veteran Families (SSVF) program provides much of this kind of support.

The VA uses a vulnerability index for assessing the housing and mental health needs of veterans. As Phipps explains, "It has questions that go on for pages. It asks questions about legal issues, interactions with the police, how long they've been homeless, the area they are staying in. Questions target how many times the homeless person has accessed crisis services, if they have been attacked, if anyone is forcing them to do something against their will." Through this tool veterans receive a score, and the most vulnerable are at highest priority for receiving services.[7]

The HUD-VASH VA initiative, Blecker says, was a dramatic game changer for those involved in fighting veteran homelessness and homelessness in general. It served as a catalyst for all kinds of community groups to shift into high gear and create broad coalitions to target veteran homelessness.

"This is when things really got cooking," Blecker recalls. "Suddenly the VA was in the housing game. Suddenly they recognized the connection between mental health and getting people off the street. This moved way beyond the traditional medical model, where doctors have no idea if their patients are impoverished, need housing or support."

As Blecker describes it, the federal subsidies also played a positive role in bringing community groups and government agencies together. "They all wanted to do a good job with this special money for rental subsidies," Blecker says. "So the VA and the housing authority and the mayor's office and the community-based organizations like Swords in San Francisco were able to come together and make real, lasting progress in reducing veterans' homelessness."

Randy Shaw, director of the Tenderloin Housing Clinic in San Francisco, could not agree more. Shaw has been running homeless programs for over thirty years. "HUD-VASH in the Obama years was the biggest new initiative providing federal money to house homeless people ever," he says. "Veterans were a popular constituency. We couldn't get federal money for other homeless people, but we could for homeless veterans. Without these HUD-VASH vouchers, veterans would have remained in a very, very long line with everyone else waiting for housing. With the money we have at least six hotels in San Francisco for homeless veterans, two of which we run."

Sam Dodge, deputy director of the Department of Homelessness and Supportive Housing for the City of San Francisco, also emphasizes that the VA was "instrumental" in reducing veteran homelessness all across the country. When the program got off the ground, Dodge recalls, there were serious logistical problems in coordinating housing efforts among the numerous parties involved. These included regional HUD administrators, local housing authorities, the local VAs, and the regional VA networks.

"Cities, through a mayor's office, were also coordinating with contracted service providers, not-for-profits like Swords to Plowshares," Dodge adds. "There were a lot of people to coordinate and get around the table, especially for vulnerable people like chronically homeless people who face multiple challenges and don't have a lot of patience to navigate a lot of barriers. You had the operational necessity to make the whole process simple, fast, and transparent and to clear hurdles within and between these departments to make things function."

The effort to end veteran homelessness is also, not surprisingly, difficult because people eligible for Section 8 or HUD-VASH vouchers are also in competition with market-rate renters. In a city like San Francisco, that competition is fierce.

"We had to find market-rate apartments and find landlords who would sign a three-party contract between the landlord, tenant, and housing authority," Dodge says. "This requires that the housing authority conduct the kind of thorough inspection that market-rate renters don't have to go through. Even when you have everyone coordinated, you're still working in a system that makes things hard to work."

The VA's entry into this effort, Dodge argues, made a difference: "We're leveraging a universal health care system for the veterans. We're able to access licensed clinical social workers and a continuum of health care that goes all the way to board-and-care facilities." HUD-VASH and SSVF, he continues, "did more than provide social and medical support. What all this did was encourage the development of a more coordinated approach between all these different levels of government and departments and nonprofits to have a unified focus on the hardest to house. There's been dramatic system redesign for how all these agencies work with people."

Dodge ticks off the resources that have been created to overcome what would have appeared to be insurmountable barriers. "We have a by-name live registry of chronically homeless veterans. It's a community-wide health registry accessible to people who work in different departments and agencies. We have data-sharing agreements and joint agreement on who needs to be housed first and why, and joint responsibility for all of them to be housed." Dodge adds that there are now landlord incentive funds, housing locators to work with landlords to find housing opportunities, and special roles for people to do repairs rapidly so apartments pass inspection.

"This joint approach," Dodge says, "reflects a deep understanding that in order to make progress with homelessness as a social phenomenon, we need to target those longest-term homeless with medical complications. We have to give them enough support and resources to make them successful in housing. That is the goal. The goal is not just to have good data or get people into shelter. The goal is to keep them housed and get them healthy."

This campaign, Dodge says, has had impressive results: a huge reduction in veteran homelessness throughout the country. Because the program has been so successful, he believes it is a model that can be applied to ending homelessness throughout the United States.

"There is now compelling evidence that these kinds of interventions can work," Dodge says. "I don't see any profound difference between veterans and the general population of people who are homeless to suggest that these interventions wouldn't work for them as well. It's a very simple truth that housing is health care. In order to be a healthy person, you need a home. Any amount of health care isn't going to overcome the fact that a person is sleeping on the street. Any complete health care system would deal with housing as the VA has done."

Between 2009 and 2014, veteran homelessness was reduced by 67.4 percent.[8] This is in large part because the VA is, as Dodge points out, a real health care system with a broad definition of both health and care. Indeed, it is the only health care system in the United States that includes a social-determinants-of-health approach in its system of care. As the World Health Organization defines them, the social determinants of health care are "the conditions in which people are born, grow, work, live, and age, and the wider set of forces and systems shaping the conditions of daily life. These forces and systems include economic policies and systems, development agendas, social norms, social policies, and political systems."[9]

Many of the leaders of prominent hospitals and health care systems give lip service to the need to attend more rigorously and systematically to the social determinants of health. Lip service is, however, usually the extent of their commitment. When I recently asked a public health care leader about the record of private-sector health care systems and their top executives in dealing with the homeless, he laughed and asked me, "Are you really, seriously, asking me that question?"

When I said yes, he replied: "Of course, they don't give a shit about the homeless and health care inequities that drive homelessness. I mean, all you have to do is look around you and see what private-sector health care systems have done to deal with the homeless to get a sense of what we can expect when it comes to the private sector and veteran homelessness. And then if the person is also a criminal, well, let's see what that does!"

San Francisco VA system director Bonnie Graham and her staff regularly attend meetings trying to persuade other local hospital leaders to do more for the homeless. As one staffer who attended a recent meeting told me, private-sector hospital leaders greeted the discussion with eye rolling rather than action.

The VHA is one of the few health care systems that—in partnership with many community, state, and national organizations—actually do anything about dealing with education, employment, housing, and legal issues that impact people's lives. In 2012 the VHA launched its Office of Health Equity to identify and reduce health care disparities. Its goal is to make sure that veterans receive "timely, high quality, personalized, safe, effective, and equitable healthcare irrespective of geography, gender, race, age, culture, or sexual orientation."[10]

A lead editorial in the *American Journal of Public Health*, which devoted an entire issue to the VA's efforts to address health care inequities, noted that "the VHA endeavors to be a leader in health equity." The special issue outlined a variety of projects and programs designed to identify and analyze—and then reduce—the causes of health care disparities that negatively impact African American, Native American, and LGBT veterans, among others. One article described an effort to make sure homeless veterans get the medical attention they need through a program that delivers text messages to remind veterans about upcoming appointments. This program has reduced patient cancellations, no-shows, emergency room visits, and hospital admissions.[11]

Through the VA, homeless veterans, like the ones Phipps monitors, are given help finding various housing options depending on their mental and physical health care needs and their ability to function independently. These options include traditional homeless shelters. To stay in a homeless shelter, veterans have to be independent, although they may get a little help getting dressed. They have to work with a social worker to establish goals and show they are progressing with those goals. There are also board-and-care homes for those who cannot live independently, which usually shelter between six and twelve people. Veterans in these homes are given three meals a day and receive help with medication, laundry, bed-changing, showering, and other activities of daily living.

"We have contract beds with various agencies where a veteran can stay up to three months," says Phipps. "We also have Grant Per Diem programs, where a veteran can stay up to two years. If a veteran has mental issues, there's a mental health contract with the Granada Hotel, where they can stay up to six months. We also have contract beds with Safe Haven, which is a harm-reduction model where a veteran who is still drinking or taking drugs can nonetheless get housing. They can't drink alcohol or take drugs in the building, but they can come in loaded. That program is run by Swords to Plowshares."

The Grant Per Diem program that Phipps mentions provides funds for state, local, and tribal governments and nonprofits "to develop and operate transitional housing—including short-stay bridge housing—and/ or service centers for veterans who are homeless." Some of the over six

hundred agencies that provide more than 14,500 beds for homeless veterans also work with community organizations that help veterans find
employment as well as the kind of social services that will help them maintain stable housing.

Yet another VA program is the Enhanced Use Lease program. It leases
underused VA property to groups that will provide approved supportive
housing to homeless veterans. Through this program the VA's community
partners also provide financial management, job training, and even computer and fitness services (or perhaps a much-needed haircut or access to
washers and dryers) to veterans in need. And then there is the Acquired
Property for Homeless Providers program. It "sells VA-foreclosed prop-
erties to homeless provider organizations at a discount for use as transitional housing for homeless veterans."[12]

The ASPIRE Center

San Francisco's homeless programs are part of an intricate web that exists
at every VA medical center and serves veterans all across the nation. In
San Diego the ASPIRE Center occupies three floors in an office building in
Old Town. The center, dedicated to preventing homelessness in veterans
from the wars in Iraq and Afghanistan with combat-related PTSD, had a
difficult birthing process. In NIMBY fashion, residents in the area were
aghast that the VA wanted to lodge homeless (or potentially homeless)
veterans in their neighborhood. For months San Diego papers and TV
news broadcasts were filled with complaints about the project. Residents
protested to the city council and their members of Congress. They envi-
sioned declining housing prices and homeless men running naked through
the streets or attacking children who went to the charter school across the
street from the proposed facility. The San Diego VA had to fight for several years to overcome neighborhood resistance. Now, says Carl Rimmele,
chief of the ASPIRE Center, "the neighborhood, residents, business owners, and interested locals have become our strongest supporters. The San
Diego City Council has had representatives on the ASPIRE Community
Council to observe and replicate the group as the city works with neighborhoods in other parts of the city to build recovery homes and programs
much like ours."

As you enter the nondescript building, you would hardly know the center was there. No homeless veterans are visible when I walk in the lobby accompanied by Cindy Butler, public affairs officer for the San Diego VA. A security guard has to punch in a code that allows the elevator to take us upstairs. Another code must be entered before you can get in the center itself. Once inside, the atmosphere is as far from the images conjured up by worried neighborhood residents as possible.

The center is painted in soothing pale creams, sage greens, and blue-grays, with hints of terracotta splashed on the walls. The lounge is furnished with comfortable white leather chairs and sofas. A pool table is next to the dining room, a pleasant, sun-filled space with round tables and black plastic and metal chairs. Adjacent to it is a kitchen where veterans take cooking classes and learn about healthy eating.

Staff offices are located along a quiet hall decorated in the same mellow tones. Huge, embossed nature photos of bridges over gently burbling water or green fields with wildflowers and intricately assembled stone walls are strategically positioned along the long corridor. When I observe the careful use of art and interior design as a means to encourage healing, I can't help but think of Jeff Miller, former chairman of the House Committee on Veterans Affairs, who lambasted the VHA for spending $5.4 million over ten years on art and decorations for facilities like the ASPIRE Center.[13] If he saw this building, would Miller immediately pick up the phone to fulminate to reporters at *USA Today* because the VHA was once again wasting taxpayer money on, God forbid, art and furnishings? Or, seeing how it helps the veterans, would he finally get it?

The point Miller and so many other members of Congress miss is that the ASPIRE Center, like so many similar organizations, is skillfully designed to soothe the angry, irritable, often terrorized veterans for whom it provides temporary shelter. The forty-bed facility—with thirty-four set aside for men and six for women—provides a safe space that allows them to integrate rather than disintegrate. Art, architecture, and interior design are central to the healing that goes on in the six months that most stay in the residential program.

In his small office, psychiatrist and medical director Lu Le outlines how the program works. Quietly impassioned about his mission, Le, who was a Navy physician for five years, explains that he helps lead a staff composed of psychiatrists, psychologists, social workers, a pharmacist, a registered dietitian, a team of nurses, a primary care nurse-practitioner, a chaplain, and specialists in vocational rehabilitation, as well as an addiction therapist and peer specialists. These last are veterans who have gone through what their patients have experienced and come out the other end. All of them work as a team to guide veterans through the three levels of the program.

Level 1, Le explains, involves evaluating the veteran, establishing trust, and figuring out what medications, therapy, and classes are appropriate. In the first part of the program, the team provides foundational classes and core concepts that will prepare the veteran for the challenging parts of processing traumatic events. Then the veteran will write about a traumatic event he or she experienced and begin a more tentative exploration of his or her responses to it.

Level 2, says Le, involves delving more deeply into the "index trauma"—the particular experience that triggered a more complex emotional reaction. This part of the program addresses how people think about the trauma they experienced, how they process it cognitively. It explores the distorted cognitions that arose from it. For example, Le says, a veteran might have been tasked as a convoy commander and lost some men because he was looking at a map and the road ahead at the moment when his men were killed.

"I'm a terrible convoy commander," he might tell himself, Le says. "But in reality, he was doing his job, which was to pay attention to the maps and the road ahead. There is a lot of forgiveness of self and others involved in the process."

Level 3, Le says, is perhaps the trickiest part of the program. It's designed to help the veterans move from the safe space of the center and transition to a new—or old—environment in which they are more independent. The idea here is not to abruptly cut the cord, but to give the veterans a lot of support so they can function effectively outside the center.

"We provide a bridge to the outside," Le says. "We provide social work support but also encourage self-initiative so people will show up at follow-up and treatment appointments. We allow veterans to pick up their own meds, and, of course, veterans continue in their therapy at the VA outside the program."

Through all the phases of the program, veterans' days are filled with individual and group therapy. Psychiatrists, psychologists, and social workers use cognitive processing therapy and prolonged exposure therapy as well as classes and courses to help the veterans learn and practice the skills and coping mechanisms necessary to help them rejoin the outside world. Veterans also get financial support to improve their credit scores. "That's a huge problem for many of these men and women," Le says. "They have poor credit scores and can't even get in the door with housing."

Le pulls up a spreadsheet and, carefully hiding veterans' names, shows me the packed schedule these men and women go through six hours a day, five days a week. There are yoga and mindfulness meditation classes and cooking classes. Veterans learn how to relate more calmly by training service dogs for others to use. Vocational rehabilitation services offer resources for jobs that can make use of the veterans' skills. They are also educated about alcohol and drugs, and they learn anger management techniques to develop emotional resilience. In what is called a PAIRS class, they role-play and learn more about psychosocial skills. This allows them to learn how to communicate better and interact in a more nuanced fashion with partners, friends, family members, or colleagues.

As in so many other aspects of VA care, the staff mirror the behaviors and attitudes they are trying to teach. Not only do they work with peer specialists, but they get together every day in multidisciplinary meetings to discuss patient progress, plan care, and share and update information.

During my visit I met up with one of the center's current cohort of patients in the quiet room. Brett Stevens* is a burly, bearded thirty-seven-year-old. It's hot out, and he's wearing a T-shirt and Bermuda shorts. His hair is regulation buzz cut, and he is covered, almost from head to toe, with tattoos.

Stevens grew up in a small town on the Texas–Oklahoma border and joined the Marines in 2000, when he was twenty. "All I was doing," he tells me, was "partying and getting into trouble. That's why I joined."

He was in Iraq twice and deployed in other countries. After ten years and a broken leg acquired while he was fast-roping, he left the service and went back home. He moved to the West Coast, got engaged, and then, he says, "everything started going downhill. I sank into a deep depression and an alcoholic rage."

He tried to kill himself twice. Once, he explains, he was going sixty miles an hour on his motorcycle and crashed into a brick wall. "I pretended that that wasn't a suicide attempt," he confides. "But it was." Finally, in 2016, at the behest of his family, he checked himself into a psych ward in Phoenix. He hated it. "I didn't like the staff," he said. "They pumped me full of pills and kept shoving them down my throat." The social worker suggested that he might be helped by the ASPIRE Center, and he agreed.

"This is one of the best things I've ever seen, hands down, for veterans," he says. "The people here are unbelievable. They totally listen to me, hear me out. There's a great pharmacist. I went through a lot of meds and finally got on ones that feel good."

It's been hard for him, he says, to ask for help.

"I grew up in an era where you just dealt with shit, you just sucked it up," he says. "Like PTSD—we didn't talk about it. If you talked about it, you were considered weak. We were supposed to be trained warriors. It would hinder you in promotions. What we did was train hard and drink excessively just to get blacked out. That was the norm. I was afraid to tell anybody. I didn't want people to judge me, to look at me differently. And then I hit rock bottom, and I was very fortunate."

When I ask Stevens what he likes best about the program, he mentions the pairs group. "One of the biggest problems we have is communicating how we're feeling," he says. "We learned ways of relating in the military that just don't work with your fiancée or the people you may be working with on a job. You just cannot treat people like you did in the Marine Corps."

It's hard, though. "You've been doing this for ten years," he says. "You don't see it as abnormal, and you just can't turn it off."

Stevens now realizes that he has to learn to shut it off and figure out how to cope with disabilities, both psychological and physical, that may trouble him throughout his life.

"I have problems with crowds," he says. "I have trouble sleeping. This morning I woke up depressed. I don't know why. Some days just nothing works. I am afraid. I now realize I have been afraid for four years."

Stevens takes a breath as if to illustrate what he tells me next. "So I do the breathing exercises I learned in meditation. I do yoga." He pauses and then remarks on his latest incarnation. "If you had told me you were doing yoga and meditation, I would have laughed and called you a hippie," he says. "I would never have thought I would be doing any of this. And yet here I am, doing all of this, going to a pairs group, reading a book with my girlfriend."

The Errera Center

Across the country is yet another center devoted to addressing the interconnected problems that veterans face with homelessness, mental illness, and poverty. I first heard about the Errera Community Care Center from my daughter, who was working as a nurse-practitioner at the West Haven VA Medical Center. You have to go to the Errera Center and see what they're doing there, she ordered me enthusiastically. I learned long ago that when your kid tells you to do something, you do it.

So I visited the Errera Center, located in a refurbished wire factory several miles from the West Haven Medical Center and only a few miles from central New Haven, which is home to Yale University and Yale Medical School. Leaving the elevator at the second floor at 7:45 a.m. on my first visit, I enter a large open space divided into a smaller waiting area with a reception desk staffed largely by veterans. Around a long table sit four veterans—three black, one white, and all patiently playing checkers and chatting. At lunchtime the dining room will be packed as veterans get a free lunch, which is planned, cooked, and served by veteran volunteers. The center also hosts a Thanksgiving dinner for about three to four hundred veterans and one that is equally well attended near the Christmas holiday.

The rest of the center's space is divided into cubicles and smaller rooms where a raft of psychiatrists, psychologists, social workers, nurses, vocational counselors, occupational therapists, case managers, primary care physicians, and housing and peer counselors (veterans who have struggled with mental illness, homelessness, and poverty) work with veterans. The nonprofit Connecticut Veterans Legal Center provides veterans with free legal services, though its attorneys do not work for the VA.

At the time of my visit, some five hundred veterans were cared for each day, with one hundred in the Psychosocial Rehabilitation and Recovery Center at this facility and another in northern New Haven. Clients at the recovery centers are not just veterans but also their family members, so that a veteran with a spouse or partner can work with marriage and family therapists.

According to Debbie Deegan, the current director of the Errera Center, the Psychosocial Rehabilitation and Recovery Center provides daily structure, teaches coping skills, helps veterans get back in school, and offers a range of classes to help veterans manage daily life and reintegrate into their community. Errera also offers a Critical Time Intervention program, which is an intensive case management program for mentally ill and homeless veterans. Staff members work with them for nine to twelve months, with the goal of providing them with permanent housing.

There is also a walk-in clinic for homeless veterans, which is open from eight to ten, five mornings a week. A social worker sits down with veterans to gather a history of medical and mental health concerns, assess their housing history, and refer them to the right housing service. The center partners with a variety of community agencies and the state. This partnership has resulted in one of the most successful state efforts to end homelessness in general—and not only veteran homelessness.

The wide variety of groups veterans can attend include Addiction Psychoeducation, Community Socialization, and Recovery Planning. There is a women's group and a group dealing with resilience, stress, and trauma. And there is one called the 3Cs—Catch It, Check It, Change It—the goal of which is to enable veterans to deal effectively with their life situation, a group a lot of us nonveterans could definitely use.

I am guided throughout my stay by Laurie Harkness, the center's longtime director, who has worked for the VHA for almost forty years and whose infectious enthusiasm seems to propel her through her days. I am catching her just months before she retires. Neat, trim, with short gray hair falling just at her ears, she talks almost nonstop about her journey and her team.

Harkness began working with veterans when she ran a PTSD program. Trained in traditional fashion to sit with a veteran in an office gathering her patient's history and listening to his story, she was struck by one particular experience that crystallized her mission and launched her on the trajectory that led to her work at the Errera Center.

"I remember this one veteran who was not getting better," she says. "He would go grocery shopping at eleven at night because no one was there in the supermarket. Not surprisingly, he had a sleep disorder. I wanted to understand what was going on, so I suggested I meet him at the supermarket."

Remember, Harkness tells me, this was decades ago, and social workers and psychologists did not leave their offices. In this instance Harkness felt she had to meet the veteran in the middle of the night. As she watched him do his shopping, she was impressed by the fact that he made good, healthy choices. She thought, "Well, this looks okay."

And then they got to the checkout counter. Someone got behind the veteran, and Harkness could immediately see the problem.

"He was out of there in a flash," she recalls. "He left his food, and I'm chasing him through the parking lot. I then understood what my work was. It was to teach him skills. How do you ride a bus with paranoia? How do you shop with anxiety? That's what we do here. We're out in the community helping people learn those skills so they can live the way they need to or want to in the community of their choice."

She and her colleagues don't spend a lot of time probing to ascertain all the factors that are contributing to the veteran's particular issues or even to arrive at an ironclad diagnosis. They're more concerned with helping the veteran cope.

"You don't hear so much about diagnosis here," she says. "What we ask are, 'What are you dreams and your hopes? What brings you here? What are the skills you need to bring you out of crisis that will equip you to do what you need and want to do?'"

To do this, Harkness and the Errera Center team have made use of a variety of funding sources and have pioneered several different therapeutic approaches. "We were one of the original sites for intensive mental health case management," Harkness says. "Initially Congress gave us $3.2 million to serve veterans who were high users of inpatient services. Five percent of veterans who were using inpatient services were consuming 20 percent of mental health resources. Our hypothesis was if you wrap around services in the community, veterans won't use hospitals as much. Guess what? It's true. If you give the right services, at the right place, at the right time, and in the right way, people use less inpatient services."

That means really getting to know and care about the veterans in your program. "We'd go to AA meetings with people, funerals with people, intensive case management," she says. "From the initial grant of $3.2 million, we showed decreased hospital utilization. So Congress funded us with $10 million, and we funded thirty programs. Then they gave us $100 million, and now every VA in the country has this program, which decreases the use of inpatient and ER services."

The center also has a full gym staffed by an exercise specialist and a health psychologist, Carol Hendricks. When I meet exercise specialist

Craig Funaro, he is down in a fully equipped but nonetheless cramped gym in the basement of the building. He explains that the gym will be expanding. It will have state-of-the-art equipment, as well as showers and a dressing room. In other words, it will be the kind of gym that many of the upper-middle-class students and faculty who go to Yale take for granted. Except in this case, it's been specifically designed for homeless, mentally ill, and indigent veterans.

To take advantage of the exercise program, veterans must be cleared by a doctor. Funaro calls the physician and then plans an exercise program. "Once we decide what's safe, I monitor them, and they can come any time they like, once a week, every day, whenever," he says.

Funaro does more than advise on what weights or machine a veteran should use. In the course of working out, veterans learn to trust Funaro and reveal their complex stories. "I've learned to use discretion and never intrude," he says. "Nonetheless, they're pretty open with me. They talk to me about their problems. If something raises a red flag, I will talk to the health psychologist, Carol Hendricks. But a lot of times, through exercise I can overcome what they're feeling."

After I meet with Funaro, I sit in on a meeting of peer support staff. The group is led by Moe Armstrong, who was at the time a lead peer specialist at the center. Armstrong, who founded Vet2Vet, is a legend in the veteran peer support community because he helped to pioneer the concept that veterans with serious mental illness could help other veterans with the same problems through peer support. He has received local, regional, and national awards for his work, Harkness tells me proudly.

In his late sixties, Armstrong is a heavyset, tall, lumbering genie with white, wispy hair flying around his bald head like one of the wizards in a Harry Potter movie. He has struggled with serious mental illness since his stint in Vietnam. A decorated combat veteran, he was a medical corpsman in the Marines, Third Recon Battalion. He was in Vietnam in 1965 and 1966 and went on more than twenty combat missions.

"I was discouraged by the time in war because we were spending all this money and not getting anything back," he says. "When we had been instructors in the Marine Corps, we were told how to build villages, do community action. Then, when we got to Vietnam, we depended on mass bombings. You've got to fight them and build them up at the same time, and we just couldn't get that together."

On his last patrol in Vietnam, he had a nervous breakdown. After he got out of the Oakland Navy hospital in 1966, his family abandoned him, and he went to live in San Francisco. Over the next few years, Armstrong became a hippie and worked with the famous San Francisco Diggers and the US Forest Service and as a street musician and singer. He even had a recording contract with Warner Brothers. He moved to the mountains of New Mexico, to London, to Colombia, and back to New Mexico. Along the way he had another breakdown and became more depressed.

"Then," he says, "the VA offered me a chance, in 1984, to get a college education at the College of Santa Fe, where I got two master's and a bachelor's degree. I wanted to help other veterans get sane, stable, safe, and sober, and so I started peer support for veterans in 1985."

Back then, with the exception of AA, people with a history of mental health problems were not given the opportunity to help one another. But Armstrong did just that, working in state mental health programs in New Mexico and Massachusetts. In 1996 and 1997, he set up a peer educators project for the entire Commonwealth of Massachusetts with the motto "Each one, reach one, teach one, get sane, stable, safe, and sober."

It was through this work that he met Harkness and eventually began doing peer support at the VA. Harkness persuaded Yale to research and evaluate the program, which eventually moved all across the country. Armstrong worked for almost a year at the San Francisco VA Health Care System, helping people like licensed clinical social worker Dan Evenhouse start a peer support program in the new Psychosocial Rehabilitation and Recovery program.

"Peer support specialists are trained and get a certification," Evenhouse says. "They have to pass a pretty serious test. But apart from what they learn, they know so much because of their own experience. They act as ambassadors who help veterans navigate the system. They also provide— not therapy, but therapeutic services."

He has high praise for Armstrong in this regard. "It's really important to have someone like Moe work with veterans who've been suicidal or are depressed or have schizophrenia," Evenhouse says. "They can share their lived experience with them. For example, somebody comes into Psychiatric Intensive Care Unit [who is] hearing voices or is suicidal. I can come in as a clinician to talk to them, and they may not respond well. I look like I have it together. I have a good job, a family, a roof over my head, and they may not think I can understand the struggle of a homeless person with serious mental illness. When he worked with us, Moe, on the other hand, would come in, and he could relate to them from his real experience." The patients, Evenhouse adds, would feel there was "someone in their corner."

And Armstrong really does understand, not only because he had problems in the past but because his life continues to be a constant struggle with mental illness. "I have PTSD, schizophrenia, and also major depression," he does not hesitate to admit. "I'm always just teetering, even though I work hard. That's how I don't fall apart. No matter how bad things are, I work."

At the time of my visit, Armstrong is working with a cohort of thirty-one peer support staff that the center has recruited. "A lot of people think people with mental illness or who were homeless can't work," Harkness says. "We've spent seven years selling our peer services throughout the hospital. People originally thought, 'They're mentally ill, they're going to fall apart, they aren't going to be able to deal with boundaries.' One staff person thought we couldn't have parties anymore because peers would be involved, and we wouldn't be able to drink." Harkness laughs, thinking of all the people whom she has worked with who are in recovery and yet still go to parties where other people drink alcohol. "Part of selling peer services," she continues, "was dealing with resistance, educating people."

I learn firsthand about this kind of resistance when psychologist Anne Klee invites me to attend an impromptu in-service with nurses at the VA hospital several miles away. They have just called to ask her to speak with some home care nurses who are in semi-revolt because of their fears for their own safety as they are asked to provide home care services to poor, mentally ill veterans in some of the area's worst public housing complexes or neighborhoods.

We go down to one of the fleet of fifty-two cars that the center has at its disposal and drive to the hospital. For the next hour, Klee listens to nurses express the tension between their professional and ethical responsibilities and the fears that have arisen because of stories they've heard or experiences they have had. A nurse was raped in New Orleans. One patient had a neighbor who turned out to be a pedophile. What do we do when people have guns or knives in their homes? they asked.

Klee proposes a series of safety measures that she says she will help arrange. They should, she says, never go into a stranger's home alone.

They should go in pairs, or be accompanied by a peer specialist, or even a medical fellow. Everyone doing home care should carry VA cell phones and prominently display VA badges. One of the nurses suggests that wearing white coats would help. Klee agrees. She also suggests that a poverty simulation as well as the VA's disruptive behavior management training might be helpful tools. What they need, all conclude, is a multipronged approach.

When we go back to the Errera Center, I see another multipronged approach when I meet with counselors in all the different programs the center runs. The center offers a variety of housing options that help veterans transition out of homelessness. These include emergency contract beds in homeless shelters that are specifically set aside for veterans. There are, at this writing, 161 Grant Per Diem beds all over the state of Connecticut. Commonly referred to as transitional housing beds, they are provided by a collaboration between the VA and community providers. Legally, a veteran can stay in one of these transitional housing beds for up to two years, and the VA or community provider will deliver case management and residential support to veterans to assist them in obtaining permanent housing. As Maureen Pasko, director of the homeless programs for VA Connecticut, explains, the focus in the state is on a ninety-day length of stay because, she says, "We want them into permanent housing sooner."

Then there is the HUD-VASH program. As we have learned, the Section 8 voucher comes with case management services and is reserved for chronically homeless and highly vulnerable veterans so they can maintain stable housing. In 2017 there were eight hundred vouchers in Connecticut, and neither income nor employment was a requirement for any services provided to veterans.

"The federal program Supportive Services for Veteran Families is another that provides outreach, case management services, help finding employment, and—more importantly for many of our veterans—rapid rehousing financial assistance," Pasko continues. "They provide a security deposit and the first month's rent. There is an individual amount given, depending on the veteran. It can be up to five months' rent, but usually it's only the first month's rent. The program can also provide people with money for furnishings or help with car repair." SSVF and the Grant Per Diem programs, Pasko points out, are also available to veterans with other than honorable discharges, who are, as we have seen, ineligible for VHA care.

Veterans can also connect with the National Call Center for Homeless Veterans line, which is located in Canandaigua, New York, or the Veterans Crisis Line. Veterans or their families who are homeless or at risk of homelessness can call an 800 number, which will connect them to VA or community resources to help get them housing and mental health or medical care, as well as employment.[14]

One of the housing options that the Errera Center is proudest of opened in 2010. Located in downtown New Haven, the Harkness House, obviously named after the center's longtime director, is a facility owned and managed by Columbus House Incorporated, which is a homeless service provider in the Greater New Haven area. The VA provided 65 percent of the $460,000 it cost to renovate the building specifically to house homeless veterans. The Grant Per Diem facility is divided into four apartments that house fourteen veterans in shared units. Veterans can stay up to two years and then hopefully transition into permanent housing using the skills and constant support that the Errera Center and VA homeless programs provide them.

As I am concluding my visit, Harkness sums up the spirit of Errera. "We're all about human connection," she says. "Our whole idea is about connecting. We connect people to community, to us, and to each other."

During my subsequent visit a year later, the new director, Debbie Deegan, shares her views on the program. "I've been here since the beginning," she says. "I have watched veterans come in here, and their lives were in a shambles. By utilizing services here and doing a great deal of work, many have transformed their lives—really regained their lives. They regain their lives, and they give back to their fellow veterans and communities."

14

ALTERNATIVES TO JAIL

Veterans' Justice Programs

On September 11, 2001, nineteen-year-old Phil Adams was living with his father, who had been a physician and was in the Air Force. When he got out of high school a year later, Adams knew exactly what he wanted to do: join the Army. Part Native American (his mother is full-blooded and lives on a reservation), part Anglo (his father is German, Irish, and who knows what else), Adams spent the next eleven years in the Army and National Guard, in the infantry and reconnaissance. He was deployed to Iraq twice—once from mid-2003 to the end of 2005, the second time from 2007 to 2008. When he left the military, he spent two years on a contract working for the DoD.

Adams's mental health problems, he told me, didn't begin till he left the service and began working for the DoD. They arrived in the form of stealth attacks—overwhelming anxiety and a racing heart that would last for an hour and disappear, only to reappear four or five months later. Adams chalked it up to being tired, or stressed, or maybe having a heart murmur. But the attacks increased in intensity and frequency.

"Finally," he said, "it got to a point where I couldn't function because I was having full-blown anxiety attacks. My contract with DoD was ending, and I didn't renew it because I knew something was wrong." By that time he had moved back to where he was born, to live with his girlfriend. While his girlfriend was at work, he would stay home alone waiting for her to return. With nothing but time on his hands, his symptoms got worse and worse.

"I thought I was breaking up," he recalls. "I had nightmares and flashbacks, feeling like I was back in combat. I never felt like I was in a safe situation. Pretty soon I figured out that alcohol was an amazing medication to treat anxiety and started drinking." He drank during the day to stave off the anxiety and at night to fall asleep. "I was having this emotional response every second of the day, every day of the week, and I was compensating with alcohol," he recalls.

After seeking help from a private-sector general practitioner, he added the highly addictive tranquilizer Xanax to his arsenal of relief. Adams says he told his physician he was a combat vet. Rather than recognizing PTSD, his doctor diagnosed an anxiety disorder. As Adams's symptoms worsened, the physician would write yet another prescription for an even higher dose of Xanax.

"In the VA," Adams later discovered, "you tell your primary care doctor or psychologist you're having anxiety and that you were a sniper, and they know right away. The civilian doctor wasn't really invested. He should have figured out I was dealing with depression and anxiety related to my service and sent me to the VA. He never mentioned it."

If his private-sector physician was not helpful in dealing either with the VHA or PTSD, Adams himself was assiduously ignoring the signs of a problem he had certainly heard a lot about. "I wasn't ready to admit to something that, in combat arms, we always saw as a significant weakness—big time," he says. "On active duty if someone started to show problems with anxiety or anger or things like that, as soon as that term PTSD was thrown out about them, they would disappear and be discharged and out of the military. They would literally be separated from us and be gone before we even knew about it. Everybody judged you. You were a risk to everybody else's safety, which was unacceptable. It's a pretty tough, testosterone-filled environment. You break a leg, and you're expected to carry on."

This was taught in boot camp. "Any type of weakness, whether physical or mental, is not tolerated," Adams says. "Every single day, in basic training and infantry school, we recited the Infantryman's Creed: You are physically tough, mentally strong, and morally straight."

On the battlefield that creed was stressed. "In combat the indoctrination is there's no place for overt weakness," he says. "Most people rise to the challenge when it comes to combat. But when you're back on base or on post, you didn't get much help if you started having problems. You vanished. I don't know if they ever sent people to get help, because we never saw anyone come back. For most of us, in between deployments, you just kept your head down. If you have to drink to take care of your problems, then you drink. You gotta do whatever you have to do to get to the next deployment and make it through that."

Adams's resistance to admitting the need for help persisted in spite of what he now recognizes as classic PTSD. "You don't trust anybody," he says. "You're not thinking things through, just acting out. I hated the police, hated anybody who looked at me wrong. I was constantly afraid for my safety, and that caused me to act in terrible ways." Finally, Adams says, his downward spiral led to legal problems, a felony charge, and jail time. "It was my attorney who told me about the VA," he says. "I had no idea about the VHA and what it had to offer. When I was in active duty we got a ten-minute spiel about what the VA was about, and that was it. I really didn't know it was an option."

His attorney told Adams that if he didn't go to the VA to get help, he would end up in prison. "Finally, I admitted I couldn't deal with it on my own," he says. "I lost my girlfriend. Once I was charged with a felony, I lost integral rights I fought for and had watched friends die for."

Forced to get help, Adams learned about the breadth of programs offered at the VA, including participation in the Veterans Treatment Court, a special court within a state judicial system designed to help veterans deal with mental health or substance abuse problems and reduce their involvement with the justice system.[1] As a condition of his treatment in the court, he started with a six-week inpatient substance abuse program. Once he was clean and sober, he went into a general mental health program for another six weeks, where he got a lot of individual therapy. Then he went into a PTSD program for combat vets. "Every day," he says, "you realize how much more you need this help." He was in the hospital for a total of five months. "The VA literally saved my life," he says.

Adams believes he could never have gotten equivalent help in private-sector health care. "The VA is an environment where they are focused 100 percent on veterans," he says. "It's unique. There is no other place where you can get that sense of stability."

After he left the inpatient program, his treatment continued, and he now does group and individual therapy every week. A team of physicians, psychologists, and psychiatrists, all of whom communicate with one another, provide ongoing care. "I have a general physician I see for blood pressure meds," he says. "I have a separate psychiatrist and psychologist, and those two can see each other's notes. My primary care physician can be called upon to make sure they are on the same page with medications and my various types of treatment. They will work together to change my medications according to where I am in treatment. So if my symptoms are on the rise, which they have been the past two or three weeks, they can adjust the medications. I can talk to all of them, and they can communicate without too many crisscrossing wires."

He has been helped by the VHA, Adams says, but it has been a very hard road, one that many vets resist even approaching. "The shame and guilt we have is really powerful," Adams says. "Nobody could talk me out of my determination to take care of this all on my own. At the point where I was at, I just kind of had to have faith it was going to help. It was my last resort, my last attempt to get my life back. And it really is tragic because in so many cases, that's what it takes to get us in the doors."

Adams is still in treatment and spends almost every minute of every day trying to get his life back. He can't work, he says, because he still can't sleep well enough at night to have enough energy during the day to adhere to a predictable schedule. With the help of the VA, he is starting community college and dreams of being a lawyer and helping veterans with the kind of legal problems he has had.

Veterans' Legal Issues

Adams is one of thousands of US veterans who have had run-ins with the law. Between 8 and 10 percent of those incarcerated in the United States are veterans, and 70 percent of them are incarcerated for nonviolent crimes. According to the Department of Veterans Affairs, "on average, veterans in jail have had five prior arrests, and 45 percent had served two or more state prison sentences. More than half of those who were incarcerated had mental illness or substance abuse disorders."[2] Of veterans who had served in Iraq or Afghanistan, 43 percent had an alcohol use disorder and 37 percent a drug use disorder.[3] Plus, 30 percent had a history of homelessness.[4] Fifty percent of homeless veterans have had some kind of encounter with the legal system.[5] According to the VA, three out of five of these veterans had substance dependency problems, almost one in three had serious mental illness, and one in five was homeless, while 60 percent had a serious medical problem.[6]

Most people who have been incarcerated face difficult challenges when they leave prison. Veterans' challenges include dealing with PTSD, military sexual trauma, "or other traumatizing events during military service that factor into prolonged or repeated justice involvement."[7]

Like Adams, many of these veterans benefit from a variety of VA programs that work in partnership with veterans' service organizations, community organizations, and state justice systems. These programs include the VA's Justice Outreach Program, the nation's growing system of Veterans Treatment Courts, medical-legal partnerships, or the Health Care for Reentry for Veterans Program. All these programs are linked to VA primary and mental health care as well as specialty care and the kind of programs that target homeless and seriously mentally ill veterans.

Medical-Legal Partnerships

When I first met Kate Richardson in 2015, the slim, dark-haired attorney was coming out of the legal clinic she was running twice a month at the San Francisco VA's downtown outpatient clinic. The legal director of Swords to Plowshares, Richardson, along with attorneys from the Inner City Law Center in Los Angeles and the Connecticut Veterans Legal Center, among others, encouraged the VA to move beyond narrow medical definitions of health care and adopt the social determinants of health perspective described in chapter 13. In 2011, the VA issued VHA Directive 2011-034, which stated that VA medical centers and staff were encouraged to make space available for legal service providers to assist veterans. The VHA could not endorse or recommend a particular provider, but it could offer this kind of assistance to veterans. The VA now has 147 pro bono legal clinics in its facilities, 16 of which are medical-legal partnerships.

Medical-legal partnerships are a product of a movement that began in 1967, when physician H. Jack Geiger, founding member and past president of both Physicians for Human Rights and Physicians for Social Responsibility, hired a lawyer in the nation's first federally funded rural health center in Mound Bayou, Mississippi. Geiger recognized that he could not disentangle his patients' food and housing problems from their medical ones. In the 1980s, at the beginning of the country's AIDS epidemic, some hospitals began to work with legal aid agencies to deal with patients' end-of-life issues. Then, in 1993, Boston Medical Center clinicians began to connect their patients' chronic asthma with mold in apartments where landlords refused to meet local sanitary regulations. To deal with these legal issues, Boston Medical College began the first medical-legal partnership in the country with Greater Boston Legal Services. In 2006, funding from the W. K. Kellogg Foundation created the National Center for Medical-Legal Partnership. As of 2014, 175 programs had been created throughout the country.[8]

In 2013, Richardson's group began down the path toward a medical-legal partnership with the VA. At first it signed a memorandum of understanding with the San Francisco VA to start a free legal clinic in its downtown clinic. The legal clinic provided assistance to veterans twice a month. In 2014, Swords to Plowshares launched legal clinics at the Palo Alto, Menlo Park, and San Francisco Fort Miley VA facilities. "These were powerful free legal clinics, but not fully integrated medical-legal partnerships," Richardson says. "There was case-by-case interaction with medical staff and the treatment provider. Fully integrated medical-legal partnerships, on the other hand, are more of a true partnership between provider and advocate. You not only get referrals from providers, but consistently and systematically work together with providers as well as with the client-patient to achieve the best outcome."

In the fall of 2016, Swords started a medical-legal partnership at the Oakland Vet Center with a Skadden Fellow, an attorney funded by the Skadden Foundation (of the firm Skadden, Arps, Slate, Meagher & Flom LLP). "This clinic provides legal services in two areas of law," Richardson explains. "One is obtaining VA eligibility through VA character-of-discharge applications and Department of Defense discharge upgrade applications for those with less-than-honorable discharges, and the other is accessing VA disability benefits for mental health conditions."

Richardson cites the example of a veteran who comes to the Oakland Vet Center for PTSD that was based on military sexual trauma. The veteran began treatment at the Vet Center,[9] even though he is not enrolled in the VHA because of the nature of his discharge characterization. Clinicians in this medical-legal partnership recognize that the veteran has legal issues that must be addressed if he is going to be able to get the treatment—both medical and mental health—that he needs. The veteran agrees to see an attorney, who then does a full legal evaluation of the veteran and feels that his case is indeed "meritorious." The attorney pursues VA eligibility by seeking a discharge upgrade with the DoD or a VA character-of-discharge determination application with the VBA, or both. Simultaneously, the attorney files a VBA disability compensation claim for the underlying mental condition. Throughout the process the attorney works with health care providers to put together evidence for a diagnosis of PTSD and how that mental health condition relates to the service member's alleged misconduct.

Veterans Justice Outreach Program

Founded in 2009, the Veterans Justice Outreach Program is designed to avoid the incarceration of mentally ill veterans. Every VA Medical Center has a veterans justice outreach specialist who "serves as a liaison with the local criminal justice system." These specialists "reach out to veterans in jails or the courts and work as case managers trying to engage them in treatment." They also assist veterans with eligibility claims and connect veterans to the VA or community services. And they provide training to law enforcement personnel about issues that are specifically relevant to veterans, such as how PTSD or TBI may be connected to their history of legal problems.[10] These specialists play a critical role in the system of Veterans Treatment Courts.[11]

When I went to the San Francisco VA's downtown clinic, I met with Kyong Yi, the veterans' justice outreach specialist for the Community Based Outpatient Clinic. Yi and her colleagues have created partnerships with law enforcement and staff at city jails who identify veterans in custody and try to link them with health care professionals who can deal with both their physical and mental problems. In order to be eligible for legal services, veterans have to be eligible for VA services, so Yi will work with legal clinics like those run by Swords to Plowshares to help veterans who are ineligible to gain access to them. Many of the veterans Yi and her colleagues work with are homeless and have problems with substance abuse and mental illness. Most are unemployed or have had long periods of unemployment. Yi also goes into the jails to help veterans gain access to a special Community of Veterans Engaged in Restoration (COVER) Pod. The goal here is to identify those in jail who have served in the military and gather them in a special pod reserved for veterans.

Veterans Justice or Treatment Courts

One of the places I never imagined I would learn about and visit (because, like so many people, I had no idea it even existed) was a veterans' court. The Honorable Robert Russell founded the first Veterans Court in the United States in 2008, in Buffalo, New York.[12] Judge Russell began to notice a troubling increase in the number of veterans who appeared on his drug and mental health dockets. When veterans who worked on his staff helped out a veteran appearing in court, Russell noticed the power of military camaraderie. He also recognized that not enough veterans were connected to needed services—services they had earned the right to access—at the VHA. Judge Russell reached out to the VA staff and veterans in his community to pioneer a special court that would deal with veterans involved with the justice system.

There are now over 220 veterans treatment courts in the United States. They are part of the "collaborative justice" movement, which includes community courts, domestic violence courts, drug courts, DUI courts, elder abuse courts, homeless courts, mental health courts, and reentry courts.[13] As the Collaborative Justice website describes it, "Collaborative justice partnerships—and the ability to share information, develop common goals, and create compatible internal policies to support those goals—have significant potential to positively impact crime, increase public confidence, and reduce costs throughout the justice system. Court community and criminal justice professionals join forces to analyze problems and create responsive solutions; and judges, court administrators, prosecutors, defense attorneys, probation and parole representatives, corrections personnel, victim advocates, law enforcement officers, and public and private treatment providers reach out to one another to forge partnerships that will enable them to address complex medical, social, fiscal, and behavioral problems that pose significant threats to the safety and well-being of our communities."[14]

As the California courts' website defines them, "Collaborative justice courts—also known as problem-solving courts—combine judicial supervision with rehabilitation services that are rigorously monitored and focused on recovery to reduce recidivism and improve offender outcomes."[15] Now part of a nationwide movement, these courts offer a variety of therapeutic treatment options, vocational and educational assistance, and financial and housing support in programs that last between one and two years. A veteran who successfully graduates from one of these treatment courts "may be eligible to receive early probation termination, case dismissal, withdrawal of the criminal complaint, diversion, deferred entry of judgment, or charge reduction."[16]

San Francisco Veterans Justice Court

The San Francisco Veterans Justice Court was launched in April 2013 as a partnership between "the Veterans Administration, District Attorney's Office, Public Defender's Office, Department of Public Health, Human Services Agency, Adult Probation Department, the San Francisco Bar Association and its defense counsel, San Francisco Sheriff's Department, and various other city agencies and community groups."[17]

On the day I visit, the court team meets in Judge Jeffrey S. Ross's chambers before the official session begins. The judge's small chambers can barely fit the number of people crowded into the room. The cast of characters includes nurse-practitioner Kristina Kim, Ken Miller, Kyong Mi, and Jeanine Odean from the Veterans Justice Office at the downtown Community Based Outreach Clinic. Jean West is with the court, Robert Clendening represents the probation office, and then there are attorneys. Maria Evangelista is with the public defender's office, John Sengal is an attorney for some of the veterans, and Gregory Mendez is with the DA's office. The group has an hour to discuss the numerous veterans who are to appear before the court that afternoon.

This is called a collaborative court, and this meeting is nothing if not collaborative. Six or seven veterans are leaving the program today, and it's the group's first graduation cohort. Two glass baking trays full of brownies sit on a nearby table. Judge Ross had made a promise to bake brownies for the graduates, and members of the team want to know if he actually made the brownies himself. The trim, gray-haired justice confesses that his wife did most of the baking, while he sifted, stirred, and washed the dishes.

After discussing the intricacies of brownie baking, the group turn their attention to the day's caseload, one of the biggest they have ever had. Some of the cases are relatively straightforward and involve only some scheduling calculations. For example, one veteran has been in compliance for four weeks and, according to the rules, will get a month taken off his probation date, so they need to figure out if he will be eligible for parole in November or December. Others are more complex. One veteran has had trouble getting into the county jail's COVER Pod reserved for veterans. Judge Ross explains that he can write an order to have the veteran transferred to the pod but has no jurisdiction over the sheriff's office. Hopefully, the sheriff will agree.

Other veterans—men who have been on the streets and chronically homeless and unemployed for years—have problems continuing treatment, taking medications, passing drug tests, and obtaining housing. In some cases members of the group strongly urge the judge to support the treatment plan prescribed. One veteran from Iraq, who has both a TBI and PTSD, is resisting the psychiatrist and social worker's recommendation that he do cognitive behavioral therapy. The judge asks what he can do to help, and Odean says he should tell the veteran, "I really want you to do this with the appropriate level of enthusiasm."

For other veterans, they want the judge to have them continue with therapy they have already started. One veteran has kicked benzodiazepines but still has serious mood problems. The psychiatrist wants him to take Depakote, a drug used for people with bipolar disorder. "Please really praise him," Odean recommends to the judge. "Tell him he's doing great, praise him about negative urine analyses, and then encourage him to take the Depakote."

For another veteran what they want is not quite a sermon but a stern admonition of concern. This veteran has failed a test for marijuana and methamphetamines. The judge heartily agrees: "I will have an honest discussion with him from the bench about this."

When we go into the courtroom, the judge greets a ragtag group of men, mostly African Americans, who are sitting in their orange jail uniforms behind a glass partition. Another group of veterans sitting in the back of the room are not in custody. Most appear to be in their fifties and sixties, are sporting baggy jeans or old track suits, and look very much the worse for wear. There is one notable exception. A young man and woman who appear to be in their late twenties are sitting together, watching the proceedings as if they are spectators, not participants. They are both neatly dressed. The young man's hair is closely cropped, and he is wearing a crisply pressed, blue-checked shirt. The woman is dressed in slacks and a sweater twinset.

As Judge Ross goes through the roster of cases, he encourages, cajoles, and sometimes literally reads people the law. He passes out brownies to graduates and ends the session. After everyone has left, he invites the young man to approach him. This is the Iraq veteran who does not want to do cognitive behavioral therapy. I overheard him talking with probation officer Clendening during a break, and I was stunned by his demeanor. This handsome, tall young man appears to be almost a ghost. His body is held with such intense tautness that you feel that a smile would shatter his emotional armor into a million jagged pieces.

Judge Ross asks the man if it is good to be home, to have his wife with him. He invites the young man's wife to approach, explaining that she is welcome to stand at his side. "Our goal is to help and support both of you," he says kindly. And then he asks the young man how he feels about his treatment plan.

As he responds to the judge, the young man has that same frozen demeanor. "It's not too bad," he says tentatively and then explains that he just doesn't want to do one more therapy—cognitive or otherwise. "I've been in therapy for so many years; there are so many redundant appointments. I've been talking so much for so many years—there's nothing more to say. I know what's wrong with me. I know how to handle it. I just have so much stress."

Judge Ross listens carefully and quietly explains that this therapy may be different, more helpful. "It's called cognitive behavioral therapy. It gives you very practical tools to deal with the stresses in your life."

The veteran listens politely, always at attention. "That is my problem now, this stress," he responds haltingly. "My wife and I talk about everything. I go to this At Ease group. It's a fifty-two-week group. Shouldn't that be adequate?"

The judge does exactly what the treatment team asked him to do in chambers. "There is a huge benefit to this twelve-week CBT program. It gives you tools to step back and not engage when someone provokes you. It's not the therapy you're already doing now. It can help."

The young man, seemingly encased in his despair, tries to explain himself to the judge. "I wish I could communicate this better. I'm pretty much a recluse. I sometimes go out for supplies. I got here because this man in the parking lot came up to me, and I pushed him away. I was trying to run away, and he punched me in the face." He adds unhappily, "I will do whatever I need to do to make the court happy."

Judge Ross tries to explain that this is not punishment. "The idea is to help you," the judge says. "We'll do everything we can to reduce the stress in your life and to support you."

Before the hearing, Judge Ross had noted: "For some people the court is an inducement to do what is good for them. For some people dealing with the court adds additional pressure, which makes things more difficult." This was clearly one of these cases.

Honolulu Veterans Treatment Court

In Honolulu I met with VA and state of Hawaii representatives who work through the Veterans Treatment Court. Marci Brown is the VA's veterans' justice outreach specialist and representative to the Veterans Treatment Court. Brown explains that, as a representative of the VA, she sits on a team with Cheryl Reavis, veterans' justice officer and Veterans Court coordinator for the state of Hawaii, trying to make sure veterans get the kind of services that will allow them to convince a judge that they are committed to treatment rather than committing more crimes or getting into more trouble. The state and the VA representatives collaborate to get a picture of the veteran's problems, needs, and thinking. This will determine the kinds of programs to which the veteran is directed.

Brown's team works with some veterans who may have the kind of discharges that give them eligibility for VA services. Some do not. The latter must seek legal help filing claims for VA services through the VA and DoD process. "Every veteran is different, and so we have to individualize their plan of treatment," Brown says. "Because they have been engaged in criminal behavior and criminal thinking, we have to have a therapeutic understanding of how their minds work, not just about addiction, but about their thinking."

Brown says that her background was in chemical dependency programs, where she learned that there is a mental health disorder called criminal thinking. Understanding these thought patterns will help guide individual treatment decisions. "We need to get veterans into intensive drug treatment, or counseling, or a new housing environment where they will not be encouraged through friends or family to engage in more criminal behavior."

Brown is in constant contact with treatment providers to see what kind of progress veterans are making in their rehabilitation. "The trick," she says, "is to match the person to the right program so that treatment is tailored to each individual veteran according to what kind of difficulties they may have and to make sure they stick with the program."

In Honolulu I observed VA outreach justice coordinators work with state court representatives and Judge Edward Kobu of the Judiciary of the State of Hawaii Veterans Treatment Court. Judge Kobu started the court in 2013. He works closely with representatives of the VA and veterans who appear in his court and their representatives.[18] As described in a brochure on the Veterans Treatment Court, eligible candidates for the court are identified, and alcohol and drug treatment, as well as mental health services, are integrated in the way cases are processed and managed. Sobriety is closely monitored, and compliance with treatment and housing recommendations determines whether veterans graduate from the program or are put in or return to jail.[19] In this program veterans work with mentors who, like AA sponsors, are specially selected and educated to make sure veterans have the support and encouragement necessary to succeed in the program.

On the unusually hot day in September when I observe the court in session, a number of mentors mill outside the courtroom, waiting for the session to begin. One of them is Donald Woods, who served in the Navy

Fleet Marine Force as a media corpsman between 1963 and 1967. He is the VA's Disabled American Veterans hospital service coordinator and transportation network coordinator. Raine Arndt, a social worker, is the mentor coordinator who interacts with the court, and Brown and Reavis are also present, as are lawyers representing other veteran clients.

As Judge Kobu questions the men who stand before him in the wood-paneled courtroom, his affect is supportive, curious, and collaborative. When he talks to the first veteran at the hearing, he demonstrates a deep familiarity with his history and current struggles. When he asks the over-weight Caucasian veteran standing at parade rest, arms tucked formally behind his back, how he is doing, the veteran beams and says proudly that his A1C marker for type 2 diabetes is down to 7.1 from 10-point-some-thing. The veteran also says he's doing some training to become a peer specialist, and the judge inquires about his progress, which is apparently hampered by his inability to find a donated computer. He asks the court in general if anyone knows where he can find a computer, and Reavis comments that they may be homing in on a laptop.

The judge asks him if he is keeping up with his mentor, and the veteran replies that yes, he is. "This is the first time during the program that I ever wanted to go to court," he says. "I really appreciate my mentor and the support I am getting. Everything is top-notch."

Judge Kobu asks him several more questions and then turns to Reavis and Brown and asks them if they have any concerns or anything they want to add. No, they say. Judge Kobu then says, "I am proud of you. We are all very proud of you."

The judge tells the next man who appears before him that he has some good news. "You have just one more session left, but talk to me about the surfing contest." The veteran tells him he was in the competition and did well. He's holding down two jobs, and the judge wants to know if that's going well. Yes, he says, as his mentor nods beside him. Judge Kobu then asks about his treatment, and the veteran tells him he has been clean and sober for 315 days as of today.

"You just threw a number at me: 315. That's wonderful," the judge responds enthusiastically. "How are your parents?" he inquires. "Is there anything we can do to assist you till we see you next?"

The veteran says he wants to leave the clean-and-sober house and move into new accommodations. Judge Kobu frowns. Being in a clean-and-sober house is part of the veteran's treatment plan. Any subsequent move must be okayed and supervised by both the judge and the treatment team. "I'm glad you asked about that," the judge responds. "I need to look at the environment to make sure it's okay. We'll get back to you."

Judge Kobu then turns to the mentor and asks for his input. "I am impressed by the support he's been getting from his parents and entire family," the mentor reports. After once again asking for input from Brown and Reavis, Judge Kobu tells the veteran he will see him at his next session.

As the session continues, the judge asks the veterans who appear before him how they are doing in treatment, whether they are going to AA meetings, if they are going to Care Hawaii. One veteran had trouble with his back, and the judge counsels him not to aggravate the pain. He suggests meditation, yoga, watching his diet. The veteran agrees. "I won't do surgery if there's only a minor improvement. I'm not going to do anything that could get me back on drugs." The judge nods approvingly.

Throughout, the judge peppers his conversation with comments like, "Hopefully, you will get through the program and, hopefully, get on with your life," or "Good things come to good people, so, hopefully, they will come to you," or "Good luck to you." One veteran announces proudly that he has gotten a job as a grounds supervisor, and his crews now drive him around. "Does that mean when you become a supervisor, you'll start gaining weight?" Judge Kobu jokes.

Although Judge Kobu's affect is unflinchingly supportive, he can be stern when the need arises. A middle-aged white veteran standing stiffly in front of the judge admits that he has not kept in touch with his sponsor and has not been attending AA meetings. He also tells the judge that he wants to move because he doesn't like his landlord, and his apartment is far from his treatment programs. In fact, he says, he has already found a new apartment.

The judge does not look pleased, pauses, and considers his response. "I like the initiative you have, but when decisions are to be made on that issue," he reminds the veteran, "I have the final say, yes or no. We have to do background checks on your new location."

The veteran looks deeply frustrated and blurts out: "I made a deposit on the apartment. No disrespect to anyone or the court, but I'm going to do what's best for me."

The judge stares intently at the veteran. He does not scold but speaks very firmly. "Now hear me out," he tells the veteran. "If you move out without court authority, you are not in compliance. If traveling is a problem, we can work things out. Don't break out ahead of command. Sometimes we don't like our landlords."

The veteran interrupts. "If the conditions of my release are that I have to suck up to my landlord—"

The judge continues. "Sometimes you have to be among people you don't like, with people no one likes. Keep your head down, your voice quiet. Stay in touch with Cheryl and Marci; we're all here to help you. Don't get ahead of us."

The judge asks the veteran's mentor to comment, and the tall, lean mentor, sixty or older, chimes in. "He's constantly in contact with me," he offers. "But I'm not always aware of his actions and what's behind his actions. My advice to him is chill, calm down. He's very rambunctious, but he wants to succeed. I want to see him calm down. He's got a lot of pride. I know he's got what it takes to succeed."

The judge then turns to Reavis and asks her if she has anything to add. "I have a lot to say," she says and turns to the veteran. "When people say you're not ready, people are saying you will be ready. We want you to be great at things, not struggle through them."

The judge notes that Brown is aching to add something and asks her to speak. "Everything is a learning experience," she advises. "You are going to bump up against things. But you can learn from them. I just want to say, 'Be kind to yourself, be patient with yourself.' Not everything everyone says is an attack on you. When the rubber hits the road and stuff comes up, learn from it. Take a good look at yourself; don't point a finger."

Judge Kobu concurs. "Don't get so busy or upset that you forget to use all your supports and resources," he says, concluding his time with this veteran. "Come back next week."

After the court adjourns, I talk with Judge Kobu in his chambers. He tells me that his father was in the Korean War and Vietnam and gets his care at the VA. His son, who was in Kuwait and Iraq, hasn't yet gone to the VA. He shows me his books on recovery. He explains that he is active in the Veterans Treatment Courts nationwide, which borrow practices from drug courts. And he explains how thorough his program is. "We carefully select veterans, pair them up with veteran mentors, and run them through with very high supervision," he says. "We see them every week, then every two weeks, then every three weeks, and they graduate in two years."

As for his own role, he reflects: "I offer positive reinforcement. My job is to persuade people in a nice way to obtain their objectives. I prefer a compassionate end rather than a big-stick approach, which I use only as a last resort." And he doesn't miss the big picture. "War changes everybody," he says. "We work as part of the recovery team."

Profile

COPS AND VETS

The Memphis Crisis Intervention Model

In mid-October 2017, I sat with twenty police officers who had come to the Memphis VA Medical Center on the second day of a week of training as members of their department's Crisis Intervention Teams (CITs). They included officers and one dispatcher from the Memphis Police Department, as well as officers from the departments in Oakland and Bartlett, Tennessee, the BNSF Railway Police, the Christian Brothers University and University of Tennessee police, and the VA police. They had spent the morning at the Memphis Mental Health Institute meeting with people who suffered from mental illness. This afternoon, they would listen to three veterans describe their experiences with PTSD and military sexual trauma.

The Memphis Police Department, working with the Universities of Memphis and Tennessee as well as the Memphis VA, created this crisis intervention training almost three decades ago. Their goal, the VA's chief psychologist Thomas Kirchberg explains, is to reframe how police officers view the mentally ill. "Officers who have been trained to view the mentally ill as they view criminals who are 'defiant or noncompliant' will approach them with escalating displays of force." The end of this road is the use of lethal force. If, however, police officers are trained to understand what mentally ill people are feeling, experiencing, and perceiving, they will be able to help them get the treatment they so desperately need.

To do this, the training uses its didactic sessions to introduce new recruits to clinical issues relating to mental illness; psychotropic medications and their side effects; mental illnesses like depression, anxiety, or schizophrenia; PTSD; TBI; and developmental disabilities. Then they meet with people who have struggled with mental illness. "We are trying to change the attitudes of police officers," Kirchberg elaborates, "to help them understand that mentally ill people are acting out of fear. They are not being defiant or noncompliant; they are out-and-out terrified." The solution to their problems is not, Kirchberg says, to throw them in jail and then send them to prison; it's to help them get treatment. When police officers talk to real, live veterans who are in recovery and who have been helped by getting treatment, Kirchberg says, "the officers get a completely different picture of veterans. They don't see Rambo in front of them. They see a human being who's been suffering and who's been helped."

There could be nothing less Rambo-like than the three veterans sitting at the front of this small VA conference room. B. J. Whit is a Vietnam veteran in his late sixties, a stocky man wearing jeans and a green, white, and maroon plaid shirt. His face is a road map of sorrow and regret. Norma Smith is in her early sixties. She is as neat as the proverbial pin. Her sandy brown hair flecked with gray is cut short, and she is dressed in dark brown pants and a vivid pink, long-sleeved shirt under a multicolored vest. When she begins to talk to the officers assembled in front of her, she is both affable and no-nonsense. She will tell her story, she informs them, but will tolerate no disrespect of herself or other veterans. That's not a threat—it's an order. Phil Wright* (he was fine with me telling his story word for word but not using his name), casually attired in plaid and jeans, is a bearded Iraq veteran who deployed several times.

The veterans are flanked by two VHA social workers, Michelle Bowen and Courtney Deviney, who work in the PTSD program. Their role in the session is to introduce the veterans, ask them questions, annotate their answers, and—most important—make sure they feel safe and that no one pressures or triggers them in any way.

Bowen begins the session by asking the veterans to tell the audience what PTSD has cost them. Wright jumps right in. "It cost me my marriage," he says, not stinting on any details. "It cost me the first six years of the life of my son. I didn't care. I wanted to be over there [in combat] rather than here. When I was here, I washed down six Percocets a day and a bottle of whiskey at night. I didn't think there was anything wrong with me. I was fine." He insisted he was "fine," he said, even though he had panic attacks that drove him into his parents' room in the middle of the night, where he would huddle on the floor in terror, creeping away before they woke up.

A lot of veterans, Deviney interjects, use substances to avoid trauma, and then they need more and more and more. However, she adds, this is not the case with all veterans. "A lot of Vietnam veterans work and work and work to escape the trauma. Then they retire, and it hits them over the head."

That's what happened to Whit. "For me, I didn't turn to alcohol and drugs. I buried myself in work. There was nothing wrong with me. I just thought I had a hot temper. I had nightmares and flashbacks, but I refused to talk about it. I shut my wife out, and she resented it. But I couldn't do it," Whit says emphatically, his voice awash in self-blame. "I just couldn't do it. It was a weakness on my part. And then I stopped working, and I couldn't deal with it anymore. I had to get help."

Looking straight at the group of men and women, about half Caucasian and half African American, he continues the heartrending calculation. "It forced me to live my life almost in a cloud. I lost so much happiness. There were days I couldn't even get out of bed. It stole all the joy from my life all those years."

Smith is the last to speak. Her husband was also in the service, on active duty in Desert Shield and Desert Storm. "When he came back," she recounts, "he was not the same person. At that time we didn't know what PTSD was. He committed suicide."

She had been in the Air Force, in and out of the Middle East, for ten years. She had been trained to handle many difficult, even life-threatening, situations. "What they don't train you for," she says, "is what happens when you are raped by some of your own people. That cost me my family and relationships. I had nightmares and flashbacks. I got to the point where I thought maybe my husband was the smart one, after all." Had someone at the VA not reached out to her, Smith says, she was more than ready to join him.

All three veterans insist that their lives, relationships, and families were saved because they went into treatment at the VA.

"Why did you stick it out?" Bowen asks.

Wright takes a stab at an answer. "I was not leaving home for six or seven months, and now I am here. I am now going to my son's games. I am taking him to the movies. Seeing that progress made me stick to it. My son needs a father, not a shell of a man."

"I have taken a lot of pills and done a lot of therapy," Smith says. "It was a lot easier to take the pills. The therapies were hard. The hardest part was processing the traumatic event—to go through it over and over again. I had the same experience whenever I did that, even the same physical reactions. You ask why I did it—honestly, I don't know. You'd have to be crazy; I don't know why I kept coming back."

Whit, too, marvels at his persistence but concludes, "My wife had been loyal to me for forty-eight years. I had to do it for her. We couldn't survive like this. It wasn't fair to her or me. I had to see what could be done and stick it out. It was very painful to have to face it down and relive it all. For me the war is never going to be over, but it has gotten easier. The treatment has allowed me to face things head-on."

The veterans want the police officers in the room to be part of the healing process. They urge them to develop an understanding of what might be going on with the veteran who may, for example, be freaking out in a parking lot at night. Whit explains that he dreads such nightly crossings more than anything else. Smith tells the male officers to be careful when they put on cologne. "I knew a woman whose attacker wore Polo cologne. If she just smelled that cologne, she would have a total panic attack."

"Don't crowd us; that scares us to death. Don't come up on us suddenly. Turn down your radio. Use your de-escalation skills. It really helps if you send a veteran, if you can," Wright suggests. "If a patrolman came and identified himself as a veteran instead of just some random dude—me, if I know you're a veteran, it makes an instant connection."

As the veterans finish talking, Kirchberg stands in front of them and addresses the group. Tearing up, he thanks them for their courage. Kirchberg has worked for the Memphis VHA since he did his internship in psychology there in 1991. He and the Memphis VA have been working with this pioneering police program almost since its inception in 1988. The program began after a mentally ill man—twenty-seven-year-old Joseph DeWayne Robinson—charged police with a knife and was shot to death. This tragic death caused the city to rethink the way the police department interacted with the mentally ill, and the police department formed a partnership with the National Alliance on Mental Illness. The department recruited psychologist Dr. Randy Dupont, now a professor of criminal justice at the University of Memphis, who, as a professor of psychiatry at the University of Tennessee, ran the city's main psychiatric emergency service at "the Med," the Regional One Medical Center. Dupont recounted the program's beginnings as we sat in one of the city's famous barbecue restaurants along with Kirchberg and Lieutenant Colonel Vincent Beasley, the program's current coordinator and a veteran of the Iraq War, and its assistant coordinator Officer James Lash, also a veteran who was recently deployed to Afghanistan.

In between bites of dry ribs and sides of beans and slaw, Dupont explained, "Police needed to understand and address the complexity of what's going on with a person with mental illness." At that time, then Lieutenant (now Major, retired) Sam Cochran of the Memphis PD took ideas from a blue-ribbon task force and worked with Dupont to train a special group of patrol officers who would form a CIT. The team would be called out when there was a hint that an encounter would involve someone with mental illness. Dupont told me the program took several years to really get off the ground. "It didn't get support from fellow officers. They thought it would put them at risk in life-or-death situations." But the group persisted, recruiting officers who themselves had experiences with mental illness in family, friends, and neighbors. The CIT concept also coincided with emerging trends like community policing.

The VA was involved very early on, Dupont told me. "I needed to work with the VA from the start because they knew a lot about PTSD, alcohol and drug issues." The group also reached out to the VA because many of the "consumers" involved with the police were and still are veterans. "Today," Beasley tells me, "many of the people we interact with are Iraq and Afghanistan veterans."

On Wednesday afternoon Kirchberg travels out to the Memphis Police Academy to teach the first course in de-escalation skills the group will receive. He begins with some personal history. Although he is not a veteran himself, his father and mother were in the Navy in World War II, and his brother was a Marine physician assistant for thirty years and served in Operations Desert Shield and Desert Storm. Then he explains precisely what it means to be in crisis, to be in a place where one simply cannot maintain any balance either physiologically or emotionally. The kind of emotions and triggers the veterans and other people struggling with mental illness have shared with the group make it imperative that police officers display empathetic understanding, genuineness, and acceptance. To intervene in a crisis means engaging in "active listening" and "emotional communication," mobilizing not only verbal communication but also the appropriate tone of voice and body language to help people in crisis understand that you are there to help, not punish.

Kirchberg teaches the group basic de-escalation techniques like restating or reflecting back a person's concerns. A desperate comment like, "I don't know what to do; my family doesn't want me back home," should not provoke, "Oh, I'm sure that's not true," as a response. Rather, the CIT officer would say, "Let me see if I understand you correctly. You're not sure where you can go when you get out of here. Your family doesn't seem to want you back home."

An enraged rant about being "sick and tired of them screwing with me" does not elicit a "Come on, calm down, now," but rather, "Let me make sure I hear what you are saying. You're sick and tired of people harassing you." All these techniques and more allow police officers to respond in a nonthreatening way, Kirchberg says.

"A lot of people we come into contact with just want to be heard," Beasley elaborates as we talk later. "They may even have been victims of a crime. They want to vent. So what do I do? I practice my listening skills, and there's nothing better than when you're yelling and screaming and cursing and I can say back to you what you just told me. Now, that means I'm listening to you, and after a while, they just lose their steam, and you can find out what's really going on."

Over the course of the training, Cochran and criminology professor K. B. Turner and psychologist Dick James of the University of Memphis repeat Kirchberg's message and add new, more advanced layers to the skill set these officers are here to master. Expert CIT officers act out real-life scenarios that their colleagues have successfully defused. In one a distraught African American woman is trying to hang herself but can't manage to tie the knot. "I can't do anything right," she raves. "Help me, Officer. I've heard of suicide by cop; please, please help me," she begs the trainees, who must figure out how to manage the scene. In another a mother calls the police because her three sons are smoking marijuana and acting up and she wants them out of her house—now! As four officers try to put their newfound skills into practice, the three "sons" (all CIT officers in the role-play) become increasingly obstreperous, the "mother" more insistent that the police "get them the hell out of here," and the scene noisier and more chaotic. Anyone who hasn't had sympathy with the situations the police confront on a daily basis would be impressed with the department's burdens and its commitment to deal with them in a nonviolent fashion. I know I certainly was. I was also impressed with the skill of the experienced CIT officers who assisted with the training.

The Memphis PD and its university and VA partners hold four training sessions each year—two in October and two in July. Between twenty and forty full-time police officers or dispatchers are in each session. One slot in each session is reserved for a VA police officer (at no charge to the VA). They all have volunteered for the program and passed through a rigorous selection process in order to attend. According to Beasley, coordinator of the program for the last five years, the records of officers who apply are scrutinized for any suggestion that they might have used excessive force or do not have the personality and character necessary to display empathy and defuse complex situations. After the weeklong training, these CIT officers take the lead on calls that involve mentally ill consumers.

Beasley explains the dynamic. "We tell other officers that the CIT officers are the subject matter experts. It's in their arena, so let them handle it. We empower them. This is your scene. And I'm telling you, you should see how the officers take this to heart. The CIT officer walks up, and it's like the waters are parting. It's like, boom! Here he comes. He's going to make this right."

The program's two leaders, Beasley and Lash, are both veterans. A tall former Navy and Air Force service member with close-cropped, receding sandy brown hair, Lash tells me how he became involved with the program. He was deployed as a military policeman in both Operations Desert Storm and Desert Shield. During his nineteen and a half years on the Memphis police force, he was exposed to CIT when he rode with partners on a CIT call. At first, Lash says, smilingly sheepishly, he thought it was all pretty much "mumbo jumbo." As he got older, he began to reconsider his stereotypical idea of police work as, he quips: "running, chasing, and locking the bad guy up. I made several of those calls where I was absolutely lost because the stereotypical Johnny Law has nowhere to go in those situations. All the avenues ahead were dead ends, with the exception of deadly force. Watching the CIT officers at work, you realize there are other avenues to get what you want."

Years later, after he was activated in the reserves post-9/11 and went to Afghanistan, he came back to the police force. "Things had progressed in law enforcement, and I was even older," he says. "I made a call one day with a veteran CIT officer of a consumer who had run away from a care home. I spotted the guy running into the woods. I did what most cops would do. I gave chase. It was summertime and felt like it was 140 degrees out. It was sweaty and sticky in the woods, and there was a lot of overgrowth, and I was beginning to get pretty frustrated." He scowls at the memory. "And then I started remembering how the CIT officer talked, and I mimicked him. And lo and behold, the guy was helping me out of the woods." Lash realized there really was more to CIT than mumbo jumbo and decided to apply to be on the CIT team.

He took the forty-hour training and admits that he still hadn't fully bought in. "I'm a kinetic learner," he jokes. "You have to beat me over the head." The morning following the training, the police got a call. "It was a doozy," he recalls. Six cars had been burgled at a hotel. "A very sturdy-framed male white whose car had been burgled had all the windows up, and I could hear him cursing."

When he got out of his car to report the theft to Lash, he was furious. "I immediately put my hands up in a surrender position, nodding my head. He continued to berate me, and I let him vent for six or seven minutes. When he allowed me to introduce myself, I said, 'You seem very angry.'" That triggered another bout of fury. "He had a lot of fuses," Lash said.

But after Lash listened to the man talk, as he had been taught in CIT, the man calmed down. "After about fifteen minutes, he wanted to write the report for me. That's when I finally bought in. There is a time for Johnny Law," Lash says. "You can't delete that from police business. But there is also a time for something else."

"Developing empathy?" I venture.

Lash laughs. "We don't use that word so much—you'd get too much pushback." But that is precisely what it's all about.

As I am leaving Memphis after observing the training, I ask Beasley if he can imagine what the program would be like without the VHA's participation. "I can't," he says emphatically. "Honestly. And let me tell you why. Most of the people we are dealing with now—the younger generation—are veterans. And I tell police officers all the time, these guys that are fresh out of the military, they are trained killers. I hate to say this, but that's how they're trained. They're in shape. They're young. They're strong. They know their job. They practice their job all the time, whereas police officers, we kind of sit around and get lazy and eat doughnuts and get fat.

"We don't want to be fighting these young military guys," Beasley, who was one of them, continues. "So we need to figure out how to deal with them. Most of the time, if we know it's a veteran, we try to send a CIT officer out who's also served in the military, in the same branch, so they can talk."

The cost of not talking, he adds, is way too high. About three years ago, in Germantown, outside of Memphis, a twenty-five-year-old active-duty service member, fresh off deployment from Afghanistan, was killed by the police. He had driven from Fort Campbell and was in his car with a high-powered rifle. He wouldn't get out of the car when asked, and when he picked up the rifle, he was shot. "Just by the grace of God it didn't happen in Memphis," Beasley says.

Some officers wanted to know why the military would let someone come home with mental health problems. Beasley completely understands. "When I was in the military, I didn't see my wife and daughter for eighteen months. So when it's time for me to come home, I want to come home, so I'm not going to tell them if anything's wrong. Because if I tell them something's wrong, like I'm hearing voices or whatever, they're going to put me in a holding cell—a unit they put you in to evaluate you. And that's another six months. So they say, 'Hey, I'm good,' and they come home, and everything starts to go south on them. And then, of course," Beasley adds, "there's a stigma attached to it, a chance I might not get promoted. There's a chance the military might kick me out if I tell them I have issues."

Beasley concludes, "We want them to be able to talk our language. I always tell them, 'If it's a veteran, say "Thank you for your service." That brings them right down.'"

By mid-October 2017, Beasley tells me as we drive from the police academy, the Memphis police had responded to 18,435 CIT calls since the previous January. Only 592 resulted in an arrest. Kirchberg, as a member of the University of Memphis Crisis Intervention Center's train-the-trainer team, has helped to do precisely that all over the United States. To name only a few sites, the team has trained police officers in Idaho, Pennsylvania, Montana, Utah, Hawaii, all of Tennessee, Mississippi, and Florida. They also traveled to Uruguay, where they worked with the Uruguayan National Police and National Prison Service.

As I talked with Beasley and Lash and observed the collaboration between the VHA and the Memphis Police Department, I was once again struck by the power of the public–public partnerships in which the VHA engages. I was also struck by the power of this model to transform relationships between police and community in a nation in which tensions between the police and those they are sworn to protect have been escalating.

When I ask participants in the CIT program if they think the Memphis model is part of the solution to larger national policing problems, Lash, Beasley, Kirchberg, and Dupont all nod furiously and argue that yes, most definitely, it is. As Kirchberg says, "There's a new movement in policing that conceptualizes police officers as guardians."

Although many officers, Kirchberg says, want to act in that capacity, it takes training to help them navigate the contradictions inherent in their work. "On the one hand, we want police officers to rush into situations and take out the criminals and terrorists, but we also want them to protect and serve, to show empathy even in life-or-death situations." Kirchberg outlines the problem. "In order to do this, they need specific training. It all comes down to dignity and respect and empathy. It takes skill to mobilize that when your life and that of others is on the line. The CIT model offers that kind of training, not only when dealing with the mentally ill but in dealing with members of the community in a variety of complex situations."

Specializing in Elder Care

The VA and Geriatrics

Just south of San Francisco, the San Bruno VA clinic sits in a sun-drenched building across the street from a large VA cemetery, its gleaming white headstones stretching out along the drought-burned hills. I am sitting in on a meeting of the PACT Intensive Management (PIM) program. The team today includes physician and medical director Jessica Eng, psychologist Nate Ewigman, social worker Angela Bodnar, registered nurse Robert Carr, and two medical students.

In 2014 the VA central office launched the PIM program with a three-year grant. Five sites were chosen to pilot an effort to reduce costs and utilization while providing high-quality care to high-risk veterans. At least half of its patients are seventy or older. Some are younger but are as complex as geriatric patients. Indeed, they are often described as having early-onset geriatric syndromes because they have memory problems, falls, and physical disabilities earlier in their lives. All these patients have a hard time navigating daily life as well as getting to appointments and following medication and treatment regimens. They thus frequently end up in the emergency room or are admitted—and then perhaps readmitted—to the hospital. This means they use a disproportionate share of health care dollars and experience a great deal of unnecessary suffering.

"PIM was started because people felt there was a group of patients in primary care who needed more intensive interaction than what a typical PACT team can provide," Eng says. These patients, she continues, have been referred by primary care providers who are concerned about their well-being. The team, with members from the disciplines of nursing, social work, psychology, and geriatrics, discusses the patients with their primary care team. Members of the PIM team then go out to the patient's home to "get a more complete picture of what the veteran is facing on a day-to-day basis," according to Eng. "We also try to find out what is important and valuable to them in their life. The primary care provider has usually known the patient for a long time but hasn't been in their house or seen their family."

Carr, on the other hand, can check their medications, see how they organize their different pills, or find out how many old bottles of medication are lying around. Bodnar figures out where the patient's money goes or who is financially dependent on the patient. On his visit, Ewigman can discover why patients are having problems getting to appointments or if they have an undiagnosed mental health issue.

After these visits the team meets to, as Eng puts it, "try and put it all together for the primary care team. We come up with a plan and communicate with the entire PACT team, trying to figure out what makes sense in terms of next steps so that we can align patients' values with perceived medical needs."

Although the PIM team may follow patients for three to six months, its job is not to take over the care of these high-risk patients but to serve as an adjunct to the primary care team. "We provide a comprehensive view to the primary care team and veteran and then, with both, help create a plan that makes sense. Then the veteran and primary care team work together over the long term," Eng says. The PIM team can also accurately ascertain whether a patient should receive care from the Home Based Primary Care (HBPC) program—which we will learn about in this chapter—or be cared for in a nursing home.

Today, for example, the team begins by reviewing a recent visit with Mr. G. He is a seventy-year-old Vietnam-era veteran with a history of

PTSD, alcohol abuse, cirrhosis of the liver, and hepatitis C. He is on a HUD-VASH voucher and interested in moving to the Veterans Home of California in Yountville, which is run by the state and has an assisted-living facility. The visit started out well, with Mr. G. welcoming the two team members into his home. However, when they asked if they could go in his bathroom and check on his medications, Mr. G. became very agitated. "Do other people let you do this?" he demanded.

He finally allowed the team to review his meds and admitted that he had been drinking again and was very anxious. He also had foot pain from plantar fasciitis. The team suggested that he visit physician Karen Seal's interprofessional pain clinic. As the team members discussed his needs, they agreed that he should be referred to the chronic pain team.

Up next was Mr. W., an eighty-three-year-old veteran referred from the Infectious Disease clinic. His primary care doctor was concerned that he was not safe at home. He scalded himself with hot tea and is on the wait-list for HBPC. He has HIV, lipodystrophy—a condition in which the body is unable to produce fat—neuropathy, type 2 diabetes, sleep apnea, heart failure, and swelling of the extremities.

After the meeting, Eng says, "Over the past three years, we've learned that the most valuable thing we offer to the patients and the PACTs is the home visit. This helps us figure out the barriers patients have to getting what they need."

She tells me that some veterans need little more than a quick visit. For example, there's the ninety-year-old veteran who is legally blind. The primary care team was informed that the veteran's live-in caregiver had quit and moved out. The primary care team, Eng says, "was very concerned everything was going to fall apart. They were sure his medical issues would worsen and he wouldn't be able to continue living on his own."

The PIM team visited him and discovered that he was actually doing very well. His children lived nearby and visited every other day. He was very organized about his medications and knew precisely where everything was. He even knew where to find his backup razor. The veteran had a system of PVC pipes affixed to the walls of his house so that he could follow them from one room to another.

"If I saw that patient in clinic," Eng confesses, "I would be scared to death about him. We helped the primary care team by reassuring them that he was really okay. We also helped make sure someone came in to visit him and that he wouldn't be lonely and isolated. Instead of guessing about the need for home-based primary care or a nursing home placement, the PIM team made a reasoned evaluation based on the facts on the ground." All it took was one visit.

Other cases are more complex. Ewigman tells me about a patient who was having a lot of dizziness and pain. He was very depressed and also had type 2 diabetes and diabetic neuropathy. Severe abdominal pain led to many emergency room visits, which were very frustrating to the patient. ER physicians suggested that the veteran see a psychologist or psychiatrist for help with the pain. The veteran, Ewigman says, felt like physicians were telling him that his pain wasn't real.

Ewigman came to visit the veteran with Carr and Bodnar. "I came to his house as just one of the team, which made him feel more comfortable and normalized the practice of behavioral health. We got to understand his values and what was most important for him. He was feeling very depressed—almost suicidal—smoking a lot, and was very unhappy that he could not get out of the house because of his pain." Ewigman did some cognitive testing and found the veteran had some mild memory issues. Most important, he found that the patient had been on long-term morphine.

Using the kind of motivational interviewing techniques we learned about earlier, Ewigman spent a lot of time talking with the veteran about his pain. The team decided to see if he would agree to a prescription of suboxone (a safer alternative to long-term morphine). This would reduce the constipation that is a side effect of morphine. He agreed.

Through the VHA's Opioid Treatment Program (OTP) clinic, he met with psychiatrist Tauheed Zaman and started on the suboxone. Because the OTP clinic often treats people with addiction problems, this particular veteran felt uncomfortable there. He was not an addict. "I talked with the psychiatrist, Tauheed Zaman, as well as pain physician Karen Seal," Ewigman recounts. "Karen Seal determined that she could take over prescribing suboxone to the veteran. This was precisely the outcome we wanted. We had originally wanted him to be treated by the Integrated Pain team, and that's what ended up happening."

Now, after three or four months, with the help of the Integrated Pain team, he is being treated in primary care. His pain practically disappeared because most of it was related to the morphine use. "The veteran,"

Ewigman adds, "really wanted an electric scooter, and we spent a lot of time talking with occupational therapy and advocating for him. He got his scooter; he's out and about and much happier—plus, he isn't going to the emergency room." When his old primary care provider retired, the PIM team transferred his care to a geriatric primary care physician who continues to manage his health-related issues over the long term.

Several weeks after I meet with the PIM team, I sit in on a meeting of the HBPC program at Fort Miley. About twenty different health care staff cram into a small room to discuss their various patients. The program is co-led by its program director, nurse-practitioner Paul Turnbo, and its medical director, Theresa Allison. The group also includes other nurse-practitioners and doctors, physical therapists, occupational therapists, social workers, dietitians, psychologists, and psychiatrists—some of whom specialize in geriatrics—as well as a dedicated pharmacist.

After the meeting I talk with Turnbo, a tall, older African American man with snowy white hair who was, for many years, an Army nurse. The HBPC program, Turnbo says, is designed to take care of veterans—most of them between seventy-five and eighty-five, with some in their nineties—who are referred by their primary care provider. They may be too sick to leave their homes. Some are paraplegic or even quadriplegic. Some can't drive and have no friends or family who can assist them. They thus have more frequent hospitalizations and ER visits. Because many patients can't take their medications without help, the HBPC sets up their medi-set pill containers.

"The entire team collaborates in making a written plan of care for each veteran and family—and that is a condition of staying in the program," Turnbo says. "The key is involving the veteran and family in making that plan. If they help write it, they are more likely to comply with it."

Turnbo usually makes the initial screening call, asking some very specific questions to ascertain if the veteran lives in a home, apartment, trailer, board-and-care home, or assisted-living facility. He also asks if the veteran has a firearm. The program then assigns a nurse-practitioner, who goes out to evaluate the patient and home environment. Social workers also visit patients to determine their financial status, need for help in bathing themselves, preparing food, and going shopping, and perhaps eligibility for a home health aide.

I go out on one of these initial visits with nurse-practitioner Carol Denise Tiggs, who is visiting Mr. O'Leary,* a seventy-five-year-old veteran with serious mental health issues. Mr. O'Leary lives in a small house he inherited when his father died, which is located in a predominantly Chinese neighborhood. Every room is crammed with the accumulated evidence of Mr. O'Leary's dual obsessions: Major League baseball and religious imagery. On every wall there are pictures of Jesus, Mary, and a variety of saints. Religious bric-a-brac—statuettes made of plastic, glass, ceramic, and wood—line the shelves that are not strewn with baseball paraphernalia.

The living room has two upholstered armchairs and a sofa, both covered with huge piles of shirts. Baseball pennants, caps, scorecards, sports-page clippings, and books on America's national pastime crowd every corner of the room. More baseball paraphernalia fill shelves in Mr. O'Leary's bedroom and another spare room. Every surface of the kitchen is covered in plastic bags, empty cartons, and boxes. In his one small bathroom, the tub overflows with old laundry detergent bottles. A lonely venetian blind stands under the shower, leaning against a pink-tiled wall. Mr. O'Leary is not malodorous when he greets us, so it's not clear how he manages to clean himself, since his tub and shower are unusable. That's just one of the mysteries Tiggs will have to unravel.

She chats with Mr. O'Leary and then takes his blood pressure and vital signs and examines a series of skin tags on his back. He is worried that they are cancer. She reassures him they are not. He is not comforted. He is covered in skin tags, he exclaims. Where is the dermatologist? What can be done, he rants, all push of speech and flight of ideas. Tiggs remains calm, assuring him that she will call the dermatology clinic and get him an appointment.

As she continues to check him out, he seems to notice his surroundings and apologizes. "I'm sorry it's not *House Beautiful*. I'd love it to be beautiful, but I just can't sort through all this. It's my collection; I want to get it in order, but I just don't have the energy anymore. And really, to tell you the truth, if I didn't have all this to sort through, I don't know what I'd do. I'd probably go crazy."

He explains that he has become increasingly socially isolated. He had a birthday recently, and his sister came to visit but not her two daughters. "I am stranded here, all alone," he says forlornly. He used to swim. He used to garden. But that's all in the past. I look out into his backyard. It is an overgrown welter of beautiful fruit trees. Peaches and apricots hang off the limbs, beckoning to be plucked and savored, canned, baked into crumbles or made into jams—not doomed to rot.

Tiggs asks about his background. His parents came from Ireland when he was a small boy. They landed in Boston and then somehow migrated out here to California. He was in the Army. His mother, he recounts, lived till she was ninety. His father died at seventy-five. He worries about what will happen to him if he gets more and more isolated and can't take care of himself. He's afraid of being put in a nursing home, where he can't wake up in the middle of the night, decide he wants a piece of watermelon, and just get up and get it. "I'm afraid I'll end up in a place where I'm confined just to die. Or worse, that I'll end up on the streets, homeless."

Again, Tiggs reassures Mr. O'Leary that the team will take care of him. She then asks him to go through his meds, and he escorts her into the cluttered kitchen. Pill bottles are arrayed on, of all places, the open door to the oven, next to an old copper fluted gelatin mold. He explains that he gets some of his prescriptions from Kaiser and some from the VA. The problem is he takes some pills from the VA and puts them in the Kaiser bottles and puts Kaiser pills in the VA bottles. Some of the pills are past their expiration date. "I am so grateful to the VA to have these; I want to use them up," he tells Tiggs.

His insistence on using expired medication is the least of her problems. On her next visit, it will take hours for her to figure out which pill is which. The social worker will also come for a visit, she tells Mr. O'Leary. He looks distressed by this news. Mr. O'Leary worries the social worker will make him move because the place is so cluttered. "No," Tiggs consoles him, "We are not here to judge you, Mr. O'Leary. We are here to help you."

Several weeks later, I follow occupational therapist Heather Freitag as she visits a pleasant house in a neat pastel parade angling down the hill toward the ocean in South San Francisco. Mr. Leonard* is a Korean War veteran who spent years drinking. He now has alcohol-related dementia and was recently hospitalized for hydrocephalus—fluid in the brain. Mr. Leonard refused to have a lumbar puncture to drain the fluid and became extremely weak during his stay in the hospital, so weak that he is now permanently bedridden. He is suffering from pressure ulcers as well as dementia and is unable to care for himself.

A chronic alcoholic, Mr. Leonard is still drinking, even though he can't do a thing for himself and can barely hold a cup or spoon. His wife is supplying him with whiskey every night. "If you tell them that they have to stop drinking, go cold turkey, they will become alienated, and not even let you in the house," Freitag tells me. "Then you won't be able to do a thing for them, and things will get a whole lot worse."

The HBPC team has decided to try harm reduction by encouraging Mrs. Leonard to water down the whiskey she gives her husband every night. They also want to assess the home situation to prevent falls, more serious bedsores, and harm to Mrs. Leonard. The obese seventy-four-year-old with health problems of her own is his lifeline. If she can no longer care for him, he will have to go to a nursing home. To make sure he can remain at home requires multiple visits from multiple health professionals. First comes the nurse-practitioner evaluation. Now Freitag examines his home to make sure Mr. Leonard gets all the equipment he needs.

When we knock, Mrs. Leonard cheerfully lets us in. The house is worn but neat, struggling under the effort of one aging person trying valiantly to take care of another. She ushers us through the kitchen and into the living room, where a sagging hospital bed lies in front of the TV. Mrs. Leonard says that her husband doesn't use this bed much anymore since it's almost impossible for her to turn him in it.

Freitag observes the bed with a practiced eye and instantly ascertains that it is both too small and too soft. She explains that she will get Mr. Leonard a bariatric bed with a special airflow mattress that will not only allow Mrs. Leonard to turn her husband easily but will take away the arduous work of getting him from bed to chair because the bed itself becomes a chair with the flick of a switch. She also goes into the bathroom and discovers that the lip at the edge of the shower makes it impossible for Mrs. Leonard to get her husband's wheelchair into the shower. His wheelchair, she discovers, also needs an upgrade.

Freitag leaves the couple and goes back to her office to order a new bed, a device that will be specially constructed to allow Mr. Leonard to get over the Everest-like edge of the shower stall, and a specially designed wheelchair. She will also order a set of eating utensils that will accommodate his tremor and a bed pad with handles that is washable and will allow his caregivers to shift him when he has had an accident without, hopefully, injuring themselves.

When the wheelchair has arrived and bed and shower device have been delivered, I go with Freitag when she returns to the Leonards' to make sure everything functions properly. Freitag does a dry run to make sure Mrs. Leonard can put the shower device together correctly. Mrs. Leonard proudly shows me how the metal pieces shift into place so that her husband can get from the wheelchair to the seat and then slide right into the shower. "He hasn't had a shower in a year. We haven't been able to wash his hair properly. We had to use these funny shower cap plastic things and give him bed baths. This is amazing," she beams as she sits on the toilet seat in the tiny bathroom explaining it all to me. The VHA has also delivered the special supersonic electric wheelchair, which will need some adjusting.

Mrs. Leonard is one of the nation's almost six million "informal" caregivers who provide over 532 million hours of unpaid care to loved ones who have Alzheimer's disease and related dementias (ADRD). Studies have documented that the health of these caregivers has a direct bearing on the health of those they care for and the cost of the care of patients with dementia. In 2012 the VA spent $3.1 billion on the care of people with ADRD.[1] To help manage these costs and also the burden on caregivers, the VA participated in Resources for Enhancing Alzheimer's Caregivers Health (REACH), which uses behavioral interventions to improve the coping skills of those taking care of patients with dementia. When researchers compared the impact of REACH II, which included caregivers of patients outside the VA, and REACH VA, they found that the interventions lowered health care costs for veterans far more significantly than for those outside the VA.[2] Investigators attributed this to the fact that patients and their informal caregivers benefited from being in an integrated health care system.

Although Mrs. Leonard was not part of this study, she is also a beneficiary of the VA's integrated system of care. And she knows and appreciates this fact. As Freitag leaves to fix her husband's wheelchair, Mrs. Leonard turns to me and says, "The help from the home health aide has really been huge. Taking care of him has been overwhelming for the past year. He's incontinent, and just dealing with that is exhausting. It's morning, afternoon, and night. Every day. Day after day. I hate to say it, but I was getting a bit testy with him, but just to have someone else around who can help has made a big difference for both of us. The other day, he asked to play a game. He hasn't asked to play a game in two years."

VA Geriatric Care in Context

The VA's geriatric programs are critical models not only for veterans but for a country with an aging population and not enough geriatricians and geriatric health care professionals to care for them. In 2008 the Institute of Medicine produced a report titled *Retooling for an Aging America: Building a Health Care Workforce*. It noted that "older adults account for about one-third of visits to physician assistants (PAs), but less than 1 percent of PAs specialize in geriatrics. Less than 1 percent of both pharmacists and registered nurses are certified in geriatrics."

When it comes to geriatric physicians, the report found that "as of 2007, there were 7,128 physicians certified in geriatric medicine and 1,596 certified in geriatric psychiatry. According to one estimate, by 2030 these numbers will have increased by less than 10 percent; others predict a net loss of these physicians because of a decreased interest in geriatric fellowships and the decreasing number of physicians who choose to recertify in geriatrics. According to the Alliance for Aging Research, by 2030 the United States will need about 36,000 geriatricians to take care of 21 million elderly Americans."[3]

To produce these geriatricians, the Alliance for Aging Research has estimated that the United States needs at least 2,400 geriatric academicians and has only about 900. This is hardly enough to produce the 36,000 trained geriatricians needed by 2030. In 2006 and 2007, there were only 253 physicians enrolled in geriatric medicine fellowships.[4] In 2016 the American Geriatric Society reported that things had not changed much in the eight years that followed the Institute of Medicine report. The number of geriatricians had barely increased.[5]

When I spoke with Louise Aronson, a geriatrician and professor of medicine at the University of California, San Francisco, she outlined the dimensions of the problem. "We have an old and rapidly aging population. If you look at the number of geriatricians proportionate to the number of old people and then compare that to the number of pediatricians in proportion to the number of kids in our society, or adult physicians in proportion to adults, the results are discouraging. Many other countries do a better job of this, but the US does not." This is true, Aronson says, not only in terms of clinical care but research into the development of older adults. "Whole blocks of research are devoted to human development in children and adults, but not in older adults."

The VA is a distinct outlier when it comes to this larger trend in American medicine. "The VA," Aronson says," has been one of the great supporters of funding geriatric programs and clinics. It is way ahead of most medical systems in this regard."

Anne Fabiny, who spent over a decade working in private health care systems before she became associate chief of staff for the San Francisco VA Health Care System, says that the VHA is light-years ahead of most other health care systems in the country. "The VA was one of the founding members of geriatrics in the US. Much of the momentum for creating geriatrics as a discipline and the investment in creating a science of gerontology and geriatrics came from the VA. The VA has been central to developing clinical geriatrics, and research in geriatric medicine, and understanding the health care needs of older adults—and also how to best serve older adults."

In "U.S. Geriatrics, an Historical Perspective," historian James S. Powers, who is also associate clinical director for the VA Geriatric Research, Education, and Clinical Centers (GRECCs) at Tennessee Valley Health Care System in Nashville and Murfreesboro, Tennessee, explains that the VA's interest in geriatrics was central to the development of the field. "The Department of Veterans Affairs showed great interest in geriatrics due to the increasing age of WW2 veterans, which by the mid-1970s equaled three times the rate of aging in the general population."[6] In 1975 Congress passed legislation to establish GRECCs to improve the health and research the problems of older veterans and educate staff about issues in aging. There are currently twenty of these VHA Centers of Excellence in Aging associated with academic medical centers in the United States.[7]

In New England, neurologist Andrew Budson[8] works in one of these GRECCs, which spans the Boston and Bedford VA Medical Centers. Budson is chief of cognitive and behavioral neurology, associate chief of staff for education, and director of the Center for Translational Cognitive Neuroscience at the VA Boston Health Care System. Budson's work in both his clinical practice and the center addresses patients with memory problems. Most of these patients are in the early stages of Alzheimer's disease or have other disorders. Some have problems with memory that stem from normal aging. "The work I do in my center," Budson says, "focuses on new strategies and techniques that individuals can use to have better memory function in daily life so they can continue to live at home and do all the things they enjoy doing."

Helping patients deal with their memory problems, Budson says, is critical for their independence not only because memory problems can negatively impact their ability to navigate daily life in general, but also because they can impact their ability to manage medical or psychological problems. "Memory problems," Budson says, "even those that are attributable to normal aging, mean veterans have missed medical appointments, take their medications at the wrong time, or forget to take them altogether." If their health suffers, this will make it more difficult for them to live independently.

The aim of the center is to take discoveries related to normal memory and apply them to individuals with aging memories and memory disorders. "We have explored using pictures, mental imagery, music, mindfulness, and simple strategies like, when you're trying to remember something, think about how it's meaningful to you, [and] put it in a sentence to improve one's memory," Budson says. He's recently put this information into a book, coauthored with one of his colleagues, that helps patients in and outside the VA.[9]

I observed Budson and his colleagues and trainees working with veterans in February 2015. After a major northeaster, the city was blanketed with snow. Budson, however, trekked in to the Jamaica Plain VA Medical Center to see the few veterans who had braved the weather to make their appointments. With his research assistant, Corie Nagle, and psychiatry resident Tai Soonsawat, Budson greeted a gentleman, Mr. Richardson,* in his mid-sixties. Nagle ran through a Montreal Cognitive Assessment memory test for dementia, asking the patient to connect dots, draw rectangles and a clock, remember words, and list numbers that he hears forward and backward. Mr. Richardson constantly apologized for not doing well on the test. When Nagle asked him about his concerns with his memory, he told his physicians about his difficulties caring for his mother, with whom he lived after his father passed away. He is determined to continue caring for his mother, even though his two sisters and a brother—who he says are no help at all—want to place her in a nursing home.

That's why he is so distressed by his memory loss. How can he continue to take care of his mother when he can't find things—the keys, the bills? "If I'm doing something and the phone rings, I don't remember what I was doing before." He finds all this particularly perplexing, since he can still take apart a motorcycle and put it back together. But what's with those keys and those conversations?

Another patient is Mr. Ford,* a seventy-five-year-old veteran who complains that everything he sees these days looks "strangely unfamiliar."

"I don't have a crisp, clear memory, like I might have had five or ten years ago," he tells Budson and his resident. "I'm going downtown on the bus, and I look out the window, and it's almost like I've never been there. It looks so different. In the last two or three months, that's what I've noticed."

As he talks to the two physicians, he mentions that he's been coming to the VA since the mid-1980s. "I've always been grateful to people here. They are kind and concerned. They helped me with headaches. I could get my teeth fixed so I don't scare everybody. There's nothing like being an old guy," he quips, "and sitting across from young people like you."

Budson and the trainees listen patiently to both these veterans as they recount their histories and concerns. After the patients leave, they discuss the tests and brain images they will seek and the strategies they will employ to help these veterans cope with their fading memories. Like so many aspects of VA care, Budson's work does not focus on cure, but rather on function. In his teaching of residents, he helps them understand that the work of a physician is not only about fixing and curing disease but about helping patients live lives that have been limited by disabilities and dysfunction. Similarly, Budson helps to educate his colleagues in primary care and geriatrics about memory problems and the strategies that can help patients live more effectively with them.

Budson's teaching is part of a national effort to educate more clinicians in geriatric medicine and health care. In 1978 the VA launched a Geriatric Medicine Fellowship to train physicians in geriatric clinical medicine, research, and education. Today the VA finances one-fourth of all geriatric medicine training slots and half of all geriatric psychiatry training slots in the country. In the mid-1990s, the Accreditation Council for Graduate Medical Education downgraded geriatric fellowship training from two years to one. Concerned that a one-year fellowship would not fully prepare geriatric physicians for leadership roles, the VA established an Advanced Fellowship in Geriatrics, which it has expanded from seven to sixteen GRECC sites.[10]

As part of the delivery of primary care, the VA has created sixty-five Geri-PACT teams all around the country. These integrate geriatric care of the high-risk older veteran into primary care. As James Powers describes it, physicians and nurse-practitioners work with pharmacists and social workers, dietitians, and psychologists or psychiatrists to deliver care to this subset of patients.

What is special about these Geri-PACTs is that they all have a registered nurse care manager. "The RN," Powers says, "is the glue that holds it all together. The RN is constantly coordinating care. The RN knows where patients are, if they have been hospitalized, if they are taking their medications. The care manager rides herd on higher-risk patients."

Powers gives an example of how the Geri-PACT works. "The patient we cared for was an eighty-five-year-old gentleman, a crusty veteran who was very independent. He was having chest discomfort and lived one hundred miles away from the VA. Yet he got in his car and drove himself to Nashville, bypassing four other hospitals as he was having a heart attack. When he got into the clinic, we rushed him right in, got an EKG, got a cardiologist, and he had surgery right then. He recovered well. But we weren't sure he liked us. I was particularly concerned that he didn't like me. He said he wasn't sure he was going to like this new doctor—me—assigned to him when our first encounter was with him having a heart attack. Well, he came back to us because he decided he really liked us. We have continued to follow him."

In following patients like the one Powers describes, one of the many areas of concern is polypharmacy, which is defined as taking more than five medications. According to one study of polypharmacy in the elderly, among seniors with a median age of 76.5 years, 35.6 percent had polypharmacy that resulted in contraindicated drug combinations and duplication of medication.[11] The VHA has been a leader in trying to protect patients from this kind of dangerous overuse of medication. "The appropriate use of medication makes a world of difference to older patients," says Powers. "The fewer the medications, the lower the doses, the better." This is true not only of patients who have problems like type 2 diabetes or high blood pressure but also of people with dementia. "Nonpharmacologic approaches to dementia are best. We should try to avoid medications with bad side effects. We need to address pain and other issues nonpharmacologically as well, even if patients can't communicate their pain to us."

The VHA, Powers says, is successful in dealing with polypharmacy and many other problems of the elderly because it has more information about its patients than almost any other health care facility in the country.

"Because we are the largest unified health care system in the country, the VA has a wonderful data set on all its patients. [There is] a group at the Duke VA called the GECDAC—Geriatric and Extended Care Data Assessment Center. There, investigators, statisticians, and programmers are using VA data to model the downstream effects of all the geriatric care models the VA has developed." When it comes to polypharmacy—to cite only one of the many things the center studies—Powers says that "if we reduce medications from thirteen to nine, it makes a huge difference to patients."

The VHA also protects its elderly patients from the kind of overuse of unnecessary treatments that is becoming an increasing threat. While I was writing this chapter, for example, the *New York Times* science section had a front-page story on the overuse of surgery and radiation for simple skin cancers like basal and squamous cell carcinomas. Private-equity firms, the *Times* reported, are now starting dermatology clinics, which recommend expensive, painful, and unnecessary treatments for elderly patients, who have been trained to believe that the doctor (or in many cases, nurse-practitioner or physician assistant) knows best and unwittingly follow the "doctor's" orders.[12]

ACE Units, GEM Units, and CLCs

Some VA hospitals, like Fort Miley, have Acute Care of the Elderly (ACE) units. These units practice the kind of teamwork that I described in the chapter on primary care. When I observed attending physician Kathryn Eubank leading morning rounds on the ACE unit, it was particularly interesting to watch how she emphasized nurses' participation in the planning of patient care. Morning rounds on the ACE unit included the usual cohort of medical students and residents, as well as a pharmacist and a social worker. The nurse assigned to care for the particular patient the team visited did not travel with the group through the wards. Instead, as the team fanned out around a patient's bed, the nurse assigned to that patient—who was almost always in some other patient's room—would interrupt his or her work and rush in to join the rounds. Whenever a nurse joined the group, Eubank briefly stopped the discussion and thanked the nurse for coming to join them.

She also made sure to ask the nurse if she or he had any concerns or input to share with the team. When the nurse expressed a concern or shared important information, the attending physician thanked the nurse for this input. And when the group was finished, the attending physician again thanked the nurse for joining the rounds.

When I asked Eubank about the thank yous that were given at each and every bedside, she explained that nurses are often reluctant to join physicians on rounds, even when invited, because to do so almost always interrupts their own work. Many may think that such interruptions aren't worth it, since they often feel that their concerns are rarely acknowledged or addressed. Saying thank you to the nurse, Eubank said, is a critical way to ensure that ward rounds are, as she put it, a "high-yield" activity for the nurse. It's important, she said, that the nurse knows that he or she is recognized and that physicians aren't just paying lip service to the idea of collaborative interprofessional practice.

The nurses I spoke with responded positively to these cues. They said that in the traditional model of medical ward rounds, they often felt that they were spectators watching physicians do "their" work. As one nurse put it, "the rounds are ours rather than theirs."

Although some hospitals, like Fort Miley, still have ACE units, others have Geriatric Evaluation and Management (GEM) units. These units care for frail, elderly patients who, with a little more time in a hospital, can be discharged to a lower level of care—to the home rather than a nursing home. A GEM patient, Powers says, may be a ninety-two-year-old veteran who had heart valve surgery. He is very weak and requires a little more time in the hospital so he can get stronger, adjust his medication. His caregiver, his wife, can get some education in how to deal with his problems at home. With an extra seven days on a GEM unit, the veteran can go home rather than to a nursing home.

I ask Powers what would have happened if that hypothetical gentleman had not been in the VA but in a private-sector hospital with Medicare as his primary insurance. "He would not get that extra seven days," Powers replies. He would go to a nursing home right after surgery. And, like 29 percent of patients discharged to post-acute care from the hospital, he might be readmitted to the hospital within twenty-eight days.

According to Charlene Harrington, professor emerita at the University of San Francisco School of Nursing and an internationally renowned expert on nursing homes and nursing home staffing, patients often fare poorly in nursing homes because "50 percent of US nursing homes don't have enough staff to meet regulatory guidelines, and 60 percent don't have enough registered nurses. Nursing homes with low staffing have higher readmission rates. They just don't have enough registered nurses to take care of people who are acutely ill after a hospitalization. When, like the VA, you have more registered nurses and better all-around staffing, you reduce readmission rates, provide better quality care, and reduce patient suffering."

In 1999 Congress passed the Veterans Millennium Health Care and Benefits Act (sometimes known as the Medicare for Veterans Act). The bill mandated that the VA "accord the highest priority for nursing home care to the most severely disabled veterans and those needing care for service-connected disabilities. . . . Veterans enrolled in the VA healthcare system receive non-institutional, extended care services, including geriatric evaluations and adult day healthcare."[13] VA programs not only include Adult Day Health Care programs to help chronically ill or frail, elderly patients—and their family caregivers—maintain their independence for as long as possible, but also include the home-based primary health services described previously and homemaker services delivered in a veteran's home.[14]

For veterans whose ability to live independently is limited because of mental or physical health conditions and who don't have any family or friends to care for them, the VA offers community residential care programs that provide room and board to veterans. A veteran may choose a residential care program outside the VA, but the VA has to inspect and approve of the facility. Veterans must pay for room and board in these facilities, but the VA pays for any visits VA health care professionals deliver in the care home.

The VA also has 134 nursing homes called Community Living Centers (CLCs), which are available to veterans for short-term stays or for the rest of their lives. As of 2017, there were 135 CLCs across the United States and Puerto Rico. Unlike most nursing homes, in which the majority of residents are female, in the VA's CLCs, most are male. The 1999 Millennium Act mandated that the VA pay for nursing home care if veterans have a 70 percent to 100 percent service-connected condition or if they are 60 percent service-connected and unemployable. Some residents may use CLCs but make co-pays.

In 2005 the VHA launched a transformation of its nursing homes. The leader in this effort was Christa Hojlo, who has a doctorate in nursing and was director of the Department of Veterans Affairs Nursing Homes and State Veterans Homes Clinical and Survey Oversight. Hojlo, who had worked at the VA for twenty-one years, fifteen of them at the VA central office, had become increasingly convinced that the VA had to change its model of nursing home care from a medical model to one driven, she told me, "by nurturance, comfort, and love."

In 2004 Hojlo created a national steering committee on nursing homes, which, for the first time, included not only physicians and high-level nurses and researchers but also nurses, nursing assistants, a recreational therapist, dietitians, physical therapists, social workers, and other health care workers. The group put together a conference, which was held in April 2005. Two hundred and fifty participants looked at every aspect of nursing home care, as well as the language used when discussing how that care would be delivered, to whom, and where. "If you keep talking about a 'patient' in a 'nursing home,' those words, that language, shapes our view of both," Hojlo explained.

The group decided to use the term "residents" and changed the name of VA Nursing Homes to Community Living Centers. In these CLCs, residents can have pets and even drink alcohol, a no-no in most nursing homes. "We have a regulation that says no alcohol on federal property," Hojlo explained. "It took me two years to work with general council to have them understand this was standard of care that was normal."

One of the most important differences between VHA CLCs and other nursing homes is their attention to adequate levels of nurse staffing, higher staff pay, and far better safety practices than private-sector nursing homes. The latter are notoriously understaffed, with employees who are also notoriously underpaid and poorly treated.

"In the VA we have a registered nurse on all shifts," Hojlo said. In VA CLCs, nurses, and particularly nursing assistants, are paid more than in most for-profit nursing homes. Employees get sick leave and vacation, benefits that nursing homes don't provide. Most important, in CLCs, nursing assistants and registered nurses have a voice in the planning and delivery of care. In every CLC there is a monthly nursing assistant call, and nursing assistants are on planning committees. In most traditional nursing homes, housekeepers have also been excluded from participating in the planning of residents' care. In the CLCs the role of the housekeeper has moved beyond cleaning, and nursing staff now understand that housekeepers know a lot about residents and have developed pocket scripts for house-keepers to help them better engage with the residents they serve.[15]

All this, Harrington argues, makes the VHA very different from private-sector nursing homes. "The VA does what it should be doing in terms of nurse staffing. Having an RN on every shift is what all experts recommend when it comes to safe, high-quality patient care. Many nursing homes don't have an RN on staff at night, for example. But patients get into trouble not just on one or two shifts. If you don't have a registered nurse available to assess that patient, the patient will suffer. Because VA nursing homes also pay staff better and provide better benefits, they also have lower staff turnover and better stability. Low wages and lack of decent benefits are associated with very high turnover, and high turnover is associated with poor patient care."

The VHA has done more than assure better nurse staffing and lower staff turnover. Since 2008, when the VA officially changed the name of nursing homes to CLCs, it has also been involved in trying to make CLCs more hospitable by assuring that newly constructed or renovated CLCs provide private bedrooms and baths for residents. In fact, the VA is pioneering a new program, Green House Model for Veterans. In seven different pilots around the country, the VHA is building smaller units for veterans who have a long-term need for skilled nursing care. Instead of a thirty-eight-thousand-square-foot nursing home, in Danville, Illinois, the VA Illiana Health Care System built a seven-thousand-square-foot residence called Freedom House that serves about 150 veterans, each with his own bedroom and bath. Freedom House has a comfortably furnished living room, dining and kitchen area, and a hearth and fireplace, around which residents are encouraged to gather. There is no fixed mealtime, and residents can design their own meals. Family and friends are invited to join residents for meals.[16]

BEST

In spring 2014 a group of clinicians at Fort Miley began meeting to discuss a problem that increasingly plagues many hospitals. As patients live longer, suffering from not only chronic illnesses but dementia and mental illness, a subset of these patients may be aggressive or violent and sometimes even a danger to hospital caregivers. They demand a disproportionate amount of time, and nursing staff have difficulty taking care of their other patients.

Such patients are also difficult to discharge from the hospital because their families—if they have any—cannot cope with their behavior, and nursing homes or other facilities will not accept them as residents. If they cannot be discharged, these patients ratchet up health care costs—taking care of an elderly demented or mentally ill patient on an inpatient hospital unit, where the costs can skyrocket to over $2,000 a day, is almost ten times what it would cost to take care of the same patient in a nursing home.

Many hospital officials wring their hands over the problem of how to cope with such patients. Some take action. Others tell registered nurses and aides that getting hurt because a patient lashes out at them is just part of the job.

In 2014 the San Francisco VA Medical Center decided to systematically address the problem by creating an interprofessional task force led by psychiatrist Bobby Singh and psychologist Michael Drexler, whom we met earlier when we visited the workplace violence prevention program. The task force produced the Behavioral Education and Support Team (BEST). When I visited the team, it included neuropsychologist Donna Rasin-Waters, psychiatric occupational therapist Karen Leigh, and psychiatrist Barbara Kamholz. As of this writing, it includes two registered nurses.

BEST works with patients whose behavior prevents discharge, who may be staying in the hospital for two hundred days or more, and who have major neurocognitive disorders like Alzheimer's disease. There is a smaller subsection with some kind of serious mental illness: schizophrenia, bipolar disorder, major depression mood disorder, personality disorder, or substance abuse history. All of this may be overlaid with PTSD. To deal with these patients, a mental and behavioral team was embedded in acute medical hospital units, getting to know patients and staff, creating individualized plans of care, and educating staff about how to carry them out.

"The nursing staff caring for patients have a huge amount of work to accomplish just to make sure patients take their medications, are clean, turned, don't develop bedsores or deep vein thrombosis or any of the other problems nurses try to prevent," Rasin-Waters explains. "Our job is to understand each patient's particular problems and limitations and figure out ways to cope with them."

The team is also trying to change a culture that may lead staff to silently accept aggressive behaviors. "We are helping staff have a much lower bar on what they are willing to tolerate: behaviors like difficult threats or sexual harassment [even when it is not verbal]. We are encouraging them to report this so we can have an accurate understanding of injuries and problems and can do something about it," Rasin-Waters says.

Although the program originally targeted patients who were outwardly aggressive and agitated, it has since moved on to incorporate what are known as "nonadherent" patients who, for example, may not do their physical therapy because they are depressed or are quietly delirious and confused. These patients may not be hitting their caregivers, but they are nonetheless extending length of hospital stay and escalating hospital costs.

The BEST model is also part of a national VHA effort to deal with complex geriatric patients. "We have a national task force that addresses the problem of complex geriatric patients," Rasin-Waters says. "We are constantly communicating with other VAs that have an interest in developing similar programs. The great thing about the VA," she adds, "is that we have the ability to disseminate best practices to other VAs who can adapt them to their facilities. The VA also shares best practices publicly. We presented at the International Association of Gerontology and Geriatrics this year."

While I was observing the group, they were working with a patient who was a World War II gunner—we'll call him Mr. Jones—who has Alzheimer's disease. Mr. Jones does not know he is in a hospital. He is certain he is in France battling the Nazis. When he looks out of his window, he does not see a magnificent view of the Pacific but rather German soldiers with their rifles aiming directly at him. His response to this threat is to try to escape.

Sometimes Mr. Jones manages to sneak out of the unit. What is known as a code green is called, and he is escorted back by security. Sometimes he approaches the nursing station and begs staff to give him bus fare so that he can go visit his mother, who is long dead, in San Francisco. Staff told the BEST team that they were unsure how to manage Mr. Jones. Nurses were frustrated at having to call multiple code greens. Plus, staff were having difficulty caring for other patients.

The BEST team discovered that Mr. Jones was a neat and organized gentleman who liked to keep things clean and tidy. They decided to utilize his natural inclinations to manage his current situation. The team brought in clothing and stored it in bags in his room. When Mr. Jones became agitated, they instructed nursing assistants to scatter clothing around the room. He would begin to clean up the mess, folding the clothes and putting them into bags.

They also learned that the patient, who had worked in construction, had always been active. Leigh visited the carpentry shop at Fort Miley, where a helpful carpenter cut her some wood blocks and provided sandpaper so Mr. Jones could occupy himself sanding the wood.

The team also helped the nursing staff understand how to care for Mr. Jones. Nursing staff have been taught to create order out of disorder—in this case, to tidy a messy room. They raise the window shades so that residents can enjoy the beautiful views of the Pacific. The team helped staff understand that, in the case of Mr. Jones, order came out of chaos, and that all Mr. Jones saw out of the window was an encroaching enemy.

As for Mr. Jones's endless desire to take the bus to visit his dead mother, the team developed an ingenious solution to what seemed an insuperable problem. They went online to find images of old bus tickets from the San Francisco Municipal Railway—MUNI—and printed up replicas. They left the "tickets" with staff to sell to Mr. Jones for five cents, the cost of a MUNI ticket when he was a young man. A sign posted at the nurses' station read "San Francisco Municipal Railway Station." When the weary old man wanted to go on a trip, nurses would sell him a ticket. The night before I visited the unit, Mr. Jones made a 2 a.m. stop at the bus station and then went back to bed.

"The key to BEST," Rasin-Waters continues, "is that it moves beyond staff 'knowing' there's a problem and helping them finding solutions to it. With this patient, staff knew that he was agitated and upset and was running away, but they didn't understand the severity of his underlying PTSD. We were able to help staff understand the individual veteran."

Rita McCrymonds, a certified nursing assistant who is taking care of Mr. Jones, told me that she is very grateful for the help the BEST team provides. "They are awesome. They give you good ideas and pointers and are really helpful. They constantly come up to me and ask me to tell them what I think. If there's something we're missing that might work better when we're around him, they share that with us. They work really closely with us, and I really like that.

"We've gone so far as to strip the bed, and then Mr. Jones and I remake it together. He likes to play checkers, and I've taught him to play

Twenty-One. He likes Doris Day and John Wayne. When he gets agitated, they told me to just take his clothes and put them on the bed and say, 'The laundry just came,' and that will get him in the flow of things."

Clerk Marina Kovolyova has become one of Mr. Jones's ticket vendors. "Mr. Jones would come up begging for money to take a bus to visit his parents," she told me. "He thinks his parents are going to pick him up when he returns. I listen to what he wants and give him a ticket for tomorrow. One of the nurses even wrote his name down in the sign-out sheet. He just keeps the ticket and knows he's going to visit tomorrow, and that is fine with him."

In the two weeks before the BEST team got involved, staff called eight code greens on this patient. At the time of my visit, the BEST plan had been implemented for two months, and there had not been a single code green. Because Mr. Jones's agitation can now be managed, there is a chance he will be accepted into a community nursing home with which the VHA has contracts. The BEST team will help educate staff in that nursing home on how to care for Mr. Jones. "We have contracts with places to make sure veterans get good care," Rasin-Waters says. "Because we have started to make visits at those nursing homes, we can make sure the transition is a smooth one."

On one of my visits, I walked into Mr. Jones's room with Kamholz. The cheerful old man dressed in red pajamas was sitting on the bed he had just remade with his aide. He smiled at me and said, "How you going, kiddo?" When Kamholz bent down to talk to Mr. Jones, he gave her a broad smile and said, "So nice to see you, dear." Then he reached out to kiss her hand and turned to me to kiss mine.

Mr. Jones ended up doing very well. He was eventually transferred to the CLC at Fort Miley, where he lived another year. Because of the education the staff there received, he never became agitated and died peacefully at age ninety-five.

KNOCKING ON HEAVEN'S DOOR

The VA and End-of-Life Care

Jim Ryan* can barely contain himself. He bounces on the edge of a hospital bed, his thick, black, curly hair flecked with hints of gray surrounding a face whose cheekbones are honed in enviable angles. His steel-gray eyes might, in other circumstances, be riveting. Here in his room on a medical ward at Fort Miley in San Francisco, the sixty-six-year-old Vietnam vet is almost electric with agitation.

Members of the medical center's inpatient palliative care team—physician Eric Widera, director of the Palliative Care and Hospice Program at the San Francisco VA Health Care System, geriatric fellow Stephanie Rogers, and social work student Chelsea Crown—have been asked to consult about Ryan.

Before entering the room, the team review his chart. The problems are legion: paranoid schizophrenia; alcohol and other forms of substance abuse, including heroin addiction; Parkinson's disease, perhaps Agent Orange related. Now Ryan is complaining about excruciating pain, the result of some as-yet-unidentified cancer.

While his oncologists and other assorted physicians try to arrive at the correct diagnosis, the palliative care team is here to try to figure out what matters to Ryan, what he understands, and what his goals are. They are also available to consult with other clinicians about what kind of treatment would be possible, given the fact, as they quickly discover, that Ryan has the worst case of "retrograde amnesia" they have ever seen. In other words, he has no ability to make informed decisions about his care because he cannot retain any information conveyed by his caregivers.

Before they enter the patient's room, the three members of the team stop to get an update from the patient's registered nurse. After she gives them a rundown of what's been going on with Ryan, she asks why the palliative care team is being consulted about her patient. Ryan, after all, is full code: he wants aggressive treatment should his heart stop. As Widera has explained to me, part of the team's mission is educating physicians, nurses, and others about palliative and hospice care, so he is happy to engage in a quick educational session with another colleague, explaining to the nurse that palliative care is about symptom management and making sure that treatment aligns with the patient's goals. The nurse nods appreciatively, and then the team enter Ryan's room.

As I will see over and over again, they do not, in traditional medical round fashion, stand looming above the patient while talking down to him. Their cardinal rule is to always gather up chairs so they can be at eye level with the patient. After taking her seat, Rogers begins by avoiding the standard medical conversation—Tell, Maybe Ask, Tell, and then Order—in favor of the reverse. In this case the conversational rule is Ask, Tell, Ask.

Rogers begins her Ask by inquiring about Ryan's pain.

"It's driving me crazy," Ryan says.

"Can you describe the pain?" Rogers asks.

"It's like being hit by a rubber bat," Ryan answers. As if to drive the point home, he jumps up off his bed and, grasping his left hand with his right, just as abruptly sits down again, stroking his hand as if he could will it back to strength. "It's the pain and the weakness, both of them," he says, staring at no one in particular, his attention rooted firmly inside his own bubble of discomfort.

"Do you want to push the PCA pump?" Rogers suggests, referring to the IV pump that snakes up his arm and into his vein to deliver patient-controlled analgesia.

In response Ryan looks at her blankly. She shows him where to push, which he does, and then he says, "No change."

"It usually takes a minute," she says.

As they wait, Rogers asks Ryan if he can tell her what happened yesterday, the day he was supposed to get a biopsy. He doesn't remember. "Do you know what that test is going to show us?" she asks, trying to figure out what information he can retain. Again he is a blank screen. Rogers explains that the doctors think he has cancer. "What do you think when you hear the word cancer?" she asks.

Without hesitation he blurts out, "I'll get over it; it's something you can find, something they can just squish, like a bug. I want to squish it so I can just go home." Going home, they quickly learn, is the one thing he is certain about. He wants to return to the trailer he bought with his own money, to his dogs, to hunting and fishing. The team listen attentively and leave, promising to return and to find a way to relieve his pain.

One of the team's next encounters is with Ryan and his family. This time, the group of clinicians includes the team's lead social worker, Sharon Ezekiel, Widera, Rogers, and two other physicians from the patient's primary medical team in the hospital. They will be meeting with Amanda,* Ryan's daughter, who has been his primary caregiver, and his ex-wife Claire.* Patched in via cell phone will be Nancy,* another ex-wife, who now lives with Ryan. The team discover that no one in the family likes Nancy, but they have to include her in any discussion of Ryan's care.

In the hallway, before the meeting, the group try to decide what the goal of the meeting will be. The physicians are not entirely sure what kind of cancer he has, but they nonetheless need to determine what Ryan and his family understand. Widera asks the physicians from the primary team if they would like to run the meeting. They say they would be very happy if the palliative care team took the lead.

The entire group take seats around Ryan's bedside. As the team navigate the shoals and narrows of this complicated group, they are guided by principles they have developed for conducting such meetings. Their goal here is again not to tell or order but, as is their practice, to "explore and respond." They ask open-ended questions about people's understanding of—or how much they want to know about—Ryan's medical condition. They also try to ascertain what the family members hope for the future. As family members express their confusion with Ryan's diagnosis, and with each other, members of the team respond patiently. Their aim here is to explore options and make recommendations, not to express certainty or relay orders: "Tell me more about that," they'll say, or "What do you mean by that?" Or they'll just listen and allow family members to reflect, vent, or grieve. What you never hear are words like, "There is nothing more we can do," "Would you like us to do everything possible?" or "withdrawal of care."

Under this patient tutelage, the medical team learn that Ryan has the loyalty of a cast of characters whom he has abused, neglected, or otherwise treated poorly. In spite of this fact, the family agree that everyone wants to help Ryan attain his clearly stated goal of being at home. Over the course of the next two weeks, the team will help manage his pain and deal with the complex issues that occur when he is finally diagnosed with end-stage cancer. Ezekiel organizes the help he will need when he receives hospice services at home, where he wanted to be from the moment he entered the hospital. And home is where he will die several months later.

Jim Ryan is one of the almost six hundred thousand veterans who die in America each year. Because of the demographics, veterans account for one in four deaths in America. And because of a decade of effort and commitment from palliative care practitioners and proponents throughout the entire VA system, many more veterans than average Americans may have a shot at getting the death that most Americans say they wish for but few actually get, which is at home or a residential hospice rather than in a hospital or nursing home.[1]

According to one recent study, "52% of older Americans with cancer were admitted to an acute care hospital, 27% had at least 1 admission to an intensive care unit, and 10% received chemotherapy."[2] In 2009 about 28 percent of older Americans—49 percent of them with dementia—died in nursing homes, where they received poor symptom management, with too many admissions to hospitals, as well as invasive treatments like mechanical ventilation, tube feeding, IV fluids, and antibiotics.[3]

I began writing about the promise—and underutilization—of palliative and hospice care in the 1990s when I spent three years on an oncology unit at Beth Israel Hospital in Boston writing *Life Support: Three Nurses on the Front Lines.* Day after day, I observed patients—on both inpatient and outpatient oncology units—who were offered torturous treatments that lasted until days before they died. Palliative and hospice care were then in their infancy. Physicians were trained to define hope as hope for a cure rather than hope for a decent death. Although things have improved since the 1990s, as we've seen from the study cited above, they have not improved enough.

As I was writing this chapter, two friends were coping with the terminal illness of a loved one. A year earlier, another friend's daughter was dying of cancer in one of the best hospitals in San Francisco under the care of a superstar oncologist. I watched, almost in agony, as these dying patients were subjected to MRIs, CT scans, and numerous other tests to measure their tumor growth and chart in excruciating detail their descent toward death. Their family members lacked support and guidance from their physicians. None of the aggressive, toxic treatments with which these patients were barraged had the slightest impact on tumor growth.

In all three cases, the last-ditch effort to buy more time—measured in weeks, not months or years—ended up sapping the patients' strength, eroding their immune systems, subjecting them to multiple infections that required still more assaultive doses of medication, which led to more infections and tethered them more firmly to IV drips. All of this required long inpatient stays or daily trips to and from the hospital.

Veterans, studies document, are more apt to live with terminal illnesses and die free of this kind of assaultive, futile care, with better pain and symptom management and attention to their quality of life. As one study reported, veterans with lung cancer were not as likely as Medicare beneficiaries to receive futile, toxic chemotherapy or be sent to the ICU in their last month of life.[4] In another study, family members of veterans who died in VA palliative care or hospice units were more satisfied with their loved one's care than were family members of those who died in CLCs; while family members of those who died in CLCs were more satisfied with care than family members of veterans who died in acute care or intensive care units in hospitals.[5]

The VHA now offers a system-wide alternative to medicine's costly fix-it/fight-it model of treatment[6] for the seriously ill, aging, and dying, as well as a model of full-throttle, team-based collaborative practice. The focus of this work is on symptom control; pain management; helping patients cope with depression, denial, despair, or anger; and figuring out patients' goals so that they can have better quality of life during whatever time—be it years, months, or days—they may have. The palliative care teams work with patients who may not be actively dying but who nevertheless will eventually die of their disease. Through the VHA's hospice services, they also work with patients whose lives are near an end.

VA palliative care teams embody Dame Cicely Saunders's eloquent description of good end-of-life care. The British nurse, who became a social worker and then physician and pioneered palliative and hospice care in the late 1960s, wrote: "The care of the dying includes the care of the family, the mind, and the spirit, as well as the care of the body. All these are so interwoven that it is hard to consider them separately."

In spite of the significant benefits of this quintessentially holistic approach, palliative care and hospice services are still radically underused and too often misunderstood. "Despite the high cost, evidence demonstrates that these patients (with serious illness or multiple chronic conditions) receive health care of inadequate quality, characterized by fragmentation, overuse, medical errors, and poor quality of life," the respected palliative care physician Diane Meier wrote in an essay in the *Milbank Quarterly*.[7]

This adds not only to patient suffering but to escalating health care costs. Even though those who are seriously ill or dying are only 10 percent of the total patient population in the United States, they actually consume over 50 percent of total health care costs. According to recent Medicare data, the average per-patient per-admission net cost saved by hospital palliative care consultation is $2,659. In her article Meier estimated that appropriate use of palliative care services could save between $1.2 billion and $4 billion per year. "Hospice care also reduces total health care costs for the majority of Medicare beneficiaries receiving it."[8]

Patients and their families would also benefit enormously from palliative and hospice care. Some studies have documented that patients with certain types of cancer live longer when they enter hospice programs than if they continue with aggressive treatment.[9] There are fewer costly and painful hospitalizations, hospital readmissions, and emergency room visits.

Yet, as Meier points out, for a number of reasons, neither patients nor our society benefit from palliative care. One reason is a lack of palliative care physicians. A study by the American Academy of Hospice and Palliative Medicine in 2010 provided a conservative estimate of a shortfall of 2,787 palliative care physicians (6,000, really, when you consider that most practice this specialty on a part-time basis).[10] Patients don't only suffer from a scarcity of clinicians who specialize in palliative care. They also suffer from the fact that many health care providers—nurses, physicians, physical therapists, psychologists—lack significant education and thus knowledge about the benefit of palliative and hospice care. Although every single patient will eventually die, not a single medical or nursing school mandates a required course in palliative care as a condition for graduation.

The structure of financial remuneration in the American health care system is also a significant barrier to appropriate care for patients with serious illnesses or who are at the end of life. In other countries, referring a patient to palliative or hospice services is usually a revenue-neutral decision for a physician. In the United States, where fee-for-service is the prevalent mode of payment, it is not. When oncologists, for example, suggest a patient forgo another round of chemotherapy, those physicians lose revenue from the fees they would collect after providing treatment. Even primary care physicians may lose money when they refer patients to hospice.

All this, as well as lack of research about the efficacy of palliative care, fuels, as Meier writes, "the lack of public knowledge of, and demand for, the benefits of palliative care and hospice."[11]

The VHA is notable in its commitment to the delivery and teaching of palliative and hospice care, as well as to conducting research into its benefits. Just as the VA pioneered geriatric programs, Meier points out that it was "also early out of the box in recognizing shifts in veteran population, first in starting an interdisciplinary postgraduate training program in palliative care that welcomed professionals from other disciplines than medicine. That is not typically how specialty training is done. It is typically done in silos, so the VA broke that pattern. There are places that are starting to co-train doctors and advanced practice nurses, but that is unusual. The VA is still ahead of the game on that."

Launching a National Initiative on Palliative Care

The VHA's progress on palliative and hospice care illustrates the dynamic we have seen over and over again throughout this book. A national champion or advocate launches an initiative and connects with other advocates at the local or regional level to deliver, teach, and research the particular innovation or program that is proposed. The palliative and hospice program at the VHA has worked so well because it has mobilized and exploited the kind of synergy—financial, clinical, educational, and ethical—that is available in an integrated health care system. In 2003, for example, the VHA changed payment structures so that more hospice and palliative care would be available to veterans. It also began working with community hospices to place more veterans in hospice care. In 2003, only 29 percent of hospitalized veterans had access to palliative care. By 2006 that figure had increased to 42 percent. Among outpatients only 8 percent used hospice services in 2003. By 2006 22 percent used such services.[12]

One of the people who helped encourage the use of palliative and hospice services was Scott Shreve. Before moving into medicine, Shreve worked as a corporate banker. After medical school and a residency in internal medicine, Shreve did a geriatric fellowship at the University of Connecticut. After completing his training, he chose to work at the VHA, he explains, because it was the only integrated health care system in America engaging in cutting-edge geriatric research and care. Over the years Shreve became convinced that the VA needed to make a systematic commitment to deliver palliative care and used his corporate experience to realize that goal.

Deeply influenced by Muhammad Yunus's model of micro-financing, Shreve was convinced that if he could get just the right amount of seed money from the national VA and distribute it to, as he puts it, people with "passion," he could develop a network of like-minded clinicians to promote the idea throughout the system. "What we needed at the time was a commitment from senior leadership that palliative teams were integral to the care of all seriously ill veterans at all medical centers," Shreve told me. "I wanted to get seed money to initiate teams and prove value to local leadership."

After developing his plan and taking it to various VA higher-ups, Shreve got a call from a high-level financial official at VA headquarters who invited him to Washington. Shreve told his boss about the invitation. "Take advantage of this interest, go to DC, and present a budget with funding adequate to the endeavor," his boss told him.

Shreve entered the office of a VA executive who had, or so he thought, no medical background. He expected that his job would be to educate the official about good end-of-life care and convince him of its importance.

Instead, the official delivered a forty-five-minute lecture on the sorry status quo in medicine. "He talked about how care is fragmented," Shreve recounted. "He complained that doctors don't listen to patients or family members. He lamented the lack of communication amongst specialists and that no one was to be there as an advocate for patients' rights, preferences, and values."

Astonished by this welcome, Shreve explained that palliative care is about remedying all the problems the official described. The VA higher-up responded, "Right, I know that, and that's why I called you in here. I want you to change the VA so we can change America, because this is my mother I'm talking about. She's not a veteran, but this is what is happening to her right now. She's getting fragmented care in a hospital right now, and it's terrible."

Shreve got the green light to move forward with his plan. Wheels were greased, he said, when he went through the various committees he had to persuade in a health care system as large as the VHA. Over and over again, he recalled, "I would go in with a budget and leave with more money than I had requested."

Shreve's business plan turned into the Comprehensive End of Life Initiative, which was launched throughout the system in 2008. It guaranteed that every veteran it served would have access to palliative care and hospice services. This program involved a huge culture change. Health care professionals who work at the VA have been socialized in the broader American medical system, where they are taught to pursue aggressive medical treatment at the end of life and during the course of a serious illness. To change their attitude and behavior, Shreve and his colleagues used the financial resources they obtained to support palliative care teams in each medical center as well as a regional leader in each VISN. Part of the mandate was to create inpatient hospice units. They recruited a palliative care program manager or champion to take ownership of the program in each VISN.

"Along the lines of Muhammad Yunus," Shreve continued, "we would offer opportunities for funding as long as people would make a commitment to achieve the goals of the funding. We made it moderately competitive. We didn't have enough money to fund everyone, but we put out a request for applications to develop new hospice and palliative care units. In order to get the money, the application had to be very specific about how they would establish a unit. If they weren't specific enough about how, it wasn't going to happen." Fifty-four of those units were funded with seed money that would cover a four-year period. Fort Miley received financing to start its outpatient palliative care clinic. The Center for Palliative Care also trained every palliative care team in the VA on how to build its program. This training also taught teams how to work with their facility leadership and demonstrate the value of palliative and hospice care.

Like most VHA initiatives, this one also had an education component. "We needed to develop curricula that were specific to veterans," Shreve says. The Comprehensive End of Life Initiative used financial resources to support palliative care teams in each medical center as well as a regional leader in each VISN. Shreve felt that building high-quality hospice programs wouldn't be accomplished through policy mandates alone.

Shreve and his colleagues also developed palliative care and hospice curricula that were specific to veterans. "We went to the best national experts we could find at the time, who were at Northwestern University, where physician Linda Emmanuel had developed what is known as EPEC [Education in Palliative and End of Life Care] and nurse Betty Ferrell developed the End of Life Nursing Education Consortium [ELNEC]." They also consulted with the Hospice and Palliative Care Association to develop a nursing assistant curriculum. "So we developed an ELNEC program for veterans, nursing assistant program for veterans, and EPIC for veterans," Shreve says. "We had each of those organizations work with VA subject matter experts to develop those curricula."

The initiative also worked on improving the implementation of the VA's bereavement survey. "We wanted teams to learn and produce actionable interventions from surveys. Finally, we wanted to develop community partnerships, which is how the We Honor Veterans collaboration with the National Hospice and Palliative Care Organization began." This nationwide program with the goal of making sure no veteran dies alone establishes hospice–veteran partnerships at the state level. It offers health care providers, hospitals, and hospices a military history checklist to help them identify patients who are veterans. It also encourages hospice providers to create vet-to-vet volunteer programs, which pair patients who are identified as veterans with veteran volunteers to make sure that "no veteran dies alone." The program has produced reams of educational as well as assessment and evaluation materials to help hospice partners and veteran volunteers identify and navigate critical issues at the end of life and deal with particular problems, like delivering hospice care in rural areas.[13]

Although the formal initiative ended in 2012, there has been continued growth in the VA's palliative and hospice care programs. Palliative care teams, like the one at Fort Miley, are embedded in all VHA medical centers. They offer assistance to patients who are in the hospital or seen by providers on an outpatient basis. These teams also educate their colleagues in nursing, medicine, social work, chaplaincy, and other disciplines throughout the hospital. They educate the health professional trainees who do rotations in the VHA and also conduct research on palliative and hospice care.

Ninety-six medical centers have residential hospice beds, most in their CLCs or nursing homes and some on inpatient acute care units. Palliative care and hospice teams also refer patients to outside community hospices that, with the VHA monitoring their services, provide care in the home or in residential hospices.

The VA's palliative care benefit is more generous and rational and far more compassionate than Medicare's hospice program. Under the Medicare hospice benefit, patients with advanced diseases like cancer face what is called a "terrible choice." They often must "forgo all active, disease-modifying cancer treatment" if they want to enroll in hospice.[14] Tragically, this kind of black-and-white approach to end-of-life care has reinforced the notion that hospice care is a death sentence, as I have recently experienced when several friends dying of end-stage cancer had to make this "terrible choice." A friend who has a glioblastoma (a terminal brain tumor) was told by Kaiser that he would not be able to be on hospice and continue with chemotherapy that was possibly slowing tumor growth. This would not happen in the VA, where what is known as "concurrent care" is delivered to veterans who are dying of cancer. They can receive palliative radiation and chemotherapy while receiving palliative and hospice care. Medicare will not pay for room and board in a nursing home or residential hospice. VA will pay for both hospice services and room and board.

The VHA has also created ongoing quality improvement programs that evaluate end-of-life care. One was originally called the Performance Reporting and Outcomes Measurement to Improve the Standard of Care at End-of-Life (PROMISE) Center and is now the National Veteran Experience

Center. Another is the Center for Health Equity Research and Promotion. Through both qualitative and quantitative measures, the VHA evaluates end-of-life care throughout the system. Its goal is to identify and reduce any unwanted variation in the kind of end-of-life care veterans receive.[15]

One of the primary tools used to accomplish this goal is the Bereaved Family Survey, which is sent out to family members of every veteran who dies in the VHA system. The short survey, designed to be taken in only ten minutes, is available in English and Spanish, each with a version that uses either female or male pronouns. It asks eighteen open-ended questions about positives and negatives of the care veterans received at the end of their lives: courtesy and information offered by staff, management of pain or patient and family stress, availability of spiritual support, and information and help with funeral arrangements, among others.[16] The VA also examines patient charts and tries to discover indicators of good end-of-life care: whether veterans had a palliative care consult in the last ninety days of their lives, whether patient or family consulted with a chaplain during the last thirty days of life, and whether family members received emotional support for up to two weeks after a veteran's death.[17]

VHA palliative and hospice care researchers have documented the progress that has been made as well as gaps and variations in care that need to be addressed in a number of research studies. Too many veterans still die in hospitals or get too much futile chemotherapy during their last days on earth. Patients with end-stage renal disease or cardiopulmonary failure are more likely to die in an intensive care unit than those with dementia.[18]

On the plus side, VHA evaluations confirm that more veterans are receiving appropriate end-of-life care than ever before, and there is more family involvement in decisions that affect how a veteran will die and far more support that improves how family members feel about the experience a loved one had while dying. Studies also document that improvements in the nursing environment and staffing in acute care VA hospitals make for a better end-of-life experience for veterans.[19] In the most recent study of end-of-life care at the VHA, Mary Ersek, professor of palliative care at the University of Pennsylvania School of Nursing and senior scientist at the National Veteran Experience Center, and her colleagues found that patient and family satisfaction with care at the end of life was very high among VA patients because they had access to palliative care and hospice services. "We have made a huge system change at the VA, and our satisfaction with care at end of life is quite high," Shreve stated proudly.

Ersek is equally proud of the kind of work the VHA is doing to promote high-quality end-of-life care. "What distinguishes the VHA from other systems is that we have a comprehensive end-of-life initiative that extends across the system. We decided that the VHA is going to do this right, and we are not only implementing these programs but establishing a system of quality improvement to make sure that what we're doing works."

Palliative and Hospice Care at Fort Miley

The Palliative and Hospice Care program at Fort Miley received one of the grants that Shreve created and Ersek and her colleagues are evaluating. When I observed the team at Fort Miley, it was led by Widera and nurse-practitioner Patrice Villars. Other members included Ezekiel, physicians Barbara Drye and Alex Smith, and chaplain Carolyn Talmadge. The team covers both inpatient and outpatient units at the medical center. Within Fort Miley's CLC there is a ten-bed residential hospice unit, and social worker Anne Kelly, nurse-practitioner Erin Bowman, and Widera work together on the hospice branch of the team.

As I watched them all work together, what I saw was an effort to remedy the problems that Meier identified in her *Milbank Quarterly* article. I often accompanied Widera on his educational missions throughout the medical center. He and his colleagues conducted daily sessions with trainees like Rogers. He also moved throughout the hospital patiently explaining the fundamentals, trying to help medical residents understand the content and value of hospice and palliative care. In one instance a resident who was planning to go into intensive care was struggling to reconcile his view that palliative and hospice care was just "all touchy-feely stuff," as he put it, with a growing sense that maybe there was, in fact, something to all this "touchy-feely stuff." It was almost amusing to see this male physician-in-training in a group of other male colleagues flush with embarrassment as he wrestled with exposing his reluctance to dismiss palliative care out of hand.

Every member of the team is involved in the educational mission. Education is essential, Villars told me, in expanding trust between clinicians who have been trained to attack every physical condition with an aggressive response. Villars, who became a nurse at age forty, explains that she feels like she found a home when she discovered work in palliative care. She loves the skill and excellence, she tells me, that a practitioner has to develop in order to communicate with patients and other caregivers as they all try to navigate the difficult trajectory and pain and symptom management and make sure that the exit we all have to take from life is negotiated with grace and dignity.

Drye, the physician who works with her to educate clinicians, has worked at the VA since 1994. In the emergency room and primary care, she felt frustrated by the emphasis on medications and performance measures. This left her little time to learn who her patients were, hear their backstories, and focus on their values to manage their symptoms and enhance their quality of life.

Both Villars and Drye have worked long and hard to convince their colleagues in various medical specialties that palliative care is beneficial and should be integrated into the care of seriously ill patients. This means bringing in palliative care specialists not just during the last two or three days of life but throughout the care of people who have advanced illnesses and conditions from which they will eventually die. Their goal, Drye says, is not to be involved in the care of every seriously ill patient—that would be impossible—but to identify patients with limited time who may change their priorities and their medical decision making. "We want to be involved," Drye says, "when routine medical care causes more burden than benefit. When I talk to patients, the first thing I tell them is that my goal is to advocate for the best medical care that you can get while avoiding unnecessary suffering. I am fortunate to work with top-notch oncologists and other specialists so that I can reassure my patients that they are getting the best and most up-to-date treatment. Some veterans believe that they need to go to a more famous cancer center. In my experience that's not an issue here because the care here is superb."

Drye, Villars, and the rest of the team are palpably proud to be part of what Drye describes as "a big culture shift." Over the course of six years, they have helped to integrate palliative care into the practice of many of the clinicians with whom they work. Six years ago, the team got a grant to start an outpatient clinic in palliative care, which was advertised to services like oncology, neurology, pulmonology, and the liver clinic, where end-stage diseases are most likely to be seen. "The majority of the consults we see," Drye tells me, "are for cancer-related illnesses, congestive heart failure, emphysema, cirrhosis of the liver, and ALS, and sometimes, but rarely, dementia."

Drye and Villars now have a clinic that is integrated into the liver and oncology clinics. Clinics are open four half-days a week, and veterans are seen in conjunction with their specialty appointments. This facilitates communication between palliative care and specialty staff.

When I first met her, Ezekiel was a full partner in all the team's efforts. She had originally planned to become a lawyer. That decision was derailed when she took care of her father, who was on dialysis and dying of end-stage renal disease. "We never had any palliative care consults," Ezekiel told me, both angry and tearful as she recalls the ordeal her family went through. "We never knew such a thing even existed. No one ever told us dialysis was a choice and that it wouldn't add to my father's quality of life, but only prolong his decline. I wanted to help people navigate through systems, and that's why I went into social work."

After doing a social work internship in the primary care clinic, she was hired to work in primary care in 2003, and then, in 2007, she began to work in geriatrics. "When I worked in primary care, I was working with older veterans." When she moved to the geriatric division, she started working with the palliative care service, where she was "working with others who have the same goals so we can make sure patients are well informed about their choices."

Ezekiel's particular role is to provide support, coordinate, and attend to things like discharge planning. For example, she figured out where Ryan would go when he left the hospital, home with hospice or visiting nurse services or to a residential hospice near where he lives. "Chelsea Crown and I spent a lot of time getting a will in place. Mr. Ryan didn't realize his time was so short."

"One of the things I do," she continues, "is assess a person's wishes and make sure they get done." In some cases this means getting oxygen in the home; in others, helping a patient deal with "existential distress." For example, a veteran needs to reconcile with a family he abandoned decades earlier or confess her regrets to a daughter she felt she had failed during an adolescent crisis.

The palliative care team must be invited in by physicians—oncologists, pulmonologists, ICU specialists—who are in charge of the patients. Ezekiel's job always involves an intricate choreography of invitations and requests. If physicians don't invite the team in, patients and families may request a palliative care consult. Nurses who are suffering because they believe patients need palliative care "may come up to me and tell me what's going on. In one case," she relates, "a nurse told me that a patient was depressed, and we figured out a behind-the-scenes way to help. The nurse was having a hard time because she felt she didn't know how to help him. Our role was to provide support to both patient and nurse."

Because Fort Miley is a teaching hospital, one of Ezekiel's other functions, she explains, is to provide continuity in an institution in which "medical residents and other learners are constantly rotating in and out. We pass on information to new providers rotating on as well as health professionals in training."

Another critical member of the palliative care and hospice team is Protestant chaplain Talmadge. She has worked at the VA either as a trainee or staff member since 2005. Some people believe her job is to preach or even evangelize for a particular form of religion or to make sure that patients return to the religious fold before they take their dying breath.

The short, blond chaplain adamantly argues that nothing could be further from the truth. To proselytize is, in fact, against ethical, professional, and VA requirements. "One of the jobs of a chaplain," she explains, "is to uphold the religious freedom of veterans. So in practice what we try to do is help veterans use whatever spiritual tools they have at this time of their life. For some people, that would be religious support, and for others it's going to take a different form. Some people do reconnect with the faith of their childhood. That's very important to them, and we definitely help facilitate that connection. Others do not."

Talmadge's job is to practice, not to preach—to help people express their spiritual or religious needs and attain their spiritual or religious goals when they are ill or dying. Sometimes, she says, this will involve praying with someone; sometimes it will involve simply listening. "We see folks who are atheists or have no religious preference but have spiritual needs. Once they learn that I am not going to evangelize, then they may open up."

What she learns when they do is varied and always fascinating. "People will tell us things they won't tell doctors." They will tell you they do or do not want treatment. They will tell you fears. They will confess to regrets, missed opportunities, or what they perceive to be sinful conduct.

"I have been visiting with one patient with Parkinson's over many years, and all we talk about is his son's meth addiction. I provide support, and we pray together. Sometimes I talk to patients about the need for advanced directives and advise them to be very specific about their preferences. If you don't want life-sustaining care, be specific."

She cites the case of a veteran who told his wife that no way did he want to end up in a nursing home. "He was adamant," Talmadge says. "He could have undergone a treatment that would have put him exactly where he didn't want to be, but she helped him avoid that. When he was dying, they took out his breathing tube, and he died peacefully. I ended up doing his funeral service."

"Sometimes," Talmadge reports, "I'll say, 'Would it help to get mental health support?' And sometimes they say yes, and sometimes they refuse, and I am okay with that." There are times when Talmadge will tell her patients that she has to report their thoughts or feelings if they are a danger to themselves or others around them.

I watch Talmadge in action on several occasions. One weekday, Drye, social worker Phyllis Larimore, and Talmadge drive three hours up to the Community Based Outpatient Clinic in rural Clearlake. They come up to the clinic every two months to deliver team-based palliative care to an area that would, without the VA, have little access to such specialized services. The team meets with five veterans and their families, offering critical support and advice on everything from treatment options and goals of care to how to make sure wills and other plans are in order. Over and over, they make their way through thickets of hope and denial and fear. One Vietnam veteran in his early seventies has end-stage lung cancer. Wearing a black shirt and black jeans held up by suspenders, he has his requisite Vietnam Vet baseball cap firmly on his head. His wife, a petite Asian woman he has been married to for decades, is dressed in perfectly pressed slacks and a pale blue twin sweater set and wears gold-studded, horn-rimmed glasses.

Harold* tells the group he can barely believe he was in the hospital recently for thirty-one days. The couple, who are childless, express their conviction that Harold will somehow make it, in spite of this hospitalization and constant tumor growth. "He's going to outlive me. I just know it," the veteran's wife asserts.

Tearing up and then weeping, Harold insists, "I'm not going to let this beat me. It's not going to control me. I'm going to continue to do what I want to do." Although Harold is trying desperately to be upbeat, he finally confesses that he gets sad and depressed because "You can't do what you used to do."

Drye talks about his symptoms and gently explains that his cancer is serious, and not curable, and tries to focus the couple on how any pain and other symptoms can be managed. The wife insists that she wants to care for her husband at home, no matter how difficult it may be for such a tiny woman to care for such a large man. "The VA has a commitment to giving you help in the home, so you can stay at home even till the bitter end. It's built into VA policy," Drye assures them.

Larimore talks to the couple about the mechanics of hospice care at home, as well as about wills and advance directives. The couple is having a difficult time with the concept of a conversation that will squarely acknowledge the husband's death. Talmadge offers reassurance. "You have planned your life together," she reminds them. "You can plan with each other. These are good conversations to have."

Drye, Larimore, and I eat lunch with CBOC staff, but Talmadge can't join us. She has another standing appointment with a veteran who sees her for social support. "Often as people age, loneliness can become a big challenge," Talmadge explains before leaving for her lunch date. "This particular veteran says he gets a lot of benefit from speaking to staff, including me as a chaplain. He's pretty isolated, and this seems to help him feel a part of the world. The VA is a place he comes for human validation and connection."

Back at Fort Miley, I accompany Talmadge as she walks through the hospital units, checking in on patients and offering support. She enters one dimly lit room where a slim man in his late fifties sits dozing in a chair, his hand draped over the hand of a large woman lying in the bed. An oxygen cannula is placed in her nose, and various lines and tubes snake from and around her body. As Talmadge comes in, he rouses, and she introduces herself as the chaplain. Roger Smith, we'll call him, explains that he is here from farther north in California because several months ago his wife complained of a worsening headache, and they discovered that she had a brain tumor. She's getting radiation at UCSF and is at Fort Miley because a recent session caused complications for which she had to be hospitalized. There is no mention of religion as Talmadge talks to the worried husband, but he expresses appreciation for her visit when she leaves.

Another stop is the bedside of a sixty-year-old man who is sitting in a chair tethered to monitoring machines, wearing a small, headband-like bandage with several odd protuberances on his bald head. He's here because he has tremors from Parkinson's and is receiving deep electrical stimulation in his brain. His neatly coiffed wife is sitting beside him intently working on a Sudoku puzzle. Again the visit consists of small talk about the veteran's hospital stay and concerns. As she is about to leave, Talmadge says, "I'll keep you in my prayers, and have a safe journey home."

Before we walk out the door, the veteran asks what I'm doing. When he hears I'm writing a book about the VA, he perks up. "I'm a very appreciative customer," he tells me. "I don't know where they get that bad press from. I don't have any evidence of that whatsoever. People here are totally professional. I had to have surgery on my hand," he begins to explain.

His wife interrupts and takes over relating the story. "Yes, he sliced it almost down to the bone when his Bowie knife fell out of his gun case."

"People complain," the veteran picks up the thread, "but I don't see the source of the complaints. The facility here is beautiful. The architecture, the setting, is gorgeous. If you can get better care anywhere, I've never seen it. I've seen a lot of private doctors, but it's not the same as here. You feel that they [the private doctors] are driven by the profit motive. Here it is total perfection—just can't say any more."

When Talmadge visits the ICU, she finds Harry Wright,* a seventy-year-old Army veteran, lying alone in the room, sunlight streaming in through a window that overlooks the sea and cliffs. Talmadge approaches the bed as usual, offering her presence. As soon as she tells Wright she is a chaplain, he begins to talk about God. God has saved him, he tells her, but he doesn't know why. His eyes well with tears, and he seems flooded with doubt and memory. "I have done so many bad things. I was in Vietnam twice. I have PTSD," he tells Talmadge. "I was hospitalized so many times. I don't know why God saved me."

Talmadge bends in and asks Wright if he would like to pray with her. "Yes," he says, grasping her hand in one with an IV insert, the tube coiling upward toward a machine that drips medication into his vein. They pray. Helping the veteran give voice to his concerns, she offers prayers thanking

God for how long he has lived, and, acknowledging his regrets, she asks for God's forgiveness for him. Wright's eyes close, seeping tears, as he is offered momentary respite from his demons.

I am not a prayerful person. In fact, I am an unabashed atheist and often describe myself as lacking even an ounce of spirituality. But I can see how Talmadge's genial offer of someone to talk to, to witness or be present—or even to intercede for them with God—can be a lifeline for many who are mired in memories. Here in this alien, antiseptic environment, with space-age machines zinging and beeping, solace has finally arrived.

The same kind of solace is offered in the CLC across the road from the main hospital buildings, where Bowman and social worker Kelly meet with palliative care attending physician Christine Ritchie and palliative care fellow Colin Scabetta to discuss their cases. The two physicians, nurse, and social worker have only half an hour, but nothing about their conversation feels rushed. There is no finger or leg tapping, no quick peeks at a wristwatch or cell phone. Like people who are comfortable working together, they manage to make time expand rather than contract.

They review the patients who are on the inpatient hospice. Bowman is concerned about one who is getting quite agitated and grabbed a nurse's arm yesterday. Another is having trouble swallowing. Another patient is very frail. His family wanted to fly him back to New York, but that seems impossible.

Throughout the conversation they inject personal notes, conversations about their own experiences with death and dying. Ritchie mentions the difficulties her mother-in-law had when her father was dying. "He was the sun around which she orbited, and when he died, she died within two weeks." There is no discomfort here about personal revelation.

When the meeting is finished, I follow Kelly and Bowman into their small office. They are trying to navigate a tricky situation. The son of a veteran who is dying is in prison and wants them to facilitate his temporary release so that he can visit his father. Problem is, his father, from whom he has been estranged for years, doesn't really want to see him. After a difficult conversation with the son, Bowman goes to check on her patients.

Mr. Arnold,* eighty-nine years old, lies in bed as a nurse and phlebotomist attend him. His veins are so fragile that the IV delivering pain medication has failed. The phlebotomist is trying to insert another but is getting nowhere. Everyone is frustrated. None of them believe that poking into the collapsed veins of a man who is actively dying and may have only hours to live makes any sense. They want to deliver effective pain medication and relieve his suffering, but they fear causing even more pain in the process.

As they anguish about what to do, the patient lies emaciated, cheeks sunken like a concentration camp survivor. Eyes fixed on the ceiling, he breathes laboriously, his body tenaciously, instinctively clinging to life. Bowman stands by as two registered nurses try to insert the IV. Finally, she tells them to stop. "We'll do it sub Q [under the skin]," she says. "We have to stop trying to stick him. It won't deliver the medication as well, but we have to stop trying, because it isn't working."

The phlebotomist leaves, apologizing for his inability to insert the IV. Bowman and the patient's nurse tell him not to apologize. The problem is the man's condition, not the phlebotomist's competence. Nothing could help at this stage of his illness.

Bowman stands by Arnold's side and begins to talk to him. "It's all right, Jack," she says, leaning over him, speaking in a near whisper. "We're all here. We're not going to poke you anymore. Everything's taken care of; there's nothing to worry about anymore." She whispers to me that she's hoping that she can help him let go. She pats his head and tells him, "It's raining—can you believe it?—still raining." The nurse also pats his hand and then lowers the bed so that she can raise its head to make him more comfortable.

Finally, Bowman visits Mrs. McCleary,* a ninety-four-year-old woman in the advanced stages of Alzheimer's who has been taken care of by devoted children, one of whom—a son—she has lived with for almost twelve years. I first saw McCleary when the inpatient palliative care team visited her and her devoted seventy-year-old son. Six weeks earlier, when she was still at home, she had a bedsore on her ankle. Her health care aide wasn't highly trained and advised soaking the ankle.

"My God," her distraught son recounts, "her foot almost fell off." An outreach registered nurse came over, took one look, and said, "We have to get her to the hospital," and so here she is.

Rogers, Widera, and Ezekiel were questioning the son about his understanding of what would happen after her hospitalization. Someone, he says, mentioned the CLC or a hospice. Please, he begs them, take her in. He can't stop the bedsores that seem to be eating her up, nor can he dress, bathe, and toilet her. "I am getting sick with all this stress," he says. "I had the flu; my health and mental health are suffering. I just need all the help I can get. I'm looking to the VA."

The team explain how hospice works—that it is all free to veterans and that they will make sure that his mother goes to the CLC, or they will find her another hospice. Before they leave the room, they ask her son what his mother likes. He tells them that she likes classical music and hates the television. "She loves to be read to," he says; "*Little House on the Prairie* or that genre of story."

When Bowman enters McCleary's room, the old woman, all skin and bones, lies calmly in her bed. There is classical music playing in the background, and a copy of *Little House on the Prairie* sits on a bedside table.

BETTER CARE WHERE?

The VHA Compared to the Private Sector

By late 2017 the concept of "choice" dominated the discussion of veterans' health care and how it should be delivered. Congress was considering multiple bills that would, in one form or another, make the Veterans Choice program permanent and relax its previous limits on using doctors or hospitals outside the VHA. In addition, some members of Congress sought to shrink the VHA's own health care network by creating a facility closing commission that would insulate Capitol Hill and the White House from unpopular decisions to shutter local medical centers and lay off staff. If that approach gained traction, veterans' reliance on the private health care industry would increase, regardless of their individual choice, because the VHA services would be curtailed.

Nevertheless, in the rosy scenario of outsourcing advocates, the VHA would remain one choice among many in a new public/private-sector marketplace for veterans' care. Private medical treatment would prove to be better, of course, the reasoning went, and less costly for taxpayers. But the VHA would supposedly still have sufficient resources and personnel to remain a "competitor" for patients. In areas where it has special expertise, it might even maintain its current "market share."

Understandably, some veterans now share this assumption that expanding Choice will give them the best of both worlds. Their expectation that private-sector care will be superior in quality and delivered faster is, however, often based on little firsthand experience. And assuming that the VHA will remain in the picture for long, as billions of dollars formerly allocated to its budget get diverted to private vendors, is wishful thinking, at best.

When I have described some of the downsides of private-sector care to veterans based on my own experience as a relatively savvy patient with ample medical insurance and many helpful contacts within the health care profession, my reality checks have been met with shock and disbelief. For example, VHA patients sometimes complained to me about being treated by too many younger doctors in training, who rotate in and out, with less continuity than longtime hospital staffers. They were invariably surprised to learn that the same experience awaits them at any university medical center in the country, which would also be filled with medical residents, psychology interns, and nursing students doing their clinical rotations.

One veteran who experienced VHA appointment delays—followed by an initial misdiagnosis of his condition—told me that no private medical practice would ever have such long waits or make a diagnostic mistake, because those doctors had smaller patient loads and could spend more time with each person. So I asked him how many patients he thought an average private-sector primary care physician had on his or her panel. Without hesitation, he told me, "Oh, three or four hundred." He was flabbergasted to learn that the actual range is twenty-one hundred to thirty-four hundred patients per provider.

A female veteran who was upset about cooling her heels for two hours in a VHA primary care clinic was similarly nonplussed to discover that overbooking of patient appointments in Boston, a city loaded with physicians, resulted in equivalent or longer waits when I sought primary care or specialist treatment there.

If veterans' frustration about administrative snafus or short staffing at the VHA is understandable, members of Congress have no excuse for not being better informed about the strengths and weaknesses of comparative health care systems in the United States. On Capitol Hill even politicians not blinded by their worship of the market and dogmatic devotion to shrinking government everywhere (except at the DoD) have too rarely raised relevant questions about the impact of Choice expansion, particularly on veterans in already underserved rural areas.

If the VHA has shortcomings—and indeed it does—how do those actually stack up against the well-documented failings of private hospital and nursing home chains, health maintenance organizations (HMOs), and for-profit medical practices? Who actually performs better or worse as measured by wait times, mental health coverage, services for homeless patients, overall medical outcomes, and accountability and transparency to patients, their families, and US taxpayers, who fund not just VHA care but Medicare and Medicaid as well?

Wait Times

Let's begin by separating myth from reality on the now infamous issue of VHA wait times and their impact, if any, on patient mortality. It's actually not easy to compare VHA wait times with those in the private sector because the VHA is the only health care system in the United States that systematically collects and publicly posts wait-time data. Merritt Hawkins, a health care industry consulting firm, does assemble broad wait-time information industry-wide. However, the results of its measuring system are released only sporadically and do not contain detail sufficient to be helpful in making individual patient decisions about accessing care sooner rather than later. In its 2017 survey of fifteen major metropolitan areas, Merritt Hawkins found that the wait times to get a first appointment with a physician are up 30 percent since 2014, with an average of 24 days, up from 19.4 in 2014.

In many parts of the country, the wait times are far longer than that, especially to see certain kinds of doctors. This is a very serious problem not only in rural areas but also in cities, including ones that are awash in medical schools and hospitals. Residents of the Boston area, for example, must spend an average of 109 days to find a family practitioner who is still taking on new patients and up to a year to get an appointment with a cardiologist.[1]

Even patients with good health insurance can face long wait times—particularly for primary care physicians and geriatricians.[2] A recent survey by the Commonwealth Fund[3] finds that one out of four Americans report that it took them six or more days to get an appointment with their primary care physician even when they were "sick or needing care."[4]

How Does This Compare with the VHA?

As Phillip Longman and I noted in a 2017 report for the American Legion,[5] according to the latest data, one in five VA patients are seen on the same day they make an appointment.[6] Though some 16 percent of VA primary care facilities are operating at over 100 percent of capacity, for the system as a whole, the average wait time to see a VA primary care doctor is five days, and for appointments with VA specialists, nine days.[7] Appointments to see a mental health professional average four days. A recent study by the RAND Corporation has found that "wait times at the VA for new patient primary and specialty care are shorter than wait times reported in focused studies of the private sector." Overall, the report concluded, VA wait times "do not seem to be substantially worse than non-VA waits."[8]

Wait times for hospital and specialty care are, of course, worse for rural Americans. Rural America's primary care shortage is far worse than that in urban areas. According to the North Carolina Rural Health Research Program, between 2010 and 2017, eighty-two rural hospitals have closed in the United States.[9] The National Rural Health Association predicts that seven hundred more rural hospitals will close in the next ten years.[10]

The discussion of VA wait times often leads to the accusation that patients are dying because they have to wait to see a VA physician. Although conservative groups like the Concerned Veterans for America have argued that forty veterans died while waiting to see a doctor at the Phoenix VA, these figures, as the *Washington Monthly* has substantiated, are misleading. The VA inspector general conducted a detailed and rigorous independent review of patient records and reported that six, not forty, veterans had died in Phoenix after experiencing "clinically significant delays" in seeing a VA doctor.

In each of these six cases, the inspector general was "unable to conclusively assert that the absence of timely quality care caused the deaths of these veterans."[11] In her *Washington Monthly* critique of mainstream media reporting on the Phoenix situation, Alicia Mundy put this finding in a context that too many journalists and politicians simply ignored—namely, that many patients, particularly those who are old and suffering from a chronic condition, die *while* waiting for a medical appointment. But that's not the same as dying *because* their scheduled appointment had yet to occur. As Mundy observed, "The reality behind the headlines had little, if any, more significance than the fact that people die every day while waiting for an appointment to see their tax accountant or lawyer."[12]

What's most important to the discussion of any alleged deaths due to VHA wait times or other problems is that such allegations invariably fail to include comparisons with preventable deaths and injuries in the private sector. What too few veterans and veterans' service groups seem to understand is that in the United States, private-sector hospitals and physicians kill hundreds of thousands of patients a year and injure many more. These sorry statistics were first widely publicized in 1999, with an Institute of Medicine report titled *To Err Is Human*, where it was reported that the US health care system killed over ninety-eight thousand patients a year.[13] In the past two decades, these statistics have hardly budged. The only progress we seem to have made is in more accurate reporting. We now know that the system kills over 250,000 (and according to some estimates, up to 440,000) patients a year because of preventable medical errors and injures 1.5 million patients.[14]

Over 75 percent of these deaths and injuries are due to failures not in competence or technical proficiency but in teamwork and communication. Only a small fraction of American hospitals have instituted teamwork training and integrated teams. The VHA is a notable exception.[15]

Mental Health Care

The private sector's record on other issues that impact veterans is no better. As we have seen, a large number of veterans suffer from mental illnesses and substance abuse problems. How they would fare in the private—or even public—sector outside the VHA depends on an accurate assessment of the US health care system's record on dealing with mental health and substance abuse issues. That record is hardly reassuring.

Consider, for example, how psychiatrist Thomas Insel described the system of mental health care in the United States when he was preparing to leave his position as director of the National Institute of Mental Health in

2015. In an NPR interview, Insel candidly concluded that "the mental health system is badly broken. The problem right now is that we have a lot of people with mental illness that are not treated at all, treated very late, or treated very inadequately." Insel called the lack of mental health services "the equivalent of a civil rights issue here, and we haven't dealt with it well."[16]

According to studies by the National Institute of Mental Health, 40 percent of people with schizophrenia and 51 percent of people with bipolar disorder go untreated in any given year.[17] It is by now well known that prisons and jails have become America's de facto mental health treatment system. People with untreated psychiatric illnesses constitute one-third, or two hundred thousand, of the nation's six hundred thousand homeless and approximately 16 percent of the total jail and prison inmate population. "People with untreated psychiatric illnesses spend twice as much time in jail as non-ill individuals and are more likely to commit suicide."[18]

A report by the Department of Health and Human Services on the state of the mental health workforce documents that 77 percent of US counties have a severe shortage of psychiatrists, psychologists, and social workers, and 55 percent of these counties—all of them rural—do not have a single psychologist, psychiatrist, or social worker.[19] This is due, in part, to a shortage of inpatient mental health facilities and mental health professionals—or professionals willing to accept insurance.[20]

Even supposedly well-insured people who live in urban areas have truncated mental health benefits and limited access to care. In many areas that are well supplied with psychiatrists, psychologists, social workers, or nurse-practitioners, these clinicians will no longer accept health insurance. In a post in 2007, the blog *Shrink Rap* wrote: "Many psychiatrists in private practice don't take insurance, or don't 'accept assignment.' They require the to patient pay [*sic*] them and then the patient can submit to his health insurance company and reimbursement is made directly to the patient. This often means that the patient, having gone Out-Of-Network, has a higher co-pay &/or a higher deductible, and the hassle of paperwork. Generally, if a patient sees an In-Network psychiatrist, they make a co-pay and the hassle of getting the rest of the money falls on the doctor. This means that access to psychiatric care is limited to those who have the money to pay up front, the wherewithal to stick their statements into an envelope and send them to the insurance company—after they've called a separate managed care company, gotten pre-authorization."[21]

In 2014, Kevin MD updated this reporting because the situation had gotten even worse. "[Current procedural terminology] codes," he said, "have changed since then, and the reasons to not take insurance have increased. Many other doctors don't take insurance now, though psychiatry remains the number one specialty where doctors don't participate in health insurance plans."[22]

In an article in *JAMA Psychiatry* in 2013, Tara F. Bishop and her colleagues documented that only 55 percent of psychiatrists, compared to 89 percent of other physicians, accept private insurance; 55 percent accept Medicare, compared to 86 percent of other physicians; and only 43 percent, compared to 73 percent of other physicians, will accept Medicaid patients. The authors concluded that "these low rates of acceptance may pose a barrier to access to mental health services."[23] Another study in *Health Affairs* reported similar problems.[24]

While researching this book, I decided to conduct my own informal survey of Bay Area therapists to see if they would accept someone like me, who has excellent health insurance, for the kind of cognitive behavioral therapy that is standard treatment for anxiety, PTSD, or other problems at the VHA. No one I called would accept either standard health insurance or Medicare. Therapists told me that if I could afford to pay up front—say, $450 for an initial evaluation and $235 a pop for weekly or biweekly visits for twenty to thirty sessions—they would be happy to provide patients with an invoice that they could submit to their insurers (but who knows how much of the bill the insurers will pay, one therapist warned).

Even when patients can access health care services, insurers often limit the number of mental or behavioral health treatments enrollees can receive in a given year and certainly restrict access to inpatient treatment. In 2008 Congress passed the Paul Wellstone and Pete Domenici Mental Health Parity and Addiction Equity Act (also known as the Mental Health Parity Law or Federal Parity Law). The law requires that insurance company coverage of services for mental health, behavioral health, and substance use disorders are comparable to physical health coverage. According to the American Psychological Association, insurance companies can and do still limit the number of visits a patient can have with a mental health professional based on what the insurer deems "medical necessity." Patients may also have to pay extremely high deductibles—from, say, $500 to

$5,000—before their health insurance kicks in. Many people don't know about this law, and insurance companies frequently violate it.[25]

Some mentally ill patients may have trouble getting access to care because they are what is euphemistically termed "disruptive." They may be angry, unruly, and "noncompliant" with treatment recommendations. As we have seen earlier, these patients can be "fired" in the private sector, but not in the VHA. Indeed, private-sector medical journals like *Medical Economics* often run articles about how physicians can ethically fire their patients. In 2014, for example, physician and attorney Barry B. Cepelewicz advised his colleagues about how to best fire their patients. If patients are noncompliant or haven't paid their bills, he advises that "you could mention those reasons in the letter, but otherwise it's best not to specify the reasons because it might make an already uncomfortable situation even worse (the reasons, however, should be memorialized in the patient's record). The letter should provide an effective date of termination and offer the patient at least 30 days to find an alternate provider during which time you will continue to treat the patient for urgent issues. . . . The patient should be advised to seek continued care and informed of the consequences if he or she fails to follow your directions."[26]

Finally, for patients who require hospitalization, access to mental health services in the private sector may be restricted because of a shortage of inpatient beds. According to a recent report from the Treatment Advocacy Center, when it comes to mental health, there is quite literally "No Room at the Inn," as its report is titled. Over the last half century, state psychiatric hospitals have closed entirely or eliminated beds. Between 2005 and 2010, state psychiatric beds decreased by 14 percent, with per capita state psychiatric bed population plunging to 1850 levels. "Thirteen states," the report says, "closed 25% or more of their total state hospital beds from 2005 to 2010. New Mexico and Minnesota closed more than 50% of their beds; Michigan and North Carolina closed just less than 50%. Ten states increased their total hospital beds but continued to provide less than half the beds. . . . The decrease in state psychiatric bed availability since 2005 is actually worse than the 14% that occurred 2005–2010. Completed or announced bed eliminations *since* 2010 will eliminate 4,471 additional beds."[27]

To put these figures in an international perspective, in the United Kingdom there were 63.2 psychiatric beds per 100,000 people in 2005; in 2010 the United States had 14.1 per 100,000.[28] According to statistics on hospital beds in Europe, countries have also decreased the number of psychiatric hospital beds, but nowhere near as significantly as in the United States. In 2013, Germany had 12.7 hospital beds per 100,000 allocated to those with psychiatric problems.[29] The Organisation for Economic Co-operation and Development reports that, among the thirty-nine OECD countries, the United States is one of the three lowest-ranking when it comes to the number of psychiatric hospital beds per thousand people. This helps to explain why our prisons and jails have become such popular inpatient psychiatric centers.[30]

In Northern California, where I live, the system that is most like the VHA, Kaiser Permanente, has been plagued by scandal because it forced patients to endure long wait times for mental health appointments. In November 2011, the National Union of Healthcare Workers (NUHW), which represents Kaiser's psychologists, social workers, and other mental health clinicians, filed a complaint that highlighted Kaiser's failure to hire sufficient mental staff. As Fred Seavey, research director of the NUHW, explained, the state of California requires an HMO to provide a first appointment for non-urgent care within fourteen days and an urgent appointment within forty-eight hours. It also requires appropriate follow-up visits. The California Department of Managed Health Care (DMHC) investigated this complaint and found that as many as 50 percent of patients at various Kaiser facilities experienced lengthy appointment delays that violated California law. In 2013 the state of California fined the system $4 million, issued a cease-and-desist order against Kaiser, and ordered the HMO to correct the problems.[31]

The state performed a follow-up survey to see whether the HMO had fixed the problems. The results were published in 2015. The thirty-three-page report, based on a sampling of hundreds of individual patient charts, revealed that, in Northern California alone, 22 percent of patients suffered excessive appointment delays. The DMHC called the violations "serious" and "significant."

On July 5, 2015, eighty-three-year-old Barbara Ragan drove from her home in Santa Rosa, parked her car on the third-floor parking lot at a Kaiser medical center, and, Kaiser card in hand, jumped to her death. Ragan, who had worked for Kaiser herself for more than two decades, had been seeking mental health care from Kaiser and faced lengthy delays and callous treatment. The *Los Angeles Times* reported: "The state Department of

Managed Health Care said it reviewed medical records of nearly 300 Kaiser patients and found a continuing problem with long waits for treatment. In Northern California, patients didn't get timely appointments in 22% of cases. In Southern California, Kaiser failed to meet the standard in 9% of cases. One Kaiser psychiatrist stated unequivocally, 'No one ever sees a therapist once a week in the Kaiser Health Plan. Not a covered benefit for the past 20-something years and will not be a benefit in the future.'"[32]

As of late 2017, Kaiser had still not corrected all its identified mental health care deficiencies and remained under investigation by the DMHC. Meanwhile, patients have filed two class-action lawsuits against the health plan. One alleges that the excessive appointment delays are a violation of civil rights statutes because they are discriminating against patients with mental health problems.

Given the record of the private sector when it comes to mental health, it is not hard to argue that the VHA has the only high-functioning mental health system in the entire country. When it comes to the integration of mental health and primary care, the VHA is unique. Similarly, when it comes to issues of substance abuse, the VHA is also one of the only health care systems that use medically assisted treatments like suboxone for substance abuse disorders.

The VA's record on delivering mental health care has been documented in myriad studies. One published in 2015 about how often appropriate drugs are prescribed to mentally ill patients found that "in every case, VA performance was superior to that of the private sector by more than 30 percent."[33] Between 2000 and 2010, rates of suicide increased by 40 percent among veterans who didn't use the VA, but declined by 20 percent among those who did.[34] Veterans with severe mental illness who receive VA care live much longer on average than their nonveteran counterparts in the US population.[35]

As we've seen earlier, the majority of mental health professionals in the United States do not have any knowledge of military-related conditions, and only 30 percent of them provide evidence-based care for their patients when it comes to PTSD and depression. In the VA the majority of providers have a deep understanding of the way military service creates, impacts, and exacerbates these problems, and the vast majority deliver evidence-based care to their patients.[36]

In March 2018, the RAND Corporation released a study titled *Ready or Not?* in which researchers examined whether private-sector health professionals in New York State had the "capacity" and "readiness" to deal with the state's eight hundred thousand veterans in need of care.[37] The conclusion? Only 2 *percent* of New York State providers met RAND's "final definition as ready to provide timely and quality care to veterans in the community."

While the majority of providers said they had room for new patients, fewer than 20 percent of them ever asked their patients if they were veterans. Fewer than half used appropriate clinical practice guidelines to treat their patients, and 75 percent didn't use the kind of screening tools commonly deployed in the VHA to detect critical problems like PTSD, depression, and risk of suicide.

Most providers had no understanding of military culture, and fewer than half said they were interested in filling such knowledge gaps. Mirroring a similar study conducted by the VA and the Medical University of South Carolina in 2011,[38] RAND found that New York State providers had little understanding of the high quality of VHA care. Informed by media reports rather than medical journals, they had a negative view of the VHA and would be unlikely to refer eligible veterans to the VHA for needed care in programs in which the VHA actually excels.

In March of 2018, the *Federal Practitioner* ran an article by VA psychologist Russell Lemle summarizing the accomplishments of the VHA in suicide prevention and dealing with other mental health problems.[39] In the same month, the prestigious National Academies of Science, Engineering, and Medicine released an evaluation of VHA mental health services for Iraq and Afghanistan veterans. It found VHA mental health care to be "comparable or superior to that in the private sector." The majority of veterans who accessed the system had "positive experiences" and appreciated VHA staff's "respect toward patients." This was despite serious shortages of mental health staff, as well as clinical and exam space, and confusion about how to access care—all of which could, and should, be improved. When veterans were asked whether needed services were provided in the VHA, 64 percent said they were. When they were asked about services they had received in the private sector, only 20 percent said they had received needed services. The report also said that the VHA mental health system could serve as a model for the nation.[40]

Services for the Homeless

In cities across the country, even progressive mayors have been criticized for their failure to reduce homelessness. In San Francisco, where skyrocketing rents and home prices have contributed to a large homeless population, VA staff play a critical role in helping veterans get off the street. I asked Michael Blecker, executive director of Swords to Plowshares, who would deliver such services if the VHA were privatized and facilities like Fort Miley, the San Francisco VA Medical Center, were closed.

"From the standpoint of health care and dealing with people's housing situation, the VA is like night and day from anyone else," Blecker told me. "I'm sure that at a private-sector provider like Kaiser, the last thing they care about is their patients' housing situation. If someone is stinking or acting out, not being nice, they probably can't even get in the door to get treated."

Blecker, of course, is a leading California foe of VHA privatization threats. When he served on the Commission on Care in 2015 and 2016, he became the sole dissenter from its final report because he believed the commission's support for further private-sector outsourcing would lead to eventual elimination of the VHA and loss of veteran access to "nonmedical" services like help for the homeless.[41]

"When everything is pushed from public to private, it becomes like the Wild West," Blecker contends. "In the private sector, there is just lawlessness and no accountability. That's the scary thing that's happening here: the more you push VA care from public to private, the more you lose any accountability." And accountability, he says, "is the whole point of the commons, of the government."

At the VA, he notes, there is always a way to get "someone's attention and to make sure a complaint gets heard. There are points of leverage that you can actually focus on and get things done. You take that away, and we have no leverage—zero, zilch."

Overall Medical Outcomes

On Capitol Hill, it's bipartisan conventional wisdom that only private-sector competition can spur the VHA to excel. But according to study after study, the VHA's own internal incentives have, in fact, led to excellence. The VHA is mission driven, not profit driven. Its caregivers have actually eschewed private-sector financial incentives because their incentive is delivering great care to veterans. Because of this, in many areas, it has already won the competition with the private sector. Here is only a sampling of the studies that document how well the VHA is delivering care that is almost consistently equal or superior to the private sector:

In 2003 the prestigious *New England Journal of Medicine* published a study that used eleven measures of quality to compare veterans' health facilities with fee-for-service Medicare. In all eleven measures, the quality of care in veterans' facilities proved to be "significantly better" than private-sector health care paid for by Medicare.[42]

In 2007 the equally prestigious British medical journal *BMJ* wrote that while "long derided as a US example of failed Soviet-style central planning," the VA "has recently emerged as a widely recognized leader in quality improvement and information technology. At present, the Veterans Health Administration offers more equitable care, of higher quality, at comparable or lower cost than private-sector alternatives."[43]

In 2010 another study documented the high quality of VHA care.[44] Although many veterans complain about the hoops they have to jump through at the VBA, patient satisfaction with the VHA is far higher than for those covered by private-sector insurance or Medicare.[45]

The Association of VA Psychologist Leaders (AVAPL) has assembled on its website an impressive accounting of the many studies on VA quality care that can be found.[46]

In 2015 an independent assessment of VHA health care quality conducted by the RAND Corporation documented all this and more. Here are some of its findings:

- Postoperative morbidity was lower for VA patients compared with nonveterans receiving non-VA care.
- Inpatient care was more or as effective in VA as in non-VA hospitals.

- VA hospitals were more likely to follow best practices in the use of central venous catheter line infection prevention, and rates of mortality declined more quickly over time in VA than in non-VA settings for specific conditions.

The report also found that veterans in nursing homes were less likely to develop pressure ulcers, outpatients and those suffering chronic conditions got better follow-up care, and VA health providers offered better mental health and obesity counseling and blood pressure control, particularly for African Americans. Importantly, income and educational disparities were smaller at VHA facilities in such areas as diabetes, heart disease, and cancer screenings.

The report confirmed that the VHA delivers what is known as "right care," defined as avoiding toxic, unnecessary tests, medications, and procedures. Elderly patients in the VHA were less likely to receive the kinds of medication that can make them sicker and sometimes even kill them, the report found. VHA patients were more likely to be spared toxic chemotherapy within fourteen days of death or admitted to an ICU thirty days before death.[47] This was attributed to the VHA's commitment to palliative and hospice care.

Health care quality expert Charlene Harrington, professor emerita of the University of California, San Francisco, called the report "really impressive, particularly given the patient mix and chronic underfunding."

As noted throughout this book, one reason why VHA quality is so high is that, unlike the fragmented care that is generally delivered in the private health care system, care in the VHA is integrated and coordinated. An example of how all this makes a difference in the lives of veterans comes from a study of cancer care published in the *Annals of Internal Medicine*. The study compared the treatment of older male veterans in the VA with that received by older men under traditional, fee-for-service Medicare. The study found that the VA offered care that was at least as good, and often better, than that offered from non-VA doctors. According to Nancy Keating, an associate professor of health care policy at Harvard Medical School and the lead author of the study, a key factor accounting for this result is that care at the VA "is much better coordinated than in most other settings." She also explains that the VA "has a good, integrated medical record. Their doctors all work together and communicate more effectively."[48]

Another study in California reported that VA patients with cancer had to wait longer to be treated after diagnosis than those with Medi-Cal or Medicare/Medi-Cal insurance. They were, however, more likely to get recommended treatment for their disease.[49] As Kenneth Kizer, one author of the study, notes, its findings are a reminder that wait times are not the only metric that should be used in evaluating care. Sometimes care is actually worth the wait.

Diabetes care is another example of the VA's superior integration. Outside the VA, diabetics are not generally cared for by teams but rather by different specialists who rarely coordinate their care. Because of this, a diabetic patient may not be effectively coached on how to take his insulin correctly, monitor blood sugar levels, get necessary foot or eye exams, or make sure he adjusts his diet and gets enough exercise. By contrast, VA patients suffering from diabetes receive care from providers who work as a team.[50] As a result, studies show the diabetics treated by the VA do far better on many critical measures than those using private insurance or Medicare.[51] AVAPL has also compiled an impressive list of all the medical innovations and discoveries the VHA has pioneered over the years.[52]

In our report for the American Legion, Phillip Longman and I explain that the VHA is able to provide services equal to or better than the private sector—at a much lower cost.[53]

Accountability and Transparency

In recent years there has been much media attention paid to VHA problems, real and exaggerated. Whether accurate or not, this reporting is greatly facilitated by the fact that the VHA is a publicly funded system. As such, it is accountable to Congress and the public for administrative errors, personnel failures, or clinical mistakes, in a way that the health care industry in general is not. In 2017, for example, the VHA launched a website listing information on all employees disciplined or fired—and for what infractions—to be transparent about substandard performance and send a strong signal that it won't be tolerated or concealed. There is no equivalent roster to be found anywhere in the private sector, and not because no one ever gets suspended or dismissed. Private-sector personnel information, including any listing of malpractice claim settlements (with accompanying nondisclosure clauses), is not available to the public or press.

In the fall of 2017, Senators Joe Manchin (D-WV) and Dean Heller (R-NV) introduced the VA Provider Accountability Act to ensure further transparency about any medical errors made by VHA providers. The Manchin–Heller bill, filed in response to a *USA Today* report that VHA mistakes were not being fully disclosed, would require the agency to report any major adverse events to the National Practitioner Data Bank and state licensing boards. If enacted, it would also prohibit the VA from reaching any settlements with fired or dismissed employees that would conceal serious medical errors or purge related disciplinary records from personnel files.[54] It's too bad this kind of accountability is unavailable to patients in the private sector and that few congressional representatives seem interested in protecting patients outside the VHA.

If a patient becomes a victim of private-sector medical malpractice, one remedy is to file a complaint with the state board of medicine or the federal Centers for Medicare and Medicaid Services (CMS). State boards have the power to discipline a physician, and Medicare can suspend a hospital—depriving it of federal reimbursement, although this step is rarely taken. In 2014 the industry publication *Modern Healthcare* reported that the prestigious Cleveland Clinic was threatened with suspension and placed on what is called "termination track" from the Medicare program in 2010, 2012, and 2013. This was because of patient safety complaints that the clinic had failed to address.

The clinic faced the loss of $1 billion in annual payments from Medicare, which would have seriously impacted the institution. The article reported that CMS had received 9,505 patient complaints—some of them very serious—from 1,638 hospitals. No matter how serious the complaint, CMS rarely suspends hospitals from the Medicare program. The ultimate goal with hospital inspections "is to ensure compliance with Medicare rules, not close down hospitals that are essential to local communities," a CMS spokeswoman said.[55] As I reported in my book *The Battle for Veterans' Healthcare*, an analysis of the 990s filed by the Cleveland Clinic shows that annual compensation of CEO Delos "Toby" Cosgrove increased from $2.3 million to $4 million between 2010 and 2014.[56] One can only imagine the drubbing a VHA hospital administrator would receive for far less serious patient safety violations.

Even if a hospital was suspended from the Medicare system and its CEO fired, this would not help a patient who suffered because of a preventable medical error or medical negligence. As a result, many patients suffer job loss, which means the loss of health insurance and potential financial ruin from the resulting medical bills. Patients are, of course, free to sue physicians or hospitals for malpractice. But malpractice cases, which are judged in state courts according to state laws, are extremely difficult to prove. In the VHA, when a veteran proves he or she has been injured because of medical error, the VHA bears the cost of all further care for the rest of the patient's lifetime—a remedy not on offer, without litigation, anywhere else.

According to an article by Daniel P. Kessler, patients must prove that "1) the patient actually suffered an adverse event; 2) the provider caused the event due to action or inaction; and 3) the provider was negligent, which essentially entails showing that the provider took less care than that which is customarily practiced by the average member of profession in good standing, given the circumstances of the doctor and the patient. Collectively, this three-part test of the validity of a malpractice claim is known as the 'negligence rule'" (citations omitted).[57]

The well-known Harvard Medical Malpractice Study found that only one in fifteen patients who suffer an injury because of medical negligence receive compensation, and five-sixths of the cases that receive compensation have no evidence of negligence. "More recent research by Studdert, Thomas, Burstin, Zvar, Orav, and Brennan largely mirrors these findings. Awards for medical malpractice claimants are subject to lengthy delays: on average, it takes around four years to resolve a malpractice claim. Moreover, for every dollar spent on compensation, 54 cents went to litigation expenses and other transaction costs" (citations omitted).[58]

As I reported in *The Battle for Veterans' Healthcare*, one of these patients was David Antoon, a Vietnam veteran who tried to sue the Cleveland Clinic and his surgeon for his botched prostate cancer surgery and failing to be in the operating room during crucial parts of the operation. The surgeon, who Antoon alleges was supervising multiple operating rooms, let a noncredentialed doctor-in-training do the surgery, even though Antoon had been assured in writing that the attending surgeon would perform the operation. As a result of the surgery, Antoon, a pilot for United Airlines, suffered severe complications and disabilities and lost his job as an airline captain. Antoon's "whistleblower" lawsuit was dismissed by the federal Sixth Circuit Court of Appeals. The court ruled that operating room logs and audit reports showing his doctor never present during his surgery did not represent "firsthand" knowledge required for standing. "Firsthand" knowledge required Antoon to have been awake and to have witnessed the absence of the surgeon during his surgery. Although Antoon prevailed in Ohio's Eighth District Court of Appeals, the Cleveland Clinic appealed to the Ohio Supreme Court, which expanded "tort reform" in overturning the appeals court ruling. In six different rulings in state and federal court, Antoon's case was not allowed to go to trial. Antoon is now cared for by the Dayton VHA. The VHA, he says, "is the model needed for this country—a system where patients and providers have the same goal—positive patient outcomes."

As for public disclosure of medical errors and negligence in the private sector, even when plaintiffs win or settle cases, in the private sector most legal settlements do not result in the kind of public disclosure Manchin and Heller demand for veterans. Most legal settlements are accompanied by nondisclosure agreements. Researchers in Texas conducted a review of settlements at the University of Texas system, which provides malpractice insurance to its six thousand physicians. The report, which was published in *JAMA Internal Medicine*, found that nine out of ten settlements included nondisclosure provisions. "All the nondisclosure clauses prohibited disclosure of the settlement terms and amount, 61 (55.5%) prohibited disclosure that the settlement had been reached, 51 (46.4%) prohibited disclosure of the facts of the claim, 29 (26.4%) prohibited reporting to regulatory agencies, and 10 (9.1%) prohibited disclosure by the settling physicians and hospitals, not only by the claimant. Three agreements (2.7%) included specific language that prohibited the claimant from disparaging the physicians or hospitals."

In an editorial accompanying the news report on the study, Michelle Mello, a professor of law and health policy at Stanford University, and attorney Joseph N. Catalano wrote, "Internal reporting and surveillance of adverse events and internal peer-review and risk-management investigations cannot be effective without a willingness to communicate openly within the organization." They also noted that "provisions that prevent families from discussing what happened to them greatly undercut the power of their advocacy and impair patient safety efforts."[59]

In a news report on the study, Mello commented further: "Nondisclosure agreements that prohibit plaintiffs from talking to regulatory bodies, like state boards of medical licensing, about what happened to them are really objectionable. Patients shouldn't have to choose between accepting compensation and acting on a perceived obligation to try to ensure the physician doesn't hurt someone else."[60]

Study after study has shown that the quality of VHA care is equal or superior to private-sector treatment, and its holistic approach tailored to the particular problems of veterans is not easily reproduced elsewhere. This is why patient safety and quality experts like Donald Berwick, former president and CEO of the Institute for Healthcare Improvement and administrator of the Centers for Medicare and Medicaid Services, recently told me that "the VHA has been—and remains—a pioneer in patient safety, geriatrics, the integration of primary and mental health care, and other important dimensions of care. For years, it has successfully addressed problems that remain unaddressed in our larger health care system. And the Veterans Health Administration manages to deliver care at much lower cost than most of the private sector. As a longtime observer of its evolution, I believe that the Veterans Health Administration is a system that should be emulated widely, not dismantled."

CONCLUSION

A System Worth Saving— and Making Even Better

In any health care system as large as the VHA, there will always be failings that require change in organizational leadership, administrative policies, or delivery of care. Finding the right solutions requires that institutional problems—once identified and analyzed—be placed in their correct historical and cultural context. Then, strategies for reform will better reflect the real needs of patients, as they perceive and express them, instead of being shaped by the ideological fixations of powerful private interests.

When it comes to dealing with the wounds of war, the independent assessment of the VHA, mandated by Congress under the Choice Act of 2014, gave our veterans' health care system high marks in many key areas, including overall quality of care. (While one of the VHA's reported shortcomings was variations in quality of care from one facility to another, that problem, the report said, is more pronounced in private health care.) The major challenges, identified by the VHA's outside consultants and other experts, involved increasing patient access, reducing bureaucratic micromanagement by officials at VA headquarters, and getting necessary funding from Congress.

In a report titled *Resources and Capabilities of the Department of Veterans Affairs to Provide Timely and Accessible Care to Veterans*, researchers "did not find evidence of a system wide crisis in access to VA care." The report instead pointed out that congressional policies were a significant barrier to improvements in the VHA. "Inflexibility in budgeting stemming from the congressional appropriation processes," as well as a hastily designed Veterans Choice program, "further complicated the situation and resulted in confusion among veterans, VA employees, and non-VA providers."[1]

Unfortunately, steps taken by Congress and the VA since then have not addressed these problems, or many others, effectively. As Senator Patty Murray told David Shulkin at a Veterans' Affairs Committee hearing in June 2017, "What's missing from the conversation is how you plan to actually build and strengthen the VA system for the long-term. There is no comprehensive plan to . . . get more frontline providers, increase appointments, expand services, build and upgrade facilities, and bring more veterans into the system."[2]

On the caregiver-hiring front, there were about thirty-four thousand VHA staff vacancies when I first started working on this book. By the time my manuscript was completed, four years later, the American Federation of Government Employees (AFGE) estimated that number to be forty-nine thousand.[3] The VA spokesperson under President Trump, Curt Cashour, contested this figure, insisting, in February 2018, that there were only 35,554 vacancies.[4] Filling these vacancies requires streamlining cumbersome hiring procedures, providing sufficient funds for new hires, and making VHA salaries more competitive, particularly to attract new primary care providers (because, as noted in chapter 3, the United States has a serious national shortage in this field).

The federal government could also relieve that shortage—for the VHA and our health care system generally—by ensuring that more taxpayer-funded residency slots are allocated every year to primary care residency programs rather than just boosting the supply of medical specialists. The VHA is able to provide some assistance with repaying medical and nursing school loans, as a hiring incentive. But Congress still won't let the VHA offer market-rate salaries in cities like Boston or San Francisco, where a physician, psychologist, or social worker stands to lose $30,000, $40,000, or even $100,000 a year by choosing to care for veterans.

Underfunding of the VA under Barack Obama, and now Donald Trump, has exacerbated understaffing. In February 2014, as chair of the Senate Veterans' Affairs Committee, Bernie Sanders requested $21 billion to improve staffing. Senate Republicans, then in the minority, opposed this effort. After the wait-time cover-up in Phoenix led to passage of the Choice Act, Congress allocated $16.1 billion in additional funding, yet only about 25 percent of that money went to the VHA itself. The rest was spent on outsourced care. In 2017 this pattern continued as Congress allocated $2.4 billion to Choice and only $1 billion to the VA. Between 2014 and 2017, funding for Choice increased by 49 percent and for the VHA by 9 percent.[5] The VHA is thus constantly playing catch-up, trying to meet expanding patient demand with ever-contracting staff and resources.

Things went from bad to worse after Republicans took control of both houses of Congress and Trump became president. Trump imposed a hiring freeze on the VA, which has been lifted for clinical staff but not for many in positions crucial to administrative functions, like billing and staff support. New budgetary infusions for the VHA mainly benefited the Choice program; it was kept afloat at the expense of other veterans' benefits or services. In the fall of 2017, while Congress considered the permanent extension of Choice, VHA hospitals and clinics around the country experienced local budget crunches that further inhibited hiring. As one medical center chief of staff told me, "We need more physicians and nurses, but our director refuses to hire needed staff because he has no idea if he can pay their salaries next year or the year after."

One factor contributing to the agency's de facto hiring freeze highlighted continuing flaws in its management culture and system of incentives. Medical and regional (VISN) directors are still being evaluated, promoted, and given bonuses based on whether they stay within their annual budgets and don't seek additional funds from VA headquarters. As a result, quality of care may suffer from understaffing, but if budgetary metrics are met, local management performance will be rewarded nevertheless.

Top-Down Control

The VA headquarters' disconnection from frontline caregiving and local administration is also highlighted in the independent assessment conducted for Congress under the Choice Act, and in Stephen Trynosky's monograph

"Beyond the Iron Triangle." The independent assessors found that the "central office does not focus on support to the field." In turn, local VHA administrators were "not fully empowered due to lack of clear authority, priorities, and goals."[6] According to Trynosky, the whistle-blowing in Phoenix, in early 2014, not only revealed a local wait-time cover-up. Its aftermath also exposed "a lack of agility in responding to oversight requests, the absence of proactive engagement to oversight bodies, and inadequate capacity at the VHA leadership level to manage crises."[7]

A veteran himself and VA staffer, Trynosky blames the agency's Office of Congressional and Legislative Affairs (OCLA) in Washington, DC. Under Obama, OCLA officials "tightened their control over internal response systems designed for an earlier era characterized by a more collegial and closed sub-government. Processes never designed for a continuous media environment or the congressional politicization of veterans' health care were rapidly overwhelmed and slowed responses at the very time more agile procedures were needed." VA headquarters found itself ill-equipped to deal with "chronic crisis mode . . . chronic panic . . . constant damage control."[8]

The VA's public relations problems are exacerbated by a severe shortage of PR staff. Major private hospital systems have large public relations departments, exclusively devoted to handling outside press inquiries and generating favorable "free media" coverage. The latter supplements the "paid media" component of their overall advertising and marketing strategy. Fortunately, the VHA does not waste taxpayer dollars on similar self-promotion for patient recruitment purposes. But the downside of its public relations reticence is now painfully clear.

Even large VHA facilities have only one or two public affairs officers, who are also assigned to do outreach to veterans. These media relations specialists routinely told me, off the record, that they felt stymied by the VA central office, which insisted they could pitch only local stories. All VHA-related stories with the potential for national press interest had to be funneled through Washington, DC. In that bureaucratic swamp, crucial news cycle deadlines were missed, promising pegs were essentially spiked, and lack of local press office autonomy made any quick response—much less being proactive—difficult, if not impossible.

For example, when Daniel Zwerdling, at National Public Radio, was preparing a story about how the VHA is an industry leader in installing lift equipment to reduce musculoskeletal injuries among bedside nursing staff, the VA occupational safety experts responsible for this initiative were instructed not to talk to him. Fortunately, Zwerdling found other staff willing to be interviewed, which greatly assisted his positive coverage.[9]

In June 2017 the VHA had an even bigger opportunity to showcase its cutting-edge role when the Government Printing Office published *Best Care Everywhere*. This 440-page compilation of clinical case studies of excellence was coedited by the secretary of the Department of Veterans Affairs himself and includes chapters by more than 170 of the agency's most respected researchers and health care practitioners. In his introduction, David Shulkin personally thanks *Washington Monthly* senior editor Phillip Longman, author of a similarly named 2013 book, for showing "us that the VA provides some of the best health care anywhere and who inspired us to disseminate our best practices and pursue the audacious goal of delivering the best care everywhere to our veterans."[10]

In *Best Care Everywhere*, Shulkin describes how the VA is "changing veterans' lives," noting that "it takes an average of 17 years for new medical evidence to reach patients in clinic or at the bedside"—a problem that all health care systems are grappling with. According to Shulkin, "VA is leading American health care in fixing it," an opinion seconded by his deputy under secretary for health Shereef Elnahal, a fellow contributor to the book. "It's difficult to exaggerate VA employees' excitement and burst of energy when they see their great ideas translated into better access and outcomes for the veterans they proudly serve," Elnahal reports. "No operational system, to our knowledge, has achieved the diffusion or consistency of best practices on a scale comparable to what we're seeing at the VA."[11]

For an agency afflicted with bad, if often unfair, press coverage (and equally uninformed congressional criticism), *Best Care Everywhere* is a PR goldmine. When I first got my copy from a VHA doctor in California, I immediately assumed the book would, at least, be widely distributed in-house to boost institutional morale and, in professional circles, help attract a new generation of VHA staff. I also expected that other journalists covering the VA would be notified about it, along with members and staff of the Senate and House Committees on Veterans' Affairs and leaders of major veterans' organizations.

Instead, seven months after its publication, *Best Care Everywhere* was still one of Washington's best-kept secrets. Nicholas Fandos, who covers veterans' affairs for the *New York Times*, told me he had never heard of the book. When I informed Longman, at the *Washington Monthly*, that it contained Shulkin's personal tribute to Longman's own trailblazing work, that was news to him, because no one had sent him a copy. When I queried Michele Hammonds at VA headquarters about the book's availability, even she seemed unaware of its existence. "What was that again?" she asked. "Did you say *Best Care Ever?*"

She told me to send her a formal e-mail request for a review copy and promised a quick response, which I never got at any speed. Sometime later, a more responsive VA headquarters staffer offered, in "Deep Throat" fashion, to send me a pdf version of the book. But only if I promised never to reveal his name. Posing as a mere member of the taxpaying public, I also placed an online order at the Government Printing Office. Only a few weeks after its publication date, *Best Care Everywhere* was already listed, mysteriously, as "back-ordered."[12] I supplied my credit card information and hoped for the best. When my own book on the VA went to press a year later, the GPO had still not shipped me a copy of Shulkin's collection (a customer service experience that might lead any other frustrated buyer to favor outsourcing to Amazon, where it is, by the way, unlisted!). Ten months later, in March, the book was finally available.

When I surveyed Capitol Hill staffers, who deal with veterans' affairs, about *Best Care Everywhere*, none had ever heard of it. I got the same response from the usually well-informed officialdom of veterans' service organizations headquartered in Washington, DC. ("Did Shulkin write a book?" one quizzical American Legion staffer asked me.) At VA headquarters not far away, one helpful insider reported that the secretary of veterans affairs had distributed *Best Care Everywhere* at a senior leadership meeting, but only selectively.

Another agency official observed that Shulkin "began this book under Obama and wanted to take credit for VA innovations. Now he's working for Trump, and he's in a bind because this is not the message the administration wants to deliver." The VA's self-defeating suppression of *Best Care Everywhere* only confirmed the sorrowful assessment of Dr. Ken Kizer, a Clinton-era predecessor of Shulkin, as VA undersecretary for health. According to Kizer, the agency's current leadership has "lost focus on the reason why there is a dedicated health care system for veterans."[13]

Bipartisan Solutions?

Among Democrats and Republicans on Capitol Hill, there has been far wider forgetfulness about why such a "dedicated health care system" was created in the first place. Congressional debate about the future of the VHA has centered, almost entirely, on expanded patient access to private doctors and hospitals. When members of Congress introduce bills with names like the "Veterans Coordinated Access & Rewarding Experiences (CARE) Act," they can appear to care about veterans in need of quality health care, while simultaneously ingratiating themselves with wealthy donors or corporate interests opposed, for reasons of ideology or financial self-interest, to any strengthening of the VHA itself.

On October 23, 2017, sixteen conservative lobbying groups issued a ringing call for immediate privatization of the VHA. Most were recipients of funding from the Koch brothers.[14] Not to be outdone by his fellow billionaires, one of the nation's most successful hedge fund managers, Steven A. Cohen, unveiled the modestly named "Cohen Veterans Network" (CVN) as a VHA competitor-in-waiting in the field of outsourced mental health treatment. With a practiced eye toward future market share, Cohen contributed $1 million to the cost of President Trump's January 2017 inauguration party and in February 2018 announced he would spend millions more to defeat Democrats in the upcoming elections.

Cohen is a controversial figure, to say the least.[15] He narrowly escaped prosecution in one of the biggest insider trading investigations in recent years, which led to a $1.2 billion penalty against his firm, SAC Capital Advisors, plus a short-term Securities and Exchange Commission ban on his managing any money other than his own.[16]

To facilitate future federal reimbursement of Cohen's network, Congressmen Mike Gallagher (R-WI) and Seth Moulton (D-MA) helpfully introduced a bill that would permit any VHA-covered veteran to seek private-sector therapy, at taxpayer expense, but without any VHA referral or coordination of care. To secure passage of this measure, CVN hired as its lobbyist former Florida congressman Jeff Miller, past chairman of the House Veterans' Affairs Committee and leading advocate of VA privatization when he served in that role.

Unfortunately for Cohen, creating a parallel, for-profit mental health system triggered a political backlash, which led to withdrawal of the proposed bill. VSOs weighed in against it, along with the Association of VA Psychologist Leaders, Fighting for Veterans Healthcare, the Nurses Organization of Veterans Affairs, the Society for Social Work Leadership in Health Care, and the American Psychological Association. Despite this setback, the CVN continues to expand, without federal subsidy. Any legislation expanding outsourcing in general would inevitably make it easier for private clinics to lure veterans out of the VHA.

Morever, in February 2018, the VA and CVN announced they had signed a memorandum of agreement (MOA)—which was actually signed in October 2017—that would initiate a collaboration between the VA and CVN around education and outreach activities for veterans with mental health issues. The MOA specifically stipulates that it should not be "construed as a partnership, joint venture, agency, employment or any other relationship between VA and CVN." It also stipulates that CVN not use the MOA to "promote or sell any products or services, except that the CVN may promote educational and outreach activities described in Section IV."[17] As soon as the deal was announced, however, both CVN and the VA announced that the two had entered a "partnership," and CVN began using the MOA to promote and advertise its services.[18]

Other efforts to privatize and outsource more VHA services include a bill, HR 4242, promoted by Congressmen Phil Roe (R-TN) and Tim Walz (D-MN);[19] another bill was introduced by the VA itself.[20] Other bills considered in the fall of 2017 and in 2018 were introduced in the Senate by Johnny Isakson (R-GA) and Jon Tester (D-MT)[21] and John McCain (R-AZ) and Jerry Moran (R-KS).[22] And lurking in the background as Donald Trump's first year in office came to a close was a potential presidential coup de grâce for the VA: the White House and Republican-backed VA Asset and Infrastructure Review (AIR) Act of 2017.[23]

If enacted, this bill would have created a nine-member commission to decide which VA facilities would be closed, in a fashion modeled after the Base Realignment and Closure process of the DoD. If the VA Commission on Care is any guide, the AIR panel would be dominated by privatization advocates and health care industry executives with a direct financial stake in outsourcing VHA services. Three slots would be reserved for VSOs, which could, of course, be outnumbered in any vote. The commission would transmit its recommendations to the White House, where they must be approved in toto, without any troublesome congressional input. Any VA facility—no matter how large or small—could be targeted, closed, and then sold off to private developers or health care industry competitors. Members of Congress would be safely insulated from any local political fallout over facility closing decisions because the commission, not Congress, was responsible.

A prime candidate for fire-sale diktat in the Trump era would be Fort Miley in San Francisco, my favorite VHA facility anywhere. It is located on the headlands outside the Golden Gate, where private real estate developers are already circling like vultures and dreaming of the day that this San Francisco jewel will soon become theirs.

What Kind of Choice?

In their press releases heralding VA "reform" bills, members of Congress celebrate "choice"—the more, the better, regardless of the future consequences for veterans. Republican congressman Doug Lamborn introduced his Veterans Empowerment Act of 2017 with the unassailable claim that "our veterans deserve the highest degree of care." According to Lamborn, "giving them options to choose their healthcare plans and doctors" is not only better public policy, it's also personally "empowering."[24] Avik Roy, president of the Koch-funded Foundation for Research on Equal Opportunity, heartily agrees. Providing veterans with "health care independence" will guarantee "the same health care options that all other Americans enjoy."[25]

The notion that the consumer is king in US health care is very appealing but more fiction than fact. It invites veterans, in highly deceptive fashion, to join an indemnity-plan party that ended long ago for most Americans with job-based insurance or policies purchased through ACA-created exchanges. Today health care options for all but the superrich (and other beneficiaries of "concierge care") are dictated, more than ever, by private insurers, the hospital and provider networks they choose to include in their plans, for-profit nursing home chains and long-term care facility owners, and Big Pharma and pharmacy retailers. Market competition and related health care industry consolidation (and accompanying hospital closures) are rarely consumer friendly, nor do they lead to expanded patient choice. With more megamergers in the works, like the $66 billion takeover of Aetna by CVS, experts now "worry that the nation's health care system will come to resemble a series of kingdoms, where consumers are locked into separate ecosystems of pharmacies, doctors, and health care clinics depending on their insurance provider."[26]

Despite these dominant trends, some VHA-related bills promise veterans that they'll be able to pick whomever they want to see—a VHA doctor or private physician—regardless of cost or quality of the outside care. In other legislative scenarios, there would be a negotiation between the VHA and an individual veteran, with the former retaining the right to approve any outside referrals. Veterans would then have the right to appeal any restriction on their access to private-sector care. Financial penalties for going outside of network are not part of proposed revisions of the Choice program now. But, since they are a standard feature of private health insurance plans and HMOs, it's not safe to assume they will be missing forever. In fact, beyond the Choice rainbow lie the same private insurance premiums, co-pays, and deductibles that nonveterans pay outside the VHA, not to mention the higher drug and medical equipment costs also found there.

In one Choice proposal, actually endorsed by Trump's VA leadership, every case-by-case decision about the merits of inside versus outside care would be preceded by a conversation (via telephone, virtually, or in person) between a veteran and his or her VHA provider. If veterans opt for private treatment, they would end up being responsible for finding a suitable doctor, hospital, or therapist on their own. The VA would be required to provide any individually selected outside providers with necessary medical records and later collect information on the course of their prescribed treatment, although the highly fragmented private health care industry currently lacks any common computerized medical record–sharing capacity like the VHA has internally.

When Secretary Shulkin testified before Congress in favor of this process, he was forced to acknowledge that seamless and quick medical record sharing was not possible anytime soon because of the many different systems used by outsourced care providers. Nevertheless, he went on to claim that all referral decisions would involve weighing data on how long the patient would have to wait for care (and what its quality would be) inside the VA versus outside of it. Unfortunately, wait-time data is collected systematically (and, post-Phoenix, more reliably) only by the VHA, not by its private-sector counterparts. As critics of nonessential VHA outsourcing note, the quality-of-care metrics cited by Shulkin are also largely nonexistent, as are measures of the performance of individual physicians or mental health providers. There is no national directory that would reveal whether a particular private-sector therapist is delivering evidence-based therapies to private PTSD patients equivalent to or better than what PTSD sufferers receive at the VHA, or whether a specialist in endocrinology affiliated with a private hospital has any experience diagnosing Agent Orange–related type 2 diabetes.

Furthermore, despite Shulkin's misleading assurance that there would be a smooth patient handoff, what busy clinician dealing with multiple veteran health problems has time to determine, on a case-by-case basis, what course of therapy or treatment delivered by the VHA is better or worse than care provided by any provider chosen by a patient with even less access to such information, where it even exists? As one harried nurse-practitioner told me, "I don't have time to figure out whether we do better colonoscopies than somewhere else. All I care about is that my patients get their colonoscopies. If they want to go to the private sector, I don't have time to deal with it."

The outsourcing model promoted by Shulkin and many in Congress also ignores obstacles to securing high-quality, coordinated care that even the most expert (and fully functioning) patients encounter when advocating on their own behalf or for family members. Professional journals have published many anguished accounts by doctors, nurses, and other practitioners who were well versed in surgical procedures, medication doses, postoperative complications, and the world of health care in general. But when they or loved ones were hospitalized, their inpatient treatment was not good, nor was their post-discharge experience. In his book *Escape Fire*, Dr. Donald Berwick, recounted the harrowing tale of his wife's hospitalization for a serious autoimmune disease at a leading Boston medical center.[27] Even having a world-renowned patient safety advocate at her side did not protect her from the kinds of problems and near misses all too common in the private sector, where coordination of care is inferior to that of the VHA. To expect that homeless, low-income, or mentally ill veterans with multiple chronic conditions—or the stressed-out family members who care for them—will be able to navigate the medical-industrial complex outside the VHA, on their own, is a cruel and irresponsible fantasy.

The Price of Choice

Magical thinking about Choice most dramatically obscures its bottom line. Since Choice was launched in 2014, on a limited basis to reduce appointment days and long trips to VA facilities, the program has had $2 billion in cost overruns. Now President Trump says his goal is increasing the percentage of patients getting some care outside the VHA from 30 to 90 percent. Unlimited outsourcing will bankrupt the VA, first eroding and then eliminating the VHA as a public option for veterans. Choice program legislation, in all its proposed forms, never includes supplemental funding to pay for private-sector care, which will cost far more. That omission is intentional because, according to one estimate obtained by the Commission on Care, if 60 percent of all eligible veterans were treated outside the VHA, the cost of their care would quadruple.

Since that assessment, the San Francisco–based advocacy group Fighting for Veterans Health Care (FFVHC, which I helped form) has carefully analyzed every congressional proposal to expand veterans' care in the private sector.[28] In each bill every dollar spent on outsourcing is absorbed by the VHA's own operating budget. No additional funds are earmarked for the exemplary in-house services showcased in Secretary Shulkin's own book, *Best Care Everywhere*. As the FFVHC predicts, the result of expanded outsourcing will be cuts in VHA programs, staff, and veterans' benefit coverage.

While Congress was still debating the future of Choice, Shulkin was already trying to cover its mounting deficits and VHA operating budget shortfalls by shifting nearly a billion dollars away from existing programs. As I reported in *American Prospect*, he floated the idea of shuttering ten Patient Safety Centers of Inquiry (PSCIs). These VHA facilities have developed innovative methods of reducing suicide and other forms of self-harm, now widely copied outside the veterans' health care system. Only after Senator Bernie Sanders called Shulkin personally, and nationally known patient safety experts like Berwick and Lucian Leape wrote personal letters of protest, did the secretary abandon (for now) any PSCI closing plans.[29] (Unfortunately, others, with PSCIs at risk in their own states, failed to respond, including Senator Elizabeth Warren and Congressman Seth Moulton, a veteran himself.)

Then, in October 2017, the VA leadership changed course again, issuing a memo giving medical center directors the green light to shift money from earmarked programs to fund general operations at the local level. This move threatened $265 million allocated for the HUD-VASH program, in which social workers find housing for homeless veterans. Other funding at risk included $30 million originally budgeted for mental health initiatives and $21 million for staff assisting Iraq and Afghanistan veterans in their transition back to civilian life.

The authorized funding shifts were expected to impact suicide prevention efforts (notwithstanding Shulkin's claim that they were a top personal priority), spinal cord injury rehabilitation programs, and post-amputation care for victims of disabling injuries on and off the battlefield. About $26 million allocated to Mental Illness Research Education and Clinic Centers was targeted for trimming. (These centers do pioneering research on the causes and treatment of mental disorders and translate this knowledge into new clinical practice with veterans.) Almost $23 million in funding for VHA occupational health and safety programs became uncertain. This led to cancellation of some already scheduled staff training on how to lift patients safely in hospital and nursing home beds and better handle those who are disruptive. In similar jeopardy were in-house programs to prevent workplace harassment or violence among coworkers, a not well-timed cut in the post–Harvey Weinstein era.

After much prodding from female veterans and groups like IAVA, the VHA had launched—just prior to Shulkin's directive regarding earmarked programs—a $6 million women's health initiative.[30] Its advocates now had to scramble to keep it afloat. As the impact of other program defunding was felt across the country—for example, among homeless veterans—both national VSOs and local advocates like Michael Blecker at Swords to Plowshares registered strong objections. Thankfully, the VA was forced to backtrack on its curtailment of services to the homeless.[31]

As the federal government, overall, is deprived of future revenue because of 2017 Trump tax cuts for corporations and the wealthy, conservatives in Congress will make a renewed effort, while they control the House and/or Senate, to curb all "entitlement programs." Veterans will not be immune from this trend, when the debate about the future of Medicare, Medicaid, and Social Security resurfaces under Trump. And the potential for VHA eligibility being curtailed or veterans being pitted against other federal benefit recipients is very great.

The VHA's emerging "death by a thousand cuts" requires official camouflage and rationales designed to mollify potential critics. Secretary Shulkin, for example, frequently implied that the agency can best survive and thrive by reorienting itself toward "foundational services" or, in some iterations, its "core mission" (i.e., caring for combat veterans).[32] In his testimony at a February 15, 2018, hearing of the House Committee on Veterans Affairs, Shulkin argued that the VA should focus only on what he called "foundational services" like primary care, mental health treatment, geriatrics, and extended rehabilitation. A wide range of other services—cardiology, oncology, urology, etc.—would no longer be integrated or comprehensive. Instead, they would be turned over to private doctors and hospitals. This is, of course, precisely what private-sector hospitals are angling for. They don't want to deal with the real wounds of war that require labor-intensive, chronic disease management or caring for suicidal or homeless veterans. They want to siphon off the high-cost, episodic treatments like colonoscopies or hip replacements.

What this strategy ignores is the fact that the unique strength of the VHA, as documented in this book, lies in its unmatched system of integrated care. Plus, it threatens to pit one category of patient against another, undermining the unusual sense of solidarity and community among veterans served by the VHA. If the agency no longer treated those without battlefield wounds (who represent about two-thirds of its current patient population), where would such an institutional reorientation leave many men and women profiled in this book?

What would it mean for sixty-year-old Susi Black, still hobbling one-legged through life, if she were deprived of VHA help because she's not a real "wounded warrior"? Or thirty-nine-year-old Demond Wilson, who would be literally flat on his back and dependent on local social service agencies or private charity without VHA assistance? Josh Oakley, who never left the continental United States while on active duty, would, according to his own account, be dead if it were not for VHA intervention. How would Norissa McLorin be faring if she became ineligible for military sexual trauma treatment because she was sexually assaulted, stateside, at a base in South Carolina (with no less trauma than if the attack by a fellow soldier had occurred in the Sunni Triangle)?

All these former service members have medical problems acquired or exacerbated during their military service. Even when those conditions developed long afterward, they were promised health coverage, if needed, when they signed up and made their decision to serve. Should funding of that commitment be withdrawn now? Or, worse yet, should millions of dollars that could be spent on direct care be siphoned off instead through the process of contracting out?

Already, the opportunities for Choice program waste, fraud, and abuse have been well documented; in the future, they may only increase, at further expense to the US taxpayer. In September 2017, for example, the inspector general of the Department of Veterans Affairs sent Shulkin a report on payments to TriWest and Health Net, whose combined reimbursement totaled $649 million.[33] Between 2014 and 2017, the VA contracted with these third-party administrators to set up networks of Choice-approved providers, schedule appointments for veterans, collect medical documentation, and pay provider-submitted bills. The IG's audits found much evidence of medical claims paid more than once, payments that didn't use the correct Medicare or contract adjusted rate, and overpayments to Health Net and TriWest totaling nearly $89 million over a two-year period.[34] Despite this unpromising start with Choice claims processing, Shulkin proceeded to hold secret discussions about merging Choice with the military's TRICARE insurance program, which covers active-duty personnel and their families and was formerly administered by TriWest.

What Veterans Want

The reaction from veterans' groups was fast and furious after the Associated Press broke this story in November 2017. As American Legion official Louis Celli pointed out, any such merger would siphon off funds from VHA hospitals and clinics and eventually shift costs directly to veterans, through co-pays and other possible out-of-pocket costs (TRICARE patients have recently started paying higher co-pays). Nevertheless, Curt Cashour, a spokesman for Shulkin, publicly defended the concept as a possible "game changer" that would save taxpayers money because it is based on "the type of businesslike, common-sense approach that rarely exists in Washington."[35]

Those trying to dismantle the VHA know that privatization is a dirty word among most veterans. So they generally go to greater lengths than

Cashour did on this occasion to obscure their real intentions or ultimate objective. As multiple opinion surveys have confirmed, veterans strongly oppose replacing the VHA with a private insurance scheme; instead, they want their existing health care system strengthened and improved. As VFW National Commander Brian Duffy explains, veterans rely on VHA facilities "for the high-quality, individualized care they provide, but there is always room for improvement, especially in the areas of information technology, scheduling, data analysis, and access to quality care out in the communities." When polled in 2017, nearly eleven thousand VFW members reported shorter waiting times, greater patient satisfaction, and other VHA improvements.[36] Like other veterans' service organizations, however, the VFW has had limited success getting the Trump administration to consider patient opinion and its own organizational expertise about "what works at the VA and . . . what needs to be fixed." In fact, in late January 2018, a Senate insider told me that it's now common knowledge inside the VA central office that when Secretary Shulkin says he wants to "fix" the VA, that's code for "privatize the VA."

Both older veterans' organizations and newer advocacy formations, like VoteVets and the San Francisco–based FFVHC and Veterans Healthcare Action Campaign, have clearly identified what real VHA reform looks like.[37] They favor spending more, not less, on VHA services and staff and filling vacancies by streamlining hiring processes and offering market-rate salaries. They support further investment in VA infrastructure, including necessary repairs and construction of new facilities where needed. VHA coverage should not be denied to men and women with so-called bad paper (other-than-honorable discharges) who were, in effect, punished for manifestations of mental health problems or other service-related conditions they developed while on active duty. And the VHA should expand its assistance program for family caregivers of Iraq War veterans to support those caring for veterans of other conflicts as well. Any additional mandates to serve more veterans and their families must be properly funded, so that resources should not be diverted from existing critical VA programs and staff. Failing to do so would pit older veterans against younger ones, which would lead to endless infighting about who is more deserving of services. As one VHA psychologist told me, some Operation Iraqi Freedom and Operation Enduring Freedom vets already have no love lost for Vietnam vets.

Veterans' care should be outsourced to the private sector only if care of equal quality is not available in a timely manner within the VHA. The VHA should have adequate funding and staff for continuing coordination and integration of patient care after outside referrals are made. If some veterans are unhappy with the VHA prioritizing in-house care of high quality and affordable cost over patient freedom of choice—to go anywhere outside the VHA, under any circumstances, at taxpayer expense—perhaps they need to remember that national health systems are designed to serve the many rather than the few.

Like such systems in the United Kingdom, Canada, and other countries, the VHA provides comprehensive, integrated care, but not all of its services are available at every site. Most primary and mental health care is delivered in large urban medical centers as well as in smaller, rural CBOCs. More specialized treatment—for polytrauma, spinal cord injuries, cognitive difficulties, or loss of sight—is provided at locations scattered across the country, with follow-up care at other sites. The VHA sends liver transplant patients to Portland, Oregon, heart transplant patients to Pittsburgh, and stem cell transplant patients to Seattle. When patients have to travel far from home, their travel and lodging expenses are reimbursed; assistance is also available if family members must accompany them. When the VHA is unable to provide a service, it has long contracted with outside hospitals to deliver care it cannot. Outsourcing for its own sake, or to fill the coffers of government contractors, whether needed or not, is a "spoils system" of a very different sort.

Needed Now: Defenders of the VA

The VHA has almost three hundred thousand employees, a third of whom are veterans. This workforce could be a far more potent force for real VHA reform. Anti-privatization activity, organized by the AFGE throughout the country, has already drawn on the helpful overlap between veterans who are patients, veterans who are union-represented VHA staff, and those who, in both cases, also belong to well-resourced veterans' advocacy organizations with millions of members. What is holding this coalition back from having great impact in a campaign that more than one veteran labor or community organizer has sized up as "very winnable"?

First, many people on the VA payroll are overly wary about the consequences of speaking up and becoming more politically active. About a third of all VA employees have voluntarily chosen to join the American Federation of Government Employees (AFGE) and other unions. This ensures workplace representation that most private-sector health care workers lack, although federal employees' rights have been curtailed since Republicans took control of the Senate and House. In addition, VHA staff are daily reminded that they must never violate the Hatch Act, passed in 1939 to curb patronage and corrupt practices in Washington. This law merely limits political activity by federal employees while on duty, wearing a government uniform, in the workplace or in a government vehicle—but too many have concluded that they can't get involved in politics at all.[38]

Ian Hoffmann, a legislative and political organizer for AFGE, spends much of his time setting the record straight among workers at the VA and other federal agencies. "They can talk about legislation on federal property during their lunch hour and can even call their members of Congress on their own phone during that time," Hoffmann points out. "When they are off the clock and off federal property, they can meet with political representatives, attend rallies, volunteer on campaigns, and speak up about political issues."

Federal employees are not allowed to solicit money for political candidates or represent their own views as official government positions. In the Trump era—ironically, in light of the president's own Twitter use—they have to exercise caution on social media. And, when talking about patient safety issues, they must be respectful of patient confidentiality guidelines. On their own time, they are free to defend the mission of their agency, lobby for and against related legislation, and talk with friends, neighbors, coworkers, and family members about political issues. As private citizens, they can write letters to the editor and address public meetings.

Within AFGE the challenge has been encouraging more rank-and-file activism in a national organization long overly reliant, like many unions, on full-time officials and staff and Washington-based lobbyists. Past organizational behavior of veterans' service organizations also needs to change if their "Save the VA" lobbying efforts are going get maximum benefit from their own grassroots membership base. VSOs have long been a force for holding the VA accountable—and helping to win expansion of VHA coverage. But they can't rest on those laurels now or shrink from defending a system whose shortcomings they have rightly criticized, in constructive fashion, in the past.

VSO leaders point out they, like unions, face some political constraints and threats to their own past influence. Not all their members are eligible for VA health care (less than half of all veterans currently qualify for and use the VHA). Many in their membership hold conservative views on public policy issues or voted for President Trump, even if they are not sympathetic to the agenda of Concerned Veterans of America, the Koch brothers' front with few actual dues payers. Since conscription was ended after the Vietnam War, many younger veterans have seen the Department of Defense utilize far greater outsourcing, in conflict zones and at home. Some may think that privatization of some government functions is a good idea and find the idea of Choice personally appealing.

As Stephen Trynosky notes in "Beyond the Iron Triangle," fewer younger veterans are signing up with old-line outfits like the Legion or VFW. As a result, traditional VSOs have lost significant membership as older veterans have died off. Newer organizations like Wounded Warrior and IAVA have gained media attention and some political influence without the same focus on building membership or providing services. In addition, their aggressive fund-raising has put them in thrall to corporate donors, including some potential beneficiaries of VHA privatization. As Trynosky reveals, both "TriWest and United Healthcare provide significant financial support to several newer veterans organizations, most notably IAVA."[39]

Among the older veterans' organizations, there is definitely a desire to stay on the good side of President Trump and his Republican allies in Congress. Because of their longtime inside-the-Beltway orientation, they can be very cautious about offending legislators or losing "a seat at the table." One former VSO staffer confided that his group and others are terrified that, with one tweet, Trump could mobilize conservative veterans and "bury us." Another, still working inside the Beltway, argued that "we have to be moderate and middle of the road" to accomplish broader organizational goals. A third VSO leader expressed strong personal opposition to VHA privatization, in any form. But, he acknowledged, if his particular subgroup of veterans (and VHA patients) was shielded from outsourcing, his organization would go along to get along. This will just have to play out, he told me, while admitting that "a lot of people will get hurt in the process."

Those most likely to "get hurt"—who have suffered the real wounds of war and of preparing for war—are not always capable of being public advocates on their own behalf. Over and over again, I have been struck by how fragile and vulnerable many VHA patients are. The very old, mentally ill, or physically weak among them will not be joining "Save the VA" protest rallies or picket lines. Homeless veterans, struggling to survive on the street, aren't likely to dash off an e-mail voicing their objections to budget cuts or proposed legislation affecting programs that assist them. Like most Americans, many veterans I met in VHA hospitals or clinics, at a campus veterans' center, or a homeless shelter weren't familiar with the name of their member of Congress (although activists among them certainly were knowledgeable and engaged constituents).

In my previous book about the VHA, I quoted a moving letter by an Iraq veteran (whom I did not name, at his request) who recounted being rescued from PTSD, alcoholism, and suicide. "There is no private health-care provider office that can offer me this type of care," he wrote to the Commission on Care. "So just fix our VA because it belongs to us, not the private sector." When I originally posted his letter on my blog, also preserving his anonymity, his wife informed me that he was dismayed to discover that his message had become a public document. When the letter writer and I finally talked by phone directly, he was outraged about Capitol Hill threats to the VA. At the same time, he couldn't imagine becoming more active in the defense of an institution that had saved his life. "I am tired of fighting," he told me. "I've already fought too long."

Not Just a Veterans' Issue

This veteran's story illustrates why it's so important that other VHA patients, their caregivers, and all concerned citizens join forces, as many have begun to do. In the Bay Area, for example, veterans and VHA staff formed the campaign group FFVHC. Its members (and I'm among them) have analyzed and critiqued pending legislation, while proposing measures that would strengthen and improve VHA programs. FFVHC created a website, which features video testimonials from veterans about the care they have received. The group designed "Save Our VA" and "I Love My VA" bumper stickers and has distributed thousands of them to veterans and their families at union halls, VHA cafeterias, and gatherings of traditional veterans' service organizations.

FFVHC has collaborated with like-minded groups both old and new, including Swords to Plowshares, the network known as Veterans for Peace, and the more recently formed VoteVets. In April 2017, FFVHC and Swords cosponsored a town hall meeting in San Francisco attended by 250 veterans, their caregivers, and elected officials like Congresswoman Nancy Pelosi. This anti-privatization protest became a model for similar rallies in other cities. AFGE has also held dozens of rallies across the country demanding more staffing for the VA and asking the public to join union members to save the VA.

This fight for veterans' health care needs the support of everyone concerned about US military and foreign policy, health care reform, or the future of our democracy. Liberals and progressives fighting for some form of national healthcare in the US and resisting privatization of public education, repeal of workplace and environmental protections, deregulation of Wall Street, and the erosion of retirement security must realize that eliminating the VHA is part of that same antigovernment agenda. Instead, I've discovered that even strong believers in government as an instrument for social progress and a force for the public good have been swayed by corporate media coverage of veterans' affairs.

"Most health care activists don't know much about the VHA and have no idea about the high quality of care it delivers," says Jason Kelley, a member of Physicians for a National Health Program who cares for veterans in northern New England. "Their views on what's going on in the Canadian or European health care systems are very up to date, but when it comes to the VA, they are closer to the public's outdated attitudes. When it comes to fighting to save America's only single-payer system, even dedicated single-payer activists aren't giving the issue much thought."

When I began this book project, my own ill-informed perspective was not much different, despite some hands-on experience as an outside consultant at one VHA hospital in California. Until I became immersed in the world of veterans' health care, I had little feel for the complex problems of its unique patient population. My grasp of the breadth and depth of VHA caregiver expertise was very limited. Nor did I fully appreciate the extraordinary sense of mission—of serving a higher cause—that motivates so many VHA caregivers like Kelley.

Bending to prevailing White House winds after January 2017 and reflecting his own private-industry background, VA Secretary Shulkin argued that veterans' care could be improved through competition between the VHA and private providers and among VHA medical centers themselves. When I hear such claims, what first comes to mind is the damage that market competition and health care industry restructuring have already done to patient–provider interaction and the quality of care in private medical practice (e.g., huge patient panels, the ten-minute office visit, etc.). Yet Phil Roe, Republican chairman of the House Committee on Veterans' Affairs and a doctor himself, is very intent on getting the VHA to increase the workloads of staff physicians and mental health professionals, so they see as many patients as primary care providers and therapists do in the private sector, a standard of care that is lower, not higher.

The VHA today—but not for long, if its adversaries succeed—is a community of caring. Its patient–provider relationships stand in stark contrast to those reshaped by fragmented, fee-for-service medicine, which too often leaves patients and caregivers alike dismayed and demoralized. The VHA's patient-driven model is not based on the cold, instrumental calculations of the marketplace. It provides solidarity, support, and a safe haven for sick and wounded people, who, in large numbers, come through the door frightened, angry, suspicious—even dangerous—but, in the end, leave deeply grateful. Ideological foes of the VHA—and those who would profit from its dismantling—know that for-profit health care can't compete with this. So they have resorted to rigging the game, booby-trapping what works well so it can be discredited and replaced by something that doesn't.

Personally, I have come to view our veterans' health care system as a national treasure. It may have a troubled past and been tarnished by local failings in recent years and require repair. As a federal agency currently endangered by powerful opponents of its basic mission, it's certainly not alone in the Trump era, which is all the more reason for all Americans—who have made a huge investment in the VHA as taxpayers and reaped unheralded rewards from that investment—to help save it from the wrecking ball. If public provision of veterans' health care does survive attempted privatization by the Right, all of us in need of a better health care system model will benefit from this inspiring victory. And then maybe "Medicare for All" will become more achievable too and, perhaps someday, a stepping-stone to something even better (also known as "VA Care for All").

I proudly display a "Save Our VA" bumper sticker on my car—and urge others to do so as well—because it provides an urgent reminder of our collective stake in the outcome of this struggle. I've been privileged to participate in this fight, even though I am not a veteran myself and no one in my family currently relies on the VHA for employment or health care. (My daughter, a Yale-trained nurse-practitioner, did spend a post-graduate year providing primary care for veterans, an experience that has greatly informed her subsequent career as a health care reform advocate in Vermont and specialist in geriatric care.) Providing the high-quality care that was promised to men and women who were drafted into—or volunteered for—military service is a societal obligation that should be equitably shared, even as we try to curb overseas conflicts that so tragically add to VHA patient loads.

As a patient myself, I have discovered belatedly (while researching this book) the personal benefits of VHA-sponsored medical research. I have the VA to thank for my shingles vaccine, and if I ever need an implantable cardiac pacemaker, I will thank it once again. I regularly use a VA-developed PTSD smartphone app; I sometimes fall asleep with assistance from its CBT-for-insomnia app. I was persuaded to try mindful meditation after observing how veterans of all ages and conditions benefited from learning this practice at the VHA. As a longtime researcher, writer, and consultant about patient safety and health care teamwork, I now appreciate how clinical rotations at the VHA have better prepared thousands of doctors, nurses, and other health care professionals for their later work throughout the industry.

Several years ago, when I was visiting the VA Medical Center in West Haven, Connecticut, where my daughter worked, I joined a meeting with visiting staff from the UK's National Health Service. The assembled British doctors, nurses, psychologists, social workers, and administrators had just trooped through one of the most prestigious teaching hospitals in the United States, the nearby Yale New Haven medical center. They were clearly grappling with the contradictions of what they had just seen. At a well-endowed institution, patients arrived in the emergency room with no insurance, they were discharged prematurely, medical specialists commanded huge salaries unheard of in their own country, primary care seemed undervalued, interprofessional training was spotty, caregivers of all kinds had no union voice, and coordination of care was, well, not exactly "world class."

And then the UK delegation toured the veterans' hospital just a few miles away from Yale New Haven. As they sat with VHA caregivers afterward, asking questions and exchanging information in a government-issue conference room, the same realization sank in: they had finally landed in a system—an actual system in the United States—that worked much like their own back home. One doctor finally asked the question on every visitor's mind. "Why," he wondered out loud, "do you have to be a military veteran to get this level of care in America? Why isn't it available to all Americans?" Why indeed.

EPILOGUE

Thank You for Your Service?

In June 2017, the White House held a signing ceremony for the VA Accountability and Whistleblower Protection Act, attended by secretary of veterans affairs David Shulkin.[1] The act, which he supported, weakened due process rights within the Department of Veterans Affairs, leading to the dismissal of hundreds of housekeepers, nursing assistants, or cafeteria workers, rather than, as intended, any top administrators guilty of wrongdoing.[2] At this event, President Trump assured Shulkin that he would never hear the words "You're fired!" like so many failed contestants did on Trump's reality TV show, *The Apprentice*.

Less than a year later, in March 2018, Shulkin learned of his own firing via a presidential tweet. As the *New York Times* noted, the Trump administration appointees behind this decision "had ties to the Koch Brothers and a group they . . . called Concerned Veterans of America."[3] The VA secretary helped pave the way for his own political downfall when he took a taxpayer-funded junket overseas with his wife and a large entourage; the VA's own inspector general found that the trip involved "serious derelictions" of duty and, of course, generated bad publicity for the agency.[4] But, once Shulkin was out of office, he became a helpful whistleblower himself. In a *New York Times* Op Ed piece, he predicted that outsourcing of care, on the scale favored by the Kochs and CVA, would overwhelm the private sector. VA privatization, he argued, is "aimed at rewarding select people and companies with profits, even if it undermines care for veterans."[5]

Trump's next personnel move at the VA rewarded the White House medical director for giving him with a clean bill of health after his annual physical. Dr. Ronny L. Jackson, the administration's first proposed replacement for Shulkin, assured the press that Trump was in great shape despite his poor diet, lack of exercise, and excess poundage.[6] ("I can't think of a more perfect puppet," one veterans' leader told me, when I asked about Jackson's nomination.) Although the Navy doctor lacked any experience relevant to running the federal government's second-largest agency, the question of his qualifications for that job soon became moot amid damaging reports of professional misconduct in his current position.[7]

Meanwhile, Trump appointed an undersecretary of defense, Robert Wilkie, to replace Shulkin on an interim basis. Wilkie served as a DOD official under the Bush administration and has been a staff member for conservative senators Trent Lott, Thom Tillis, and Jesse Helms. As acting VA secretary, he quickly issued a press release titled "Debunking the VA Privatization Myth." There was, Wilkie said, "no effort to privatize the VA, and to suggest otherwise is completely false and a red herring designed to distract and avoid honest debate on the real issues surrounding Veteran's health care."[8] In another press statement, however, Wilkie suggested that the way to address one veteran's complaint about the cleanliness of a VA facility in Salt Lake City was to outsource more care to the private sector.[9]

During this period of post-Shulkin leadership turmoil and uncertainty, I began to hear from many stressed out, overworked, or demoralized VA caregivers; often, they were making plans to retire or seek work elsewhere because of deteriorating working conditions and plummeting morale. In an interview with the *New York Times*, the American Legion's Louis Celli confirmed there was a "corrosive culture building" within the VA. "What we're hearing, by and large, from the rank-and-file employees is that this is the worst it has ever been."[10]

While Wilkie awaited Senate confirmation of his nomination to permanently replace Shulkin, he and other Trump administration officials made matters worse by securing bipartisan passage of the VA Mission Act in late May 2018. Backed by the Legion and other VSOs—plus their AstroTurf rival, the CVA—this legislation replaces the federal government's four-year-old experiment with Veterans' Choice. "The Choice program has been a wreck," admitted Senator Jon Tester (D-Montana). "Every veteran up here will tell you that." Nevertheless, Tester and his colleagues went ahead and expanded VHA outsourcing, under new rules. According to Tester, "the best defense against any effort to privatize the VA . . . is to make sure the VA lives up to its promise."[11]

Simply maintaining the system of veterans' care described in this book—much less achieving its full potential—will become more difficult under the Mission Act. The Congressional Budget Office estimates that the total cost of its implementation will be $46 to $50 billion over five years. The act enables veterans to seek almost unlimited care from walk-in clinics without a referral, thus fragmenting the VHA's integrated care model and creating vast new opportunities for privatizers such as the Cohen Veterans Network. It also takes the positive step of making older veterans, from all eras, eligible for financial assistance for home-based care by their family members. However, that much-needed expansion of coverage came with no additional earmarked funding for the agency's caregiver support program—not even for additional oversight staff. So all the new mandated spending on "community care"—whether outsourced to private sector providers or taking the form of family caregiver subsidies—could occur at the expense of existing VHA programs. The result would be insufficient money to fill thousands of hospital or clinic job vacancies or pay for infrastructure repair.

The Mission Act greatly increases the administrative and clinical burdens already created by Choice since 2014. VHA staff will now be asked to set up more outside appointments for veterans and coordinate care with their often uncooperative private sector providers. Nothing in the new law requires that outside providers receive any special training to qualify as caregivers for complex veterans.

Meanwhile, siphoning off patients, neglecting infrastructure improvements, and leaving the VHA understaffed in a way that adversely affects the quality of its care will generate more pressure for facility closings.

The Mission Act contains a major tool for achieving that objective. It authorizes the appointment of a nine-member presidential commission on "Asset and Infrastructure Realignment." The commission will recommend which VHA facilities should be closed and which should be rebuilt or improved. The latter options are likely to get short shrift from an administration already committed to a massive shift toward outsourcing. The commission's decisions are also largely insulated from congressional input.[12]

For this reason and others, a vocal minority on Capitol Hill opposed the Mission Act, despite the veteran organization lobbying on its behalf. Led by Nancy Pelosi, seventy Democrats in the House voted against the VA financing package. According to Pelosi, the Mission Act will facilitate "VA privatization during a time when the Department has zero leadership. By handing the Trump Administration's ideologues and Koch Brothers the keys to an underfunded VA, Republicans are pushing forth their campaign to dismantle veterans' health care."[13] Only a handful of Senators joined the former chairman of the Senate veterans affairs committee when he voted no. According to Bernie Sanders, the Mission Act does "nothing to fill the vacancies at the VA. . . . My fear is that this bill will open the door to the draining, year after year, of much-needed resources for the VA."[14]

Two days after passage of the act, President Trump took aim again at one of the main sources of opposition to VA privatization—namely, union members. He issued a series of executive orders, very much in the spirit of the VA Accountability Act, designed to weaken the labor organizations, which bargain for federal workers and provide day-to-day representation on the job.

After signing the Mission Act on June 6, 2016, President Trump further rattled the saber of his executive authority. He issued a signing statement asserting that he alone had the right to determine the composition of the Asset and Infrastructure Realignment Commission created by the act. The legislation specifies that its members include several VSO representatives. Trump would be happy to replace them with health care industry executives who would benefit from VA privatization. He also asserted his authority over the creation of pilot programs that could send more veterans to private sector care.[15] Of greater concern, the White House opposed a bipartisan effort to fund the new legislation, arguing for cuts in other VA or federal spending instead. Congressman Tim Walz, who voted against the act, reported a "stark picture of a VA forced to cannibalize itself in order to pay for private care."[16]

The defense of veterans' care is, thus, turning out to be a series of skirmishes, on multiple fronts, in a long political war. The momentum at the moment definitely favors those who do *not* view the VA as a national treasure. As always, divide and conquer is a big part of the so-far winning strategy of the agency's powerful detractors and would-be dismantlers. Hopefully, veterans and their organizations, VA patients and their families, VA caregivers and their unions, plus their real political allies, will display greater unity and common purpose in the future. Under a different Congress and a better president, there will be new opportunities to keep health, healing, and the giving of hope in the hands of those who truly care about veterans.

NOTES

Introduction

1. The federal Department of Veterans Affairs (VA) employs people engaged in providing direct health care services *and* processing claims for veterans' pension, health care, and burial benefits. Direct care is the work of the VHA—the Veterans Health Administration, the largest of three VA subdivisions, which employs a staff of three hundred thousand, the bulk of the VA's total workforce. However, when VHA patients and providers refer to the agency that cares for or employs them, they both generally use the abbreviation "VA," rather than the more specific "VHA." Because the bureaucratic distinction is important, as noted later in this introduction, I have opted for using "VHA" as much as possible when the subject matter is health care and "VA" when referring to the overall agency, with its cabinet-level director and other, non–health care functions, like making benefit determinations and maintaining cemeteries. Any quotes in this book by a person using "VA" when he or she was actually referring to the VHA have been left in their original form. After several years immersed in VA circles, even I have a tendency to use the two abbreviations interchangeably in everyday conversation, as the text of this book sometimes reflects.

2. This is a pseudonym. For the rest of the book, an asterisk indicates a pseudonym, used in cases where the veteran requested anonymity.

3. US Department of Veterans Affairs, Office of the Inspector General, Veterans Health Administration, "Review of Alleged Patient Deaths, Patient Wait Times, and Scheduling Practices at the Phoenix VA Health Care System," August 26, 2014, https://www.va.gov/oig/pubs/VAOIG-14-02603-267.pdf.

4. Few media reports highlighted the fact the Phoenix VA is flooded with over twenty-five thousand snowbird veterans who fly in for three or four months and then leave when the snow starts melting. It is a real challenge to staff hospitals and clinics serving such a transient population.

5. Phillip Longman, *Best Care Anywhere: Why VA Health Care Would Work Better for Everyone* (San Francisco: Barrett-Koehler, 2012).

6. RAND Corporation, Assessment B (Health Care Capabilities), September 1, 2015, https://www.va.gov/opa/choiceact/documents/assessments/assessment_b_health_care_capabilities.pdf.

7. Dave Philipps, "In Unit Stalked by Suicide, Veterans Try to Save One Another," *New York Times*, September 19, 2015, https://www.nytimes.com/2015/09/20/us/marine-battalion-veterans-scarred-by-suicides-turn-to-one-another-for-help.html.

8. Dave Philipps, "At Veterans Hospital in Oregon, a Push for Better Ratings Puts Patients at Risk, Doctors Say," January 1, 2018, https://www.nytimes.com/2018/01/01/us/at-veterans-hospital-in-oregon-a-push-for-better-ratings-puts-patients-at-risk-doctors-say.html.

9. Fox News, "Opioid Crisis Takes Heavy Toll on US Veterans," http://www.foxnews.com/health/2017/11/10/opioid-abuse-crisis-takes-heavy-toll-on-us-veterans.html.

10. Scott Bronstein, Nelli Black, and Drew Griffin, "Veterans Dying Because of Health Care Delays," CNN, January 30, 2014, http://www.cnn.com/2014/01/30/health/veterans-dying-health-care-delays/index.html.

11. Jonathan Saltzman and Andrea Estes, "At a Four-Star Veterans' Hospital: Care Gets 'Worse and Worse,'" *Boston Globe* Spotlight, July 15, 2017, https://www.bostonglobe.com/metro/2017/07/15/four-star-case-failure-manchester/n9VV7BerswvkL5akCgNzvK/story.html.

12. Allison Jaslow, "Cultural Change Needed at VA to Support Women Veterans," *Philadelphia Inquirer*, June 6, 2017.

13. Cary W. Akins, "Keeping Our Promise to Veterans," *Boston Globe*, September 1, 2017, https://www.bostonglobe.com/opinion/2017/09/01/keeping-promise-veterans/7JrLUswmpPNk8bf9c4PdgL/story.html.

14. Nicholas Fandos, "With Fight on Health Law Stalled, Conservatives Turn to Veterans Care," *New York Times*, November 10, 2017, A18, https://www.nytimes.com/2017/11/09/us/politics/obamacare-veterans-affairs-koch-brothers-health.html.

15. David Shulkin, Shereef Elnahal, Ellen Maddock, and Megan Shaheen, *Best Care Everywhere* (Washington, DC: US Department of Veterans Affairs, 2017), xi.

16. Joe Davidson, "VA in 'Critical Condition, Requires Intensive Care,' but Improving, Says Boss," *Washington Post*, May 31, 2017, https://www.washingtonpost.com/news/powerpost/wp/2017/05/31/va-in-critical-condition-requires-intensive-care-but-improving-says-boss/?utm_term=.0230d9e9356b.

17. Dennis Wagner, "Arizona-Based VA Contractor Collected 'Tens of Millions' in Overpayments, Federal Audit Says," *Arizona Republic*, November 13, 2017, https://www.azcentral.com/story/news/local/arizona-investigations/2017/11/13/va-inspectors-question-millions-dollars-paid-triwest-veterans-healthcare-contract/737341001/.

18. Dave Philipps and Nicholas Fandos, "New Veterans Affairs Chief: A Hands-On Risk Taking 'Standout,'" *New York Times*, May 9, 2017, https://www.nytimes.com/2017/05/09/us/politics/new-veterans-affairs-chief-a-hands-on-risk-taking-standout.html. For another view of optometry services in the malls of America see Suzanne Gordon, "VHA Must Not Outsource to LensCrafters," *Beyond Chron*, May 30, 2017, http://www.beyondchron.org/vha-must-not-outsource-lenscrafters/.

19. As Phillip Longman reports in *Best Care Anywhere*, the VHA was the first US health care system to develop and implement health care information technology that connects

all of its far-flung facilities to one another. Its user-friendly system for electronic medical record keeping and sharing created a new industry standard still not being met by some of the private-sector firms that veterans would be turned over to if VHA privatization succeeds. Longman, *Best Care Anywhere*, 23–44.

20. Rajiv Leventhal, "Report: VA-Cerner EHR Contract to Be Awarded within 30 Days," *Healthcare Informatics*, October 2, 2017, https://www.healthcare-informatics.com/news-item/ehr/report-va-cerner-ehr-contract-be-awarded-within-30-days-0.

21. House Veterans Affairs Committee, US Department of Veterans Affairs Budget Request for Fiscal Year 2019, February 15, 2018, https://veterans.house.gov/calendar/eventsingle.aspx?EventID=2041.

22. Rajiv Jain, "Not the Usual Suspects," in *Collaborative Caring: Stories and Reflections on Teamwork in Healthcare*, ed. Suzanne Gordon, David Feldman, and Michael Leonard (Ithaca, NY: Cornell University Press, 2014), 229–34.

23. Rebecca Shunk, "Coaching the Huddle," in Gordon, Feldman, and Leonard, *Collaborative Caring*, 145–48.

24. For an assessment of the VA's own expanded whistle-blower protection and complaint investigation office, created by Trump administration executive order in April 2018, see Donovan Slack, "New VA Office Gets Mixed Reviews," *USA Today*, January 18, 2018, 3A, https://www.pressreader.com/usa/usa-today-us-edition/20180118/281492161729954.

25. Suzanne Gordon, *The Battle for Veterans' Healthcare: Dispatches from the Frontlines of Policy Making and Patient Care* (Ithaca, NY: Cornell Publishing, 2017).

26. Brie Zeltner, "Cleveland Clinic Faces $650,000 Fines for Marymount Hospital Lab Violations; Patients in 'Immediate Jeopardy,' CMS Says," September 11, 2015. http://www.cleveland.com/healthfit/index.ssf/2015/09/cleveland_clinic_faces_600000.html.

27. Christine Kern, "HHS Fines Hospitals with Highest Infection Rates," Health IT Outcomes, https://www.healthitoutcomes.com/doc/hhs-fines-hospitals-with-highest-infection-rates-0001.

28. Eric Heisig, "Cleveland Clinic to Pay $1.6 Million to Federal Government to Settle Accusations over Heart Procedures," Cleveland.com, February 17, 2016, http://www.cleveland.com/court-justice/index.ssf/2016/02/cleveland_clinic_to_pay_16_mil.html.

29. US Department of Veterans Affairs, Veterans Benefits Administration, https://www.benefits.va.gov/benefits/.

30. US Department of Veterans Affairs, Veterans Benefits Administration Reports, Claims Backlog, accessed December 1, 2017, https://www.benefits.va.gov/reports/mmwr_va_claims_backlog.asp.

31. US Department of Veterans Affairs, Office of Research & Development, "The Million Veteran Program," https://www.research.va.gov/mvp/.

32. US Department of Veterans Affairs, Office of Research & Development, "Timeline of Accomplishments," accessed November 29, 2017, https://www.research.va.gov/about/history.cfm.

33. US Department of Veterans Affairs, Office of Research & Development, "VA Research News Briefs," accessed November 29, 2017, https://www.research.va.gov/in_brief.cfm.

34. Suzanne Gordon, "Will Trump Jeopardize VA Prostate Cancer Research?," *Beyond Chron*, January 3, 2017, http://www.beyondchron.org/will-trump-jeopardize-va-prostate-research/.

35. Justice for Vets, "What Is a Veterans' Treatment Court?," https://justiceforvets.org/what-is-a-veterans-treatment-court/.

36. At the risk of being a nitpicker, I try to avoid the use of the term "health care system" to refer to health care as it is delivered in the United States. Many years ago, Walter Cronkite stated that "America's health care system is neither healthy, caring, nor a system." See https://www.goodreads.com/quotes/74350-america-s-health-care-system-is-neither-healthy-caring-nor-a.

1. Promises Broken and Kept

1. Richard Severo and Lewis Milford, *The Wages of War: When America's Soldiers Came Home—from Valley Forge to Vietnam* (New York: Simon & Schuster, 1989).

2. Severo and Milford, 64–79.

3. Abraham Lincoln, "Second Inaugural Address," March 4, 1865, http://www.bartleby.com/124/pres32.html.

4. Severo and Milford, *Wages of War*, 129.

5. Severo and Milford, 130.

6. US Department of Veterans Affairs, "About VA," http://www.va.gov/about_va/vahistory.asp.

7. US Department of Veterans Affairs, "VA History in Brief," 12, https://www.va.gov/opa/publications/archives/docs/history_in_brief.pdf.

8. Severo and Milford, *Wages of War*, 275.

9. Severo and Milford, 267–79.

10. Severo and Milford, 278.

11. Wikipedia, s.v. "Bonus Army," last modified January 31, 2018, https://en.wikipedia.org/wiki/Bonus_Army.

12. US Department of Veterans Affairs, "VA History in Brief."

13. US Department of Veterans Affairs, "Veterans," http://www.benefits.va.gov/persona/veteran-vietnam.asp.

14. Severo and Milford, *Wages of War*, 347–71.

15. Severo and Milford, 356.

16. Phillip Longman, *Best Care Anywhere: Why VA Health Care Would Work Better for Everyone* (San Francisco: Barrett-Koehler, 2012), 18–22.

17. US Department of Veterans Affairs, "Vet Center Program," http://www.vetcenter.va.gov/About_US.asp.

18. Longman, *Best Care Anywhere*, 23–44.

19. George Timson, "The History of the Hardhats," accessed July 14, 2016, http://www.hardhats.org/history/hardhats.html.

20. Longman, *Best Care Anywhere*, 47.

21. Bill McAllister, "VA Hospitals Face Competition under Clinton Proposal," *Washington Post*, September 18, 1993, http://articles.latimes.com/1993-09-18/news/mn-36483_1_clinton-health.

22. Kenneth W. Kizer, foreword to *The Battle for Veterans' Healthcare: Dispatches from the Frontlines of Policy Making and Patient Care*, by Suzanne Gordon (Ithaca, NY: Cornell Publishing, 2017).

23. Kenneth W. Kizer, "Vision for Change: A Plan to Restructure the Veterans Health Administration," March 17, 1995, https://www.va.gov/HEALTHPOLICYPLANNING/VISION/2CHAP1.pdf.

24. Kenneth W. Kizer, "Healthcare Not Hospitals: Transforming the Veterans Health Administration," in *Straight from the CEO*, by Price Waterhouse Cooper (New York: Fireside, 1998), 117.

25. Barbara Starfield, Thomas A. Parrino, Elwood Headley, Carol Ashton, and Kenneth Kizer, *Primary Care in VA Primer*, Management Decision and Research Center, Health Services Research and Development Service, in collaboration with Foundation for Health Services Research, http://www.hsrd.research.va.gov/publications/internal/pcprim.htm.

26. Institute of Medicine, *To Err Is Human: Building a Safer Health System* (Washington, DC: National Academies, 1999).

27. Lucian L. Leape and Donald M. Berwick, "Five Years after *To Err Is Human*: What Have We Learned?," *JAMA: The Journal of the American Medical Association* 293, no. 19 (2005): 2386.

28. Longman, *Best Care Anywhere*, 56.

29. David Stires, "Technology Has Transformed the VA," *Fortune*, May 11, 2006, http://archive.fortune.com/magazines/fortune/fortune_archive/2006/05/15/8376846/index.htm.

30. "The Best Medical Care in the US," *Bloomberg Businessweek*, July 16, 2006, https://www.va.gov/opa/choiceact/documents/assessments/assessment_b_health_care_capabilities.pdf.

31. Amy C. Edmondson, Brian R. Golden, and Gary J. Young, "Turnaround at the Veterans Health Administration (A)," Harvard Business School Case 608-061, *Harvard Business Review*, July 2007 (revised January 2008), http://www.hbs.edu/faculty/Pages/item.aspx?num=34818.

32. US Department of Veterans Affairs, "Health Benefits," https://www.va.gov/healthbenefits/apply/veterans.asp.

33. US Department of Veterans Affairs, "Health Benefits."

34. US Department of Veterans Affairs, "Health Benefits: Priority Groups," https://www.va.gov/healthbenefits/resources/priority_groups.asp.

2. Those Who Have Borne the Battle

1. Which makes it particularly tragic that VA secretary David Shulkin has proposed eliminating comprehensive hearing care in the VHA.

2. Patricia Murphy, "The Weight of War: Soldiers' Heavy Gear Packs on Pain," NPR, March 12, 2011, http://www.npr.org/2011/04/10/134421473/weight-of-war-soldiers-heavy-gear-packs-on-pain.

3. Stephen W. Marshall, Michelle Canham-Chervak, Esther O. Dada, and Bruce H. Jones, "Military Injuries," in *The Burden of Musculoskeletal Diseases in the United States*, http://www.boneandjointburden.org/2013-report/military-injuries/vi5.

4. Robin L. Toblin, Phillip J. Quartana, Lyndon A. Riviere, Kristina Clarke Walper, and Charles W. Hoge, "Chronic Pain and Opioid Use in US Soldiers after Combat Deployment," *JAMA Internal Medicine* 174, no. 8 (2014): 1400–1401, doi: 10.1001/jamainternmed.2014.2726, http://jamanetwork.com/journals/jamainternalmedicine/fullarticle/1885986.

5. Annette M. Boyle, "Research Finds Unexpectedly High Rates of Pain, Opioid Use in Recently Deployed Soldiers," *U.S. Medicine*, September 2014, http://www.usmedicine.com/agencies/department-of-defense-dod/research-finds-unexpectedly-high-rates-of-pain-opioid-use-in-recently-deployed-soldiers/.

6. US Department of Veterans Affairs, "Veterans Diseases Associated with Agent Orange," accessed April 27, 2017, https://www.publichealth.va.gov/exposures/agentorange/conditions/.

7. US Department of Veterans Affairs, "Gulf War Veterans' Medically Unexplained Illnesses," accessed April 27, 2017, https://www.publichealth.va.gov/exposures/gulfwar/medically-unexplained-illness.asp.

8. Joseph Hickman, *The Burn Pits: The Poisoning of America's Soldiers* (New York: Hot Books, 2016), 31.

9. RAND Corporation, "Special Feature: The Cost and Quality of VA Mental Health Services," http://www.rand.org/health/feature/veterans-mental-health.html.

10. Veterans Administration, "VA Mental Health Care Fact Sheet," accessed April 2016, http://www.mentalhealth.va.gov/suicide_prevention/.

11. RAND Corporation, *Veterans Health Administration Mental Health Program Evaluation*, Capstone Report, 2011, 26, http://www.rand.org/content/dam/rand/pubs/technical_reports/2011/RAND_TR956.pdf.

12. David Finkel, *Thank You for Your Service* (New York: Farrar, Straus and Giroux, 2013).

13. Veterans Administration, "Military Sexual Trauma," accessed August 1, 2016, http://www.mentalhealth.va.gov/msthome.asp.

14. "Military Sexual Trauma," *PTSD Research Quarterly* 20, no. 2 (Spring 2009), http://www.ptsd.va.gov/professional/newsletters/research-quarterly/v20n2.pdf.

15. Monica Roy, "Healthcare for Women Military Veterans," in *The Praeger Handbook of Veterans' Health: History, Challenges, Issues, and Developments*, ed. Thomas W. Miller (Santa Barbara, CA: Praeger), 126–27.

16. M. A. Reger, D. J. Smolenski, N. A. Skopp, M. J. Metzger-Abamukang, H. K. Kang, T. A. Bullman, S. Perdue, and G. A. Gahm, "Risk of Suicide among US Military Service Members following Operation Enduring Freedom or Operation Iraqi Freedom Deployment and Separation from the Military," *JAMA Psychiatry* 72, no. 6 (2015): 561–69, doi: 10.1001/jamapsychiatry.2014.3195, https://www.ncbi.nlm.nih.gov/pubmed/25830941.

17. Sally C. Curtin, Margaret Warner, and Holly Hedegaard, "Increase in Suicide in the United States, 1999–2014," National Center for Health Statistics Brief Number 241, April 2016, 1, http://www.cdc.gov/nchs/data/databriefs/db241.pdf.

18. Sabrina Tavernise, "US Suicide Rate Surges to a 30-Year High," *New York Times*, April 22, 2016, http://www.nytimes.com/2016/04/22/health/us-suicide-rate-surges-to-a-30-year-high.html?_r=0.

19. Sally C. Curtin, Margaret Warner, and Holly Hedegaard, "Increase in Suicide in the United States 1999–2014," NCHS Data Brief, No. 241, April 2016, https://www.cdc.gov/nchs/data/databriefs/db241.pdf.

20. US Department of Veterans Affairs, Office of Suicide Prevention, "Suicide among Veterans and Other Americans," August 3, 2016, https://www.mentalhealth.va.gov/docs/2016suicidedatareport.pdf.

21. Commonwealth Club of San Francisco, "Art and Soul of Combat," Podcast, November 1, 2013, https://www.commonwealthclub.org/events/archive/podcast/art-and-soul-combat-veterans.

22. Gerry Everding, "Military Service Changes Personality, Makes Vets Less Agreeable," *Source*, Washington University in St. Louis, February 9, 2012, https://source.wustl.edu/2012/02/military-service-changes-personality-makes-vets-less-agreeable/.

23. J. J. Jackson, F. Thoemmes, K. Jonkmann, and U. Trautwein, "Military Training and Personality Trait Development: Does the Military Make the Man, or Does the Man Make the Military?" *Psychological Science* 20, no. 10 (2012): 1–8, http://www.human.cornell.edu/hd/qml/upload/Jackson_Thoemmes_2012.pdf.

24. Everding, "Military Service."

25. Anthony Swofford, *Jarhead: A Marine's Chronicle of the Gulf War and Other Battles* (New York: Scribner, 2003), 28.

26. Military Authority, US Army, "The Infantryman's Creed," http://www.militaryauthority.com/wiki/military-creeds/us-army-the-infantrymans-creed.html.

27. Erin P. Finley, *Fields of Combat: Understanding PTSD among Veterans of Iraq and Afghanistan* (Ithaca, NY: Cornell University Press, 2011), 83.

28. Jonathan Shay, *Achilles in Vietnam: Combat Trauma and the Undoing of Character* (Simon & Schuster, 1995), 53.

29. "Parris Island Hazing Scandal: Three Marines Face Court-Martial," *Marine Corps Times*, December 13, 2016, http://www.marinecorpstimes.com/search/hazing+scandal+parris+island/?q=hazing+scandal+parris+island.

30. J. L. Thomas, J. E. Wilk, L. A. Riviere, D. McGurk, C. A. Castro, and C. W. Hoge, "Prevalence of Mental Health Problems and Functional Impairment among Active Component

and National Guard Soldiers 3 and 12 Months following Combat in Iraq," *Archives of General Psychiatry* 67, no. 6 (2010): 614–23, doi: 10.1001/archgenpsychiatry.2010.54, https://www.ncbi.nlm.nih.gov/pubmed/20530011.

31. M. Jakupcak, D. Conybeare, L. Phelps, S. Hunt, H. A. Holmes, B. Felker, M. Klevens, and M. E. McFall, "Anger, Hostility, and Aggression among Iraq and Afghanistan War Veterans Reporting PTSD and Subthreshold PTSD," *Journal of Traumatic Stress* 20, no. 6 (2007): 945–54.

32. Shay, *Achilles in Vietnam*; Jonathan Shay, *Odysseus in America: Combat Trauma and the Trials of Homecoming* (New York: Scribner, 2002).

33. Shay, *Odysseus in America*, 4.

34. Shay, *Odysseus in America*, 240.

35. Shay, *Odysseus in America*, 21–22.

36. US Army, "The Army Values," accessed July 26, 2016, http://www.army.mil/values/.

3. Primary Care the Way It Should Be

1. Institute of Medicine, *Crossing the Quality Chasm: A New Health System for the 21st Century* (Washington, DC: National Academies, 2001).

2. Thomas Bodenheimer and Hoangmai H. Pham, "Primary Care Crisis: Current Problems and Proposed Solutions," *Health Affair* 29, no. 5 (2010): 799–805.

3. US Department of Health and Human Services, "Defining the PCMH," Agency for Healthcare Research and Quality, Patient Centered Medical Home Resource Center, accessed October 26, 2016, https://pcmh.ahrq.gov/page/defining-pcmh.

4. Thomas Bodenheimer, "Primary Care: Will It Survive?," *New England Journal of Medicine* 355 (2006): 861–64.

5. Phillip Longman, "First Teach No Harm," *Washington Monthly*, July/August 2013, http://washingtonmonthly.com/magazine/julyaugust-2013/first-teach-no-harm/.

6. Association of American Medical Colleges, "New Research Confirms Looming Physician Shortage," April 5, 2016, https://www.aamc.org/newsroom/newsreleases/458074/2016_workforce_projections_04052016.html.

7. Zitui Song, Vineet Chopra, and Laurence F. McMahon Jr., "Addressing the Primary Care Workforce Crisis," *American Journal of Managed Care* 21, no. 8 (2015): e452–54, https://www.readbyqxmd.com/read/26618225/addressing-the-primary-care-workforce-crisis.

8. Thomas Bodenheimer, Amireh Ghorob, Rachel Willard-Grace, and Kevin Grumbach, "The 10 Building Blocks of High-Performing Primary Care," *Annals of Family Medicine* 12, no. 2 (2014): 166–71, http://www.annfammed.org/content/12/2/166.full.

9. Perspective Roundtable: Redesigning Primary Care, *New England Journal of Medicine*, September 13, 2008, https://www.jhsph.edu/research/centers-and-institutes/johns-hopkins-primary-care-policy-center/Publications_PDFs/A234.pdf.

10. H. P. Rodriguez, L. S. Meredith, A. B. Hamilton, E. M. Yano, and L. V. Rubenstein, "Huddle Up! The Adoption and Use of Structured Team Communication for VA Medical Home Implementation," Research Gate, October 2015, https://www.researchgate.net/publication/263970677_Huddle_up_The_adoption_and_use_of_structured_team_communication_for_VA_medical_home_implementation.

11. Much of this section on huddles comes from the video *How to Huddle: Teaching Teamwork Skills to Improve Patient Safety*, produced by Suzanne Gordon and directed by Edwin Herzog, https://suzannecgordon.com/lectures-and-workshops/how-to-huddle/.

12. US Department of Veterans Affairs, VA Patient Centered Care, https://www.va.gov/patientcenteredcare/.

13. Christopher J. Koenig, Shira Maguen, Aaron Daley, Greg Cohen, and Karen Seal, "Passing the Baton: A Grounded Practical Theory of Handoff Communication between Multidisciplinary Providers in Two Department of Veterans Affairs Outpatient Settings," *Journal of General Internal Medicine* 26, no. 10 (2011): 48.

14. US Department of Veterans Affairs, "VA Research on Diabetes," https://www.research.va.gov/topics/diabetes.cfm; Eve Kerr, "VA System Superior for Diabetes Care," *Issues in Diabetes*, http://www.diabeticmctoday.com/HtmlPages/DMC1004/PDF%20FILES/dmc1004_Kerr.pdf; Association of VA Psychologist Leaders, Fact Sheet Comparison of VA to Community Healthcare, Summary of Research 2000–2016, 2, http://advocacy.avapl.org/pubs/FACT%20sheet%20literature%20review%20of%20VA%20vs%20Community%20Heath%20Care%2003%2023-16.pdf.

15. 18 Reasons, https://18reasons.org/.

16. William R. Miller and Stephen Rollnick, *Motivational Interviewing: Helping People Change* (New York: Guilford, 2013).

4. Healing Minds and Bodies

1. Delilah O. Noronha, "Primary Care–Mental Health Integration," in *The Praeger Handbook of Veteran's Health: History, Challenges, Issues, and Developments*, vol. 3, *Mental Health Treatment and Rehabilitation*, ed. Thomas S. Miller (Santa Barbara, CA: Praeger, 2012), 4.

2. Noronha, "Primary Care," 13–16.

3. US Department of Veterans, Fact Sheet: VA Mental Health Care, July 8, 2016, 3, accessed August 15, 2017, http://www.mentalhealth.va.gov/ http://www.mentalhealth.va.gov/suicide_prevention/.

5. Dealing with a World of Hurt

1. Optum, "Origins of the Opioid Epidemic: Best Intentions Gone Awry," https://www.optum.com/resources/library/origins-opiod-epidemic.html.

2. Johns Hopkins Bloomberg School of Public Health, "The Prescription Opioid Epidemic: An Evidence-Based Approach," November 2015, http://www.jhsph.edu/research/centers-and-institutes/center-for-drug-safety-and-effectiveness/opioid-epidemic-townhall-2015/2015-prescription-opioid-epidemic-report.pdf on 05.02.2016.

3. US Department of Veterans Affairs, "Pain as the Fifth Vital Sign Toolkit," 5, http://www.va.gov/PAINMANAGEMENT/docs/Pain_As_the_5th_Vital_Sign_Toolkit.pdf.

4. R. L. Toblin, P. J. Quartana, L. A. Riviere, K.C. Walper, and C. W. Hoge, "Chronic Pain and Opioid Use in US Soldiers after Combat Deployment," *JAMA Internal Medicine* 174, no. 8 (2014): 1400–1401, doi: 10.1001/jamainternmed.2014.2726, http://jamanetwork.com/journals/jamainternalmedicine/fullarticle/1885986.

5. Annette Boyle, "Research Finds Unexpectedly High Rates of Pain, Opioid Use in Recently Deployed Soldiers," *US Medicine*, September 2014, http://www.usmedicine.com/agencies/department-of-defense-dod/research-finds-unexpectedly-high-rates-of-pain-opioid-use-in-recently-deployed-soldiers/.

6. VHA Pain Management, "Opioid Safety Initiative," https://www.va.gov/PAINMANAGEMENT/Opioid_Safety_Initiative_OSI.asp.

7. US Department of Veterans Affairs, Office of the Inspector General, *Opioid Prescribing to High-Risk Veterans Receiving VA Purchased Care*, Report No. 17-01846-316, July 31, 2017.

8. Adriaan Louw, Kory Zimney, Emilio J. Puentedura, and Ina Diener, "The Efficacy of Pain Neuroscience Education on Musculoskeletal Pain: A Systematic Review of the

Literature," *Physiotherapy: Theory and Practice* 32, no. 5(2016): 332–55, https://www. tandfonline.com/doi/abs/10.1080/09593985.2016.1194646?journalCode=iptp20.

9. Michael Babyak, James A. Blumenthal, Steve Herman, Parinda Khatri, Muraji Doraiswamy, Kathleen Moore, Edward W. Craighead, Teri T. Baldewicz, and K. Ranga Krishnan, "Exercise Treatment for Major Depression: Maintenance of Therapeutic Benefit at 10 Months," *Psychosomatic Medicine* 62 (2000): 633–38, http://www.hibody.co.uk/ Exercise%20treatment%20for%20major%20depression.pdf.

10. Katherine E. Watkins, Harold Alan Pincus, Brad Smith, Susan M. Paddock, Thomas E. Mannle Jr., Abigail Woodroffe, Jake Solomon, et al., *Veterans Health Administration Mental Health Program Evaluation*, Capstone Report, 2011, RAND Health.

6. When Wounded Warriors Are Women

1. Allison Jaslow, Statement of Allison Jaslow, Executive Director of Iraq and Afghanistan Veterans of America, before the Senate Veterans Affairs Committee, May 17, 2017, https://iava.org/wp-content/uploads/2017/07/IAVA-5.17.17.pdf.

2. Allison Jaslow, "Cultural Change Needed at VA to Support Women Veterans," *Philadelphia Inquirer*, June 6, 2017, http://www.philly.com/philly/opinion/commentary/20170605_ Cultural_change_needed_at_VA_to_support_women_veterans.html.

3. Monica Roy, "Healthcare for Women Military Veterans," in *The Praeger Handbook of Veteran's Health: History, Challenges, Issues, and Development*, vol. 2, *Programs of Care Groups with Special Needs*, ed. Thomas Miller (Santa Barbara, CA: Praeger, 2012), 313–17.

4. Paul Harris, "Women in Combat: U.S. Military Officially Lifts Ban on Women Soldiers," *Guardian*, January 25, 2013, https://www.theguardian.com/world/2013/jan/24/us-military-lifts-ban-women-combat.

5. US Department of Veterans Affairs, "Study of Barriers for Women Veterans to VA Healthcare, Final Report," April 2015, 1, https://www.womenshealth.va.gov/ WOMENSHEALTH/docs/Womens%20Health%20Services_Barriers%20to%20Care%20 Final%20Report_April2015.pdf.

6. Roy, "Healthcare for Women," 317.

7. US Department of Veterans Affairs, "Study of Barriers," 3–10.

8. Russell B. Lemle, "Choice Program Expansion Jeopardizes High-Quality VHA Mental Health Services," *Federal Practitioner* 35, no. 3 (March 2018): 18–24, https://www. fedprac-digital.com/federalpractitioner/2018?pg=NaN#pgNaN.

7. Mental Health the Way It Should Be

1. Harold Kudler and Rebecca Porter, "Building Communities of Care for Military Children and Families," *Military Children and Families* 23, no. 2 (2013): 164.

2. Terri Tanielian, Coreen Farris, Caroline Batka, Carrie M. Farmer, Eric Robinson, Charles C. Engel, Michael Robbins, and Lisa H. Jaycox, *Ready to Serve: Community-Based Capacity to Deliver Culturally Competent, Quality Mental Health Care to Veterans and Their Families*, RAND Corporation, 2014, 14–18, http://www.rand.org/content/dam/rand/pubs/ research_reports/RR800/RR806/RAND_RR806.pdf.

3. US Department of Veterans Affairs, VA Caregiver Support, https://www.caregiver. va.gov/support/support_benefits.asp.

4. "Make the Connection," accessed August 1, 2016, http://maketheconnection.net/veterans.

5. Association of VA Psychologist Leaders, "Fact Sheet: Comparison of VA to Community Healthcare; Summary of Research 2000–2016," accessed August 14, 2016, http:// advocacy.avapl.org/pubs/FACT%20sheet%20literature%20review%20of%20VA%20 vs%20Community%20Heath%20Care%2003%2023-16.pdf.

6. Tanielian et al., *Ready to Serve*, 2.

7. Tanielian et al., 11.

8. US Department of Veterans Affairs, Office of Research and Development, "Anthropologists Provide Unique Perspective for VA Studies," May 22, 2014, https://www.research.va.gov/currents/spring2014/spring2014-39.cfm.

9. Elisa J. Sobo, "Anthropologists in the VA: A Generative Force," *Somatosphere*, October 14, 2014, http://somatosphere.net/2014/10/anthropology-goes-public-in-the-va-a-special-issue-of-the-annals-of-anthropological-practice.html.

10. Lizzie Johnson, "Yountville Killings Claim Young, 'Super Smart' PTSD Expert Jennifer Gonzales," *SF Gate*, March 11, 2018. https://www.sfgate.com/bayarea/article/Yountville-killings-claimed-young-super-12743676.php.

11. Elahe Izadi, Dan Lamothe, and Emily Wax-Thibodeaux, "FBI: El Paso Clinic Victim Was VA Doctor Who Had Filed Complaint Against Alleged Killer," *Washington Post*, January 7, 2015, https://www.washingtonpost.com/news/post-nation/wp/2015/01/06/doctor-shot-presumed-shooter-found-dead-at-el-paso-va-clinic/?utm_term=.cff081511b6f.

12. US Attorney's Office, District of Colorado, "Man Who Held Nurse Practitioner Hostage at VA Hospital Charged and Arrested," December 8, 2015, https://www.justice.gov/usao-co/pr/man-who-held-nurse-practioner-hostage-va-hospital-charged-and-arrested.

13. US Department of Veterans Affairs, "Vet Center Program, Eligibility," accessed May 27, 2016, http://www.vetcenter.va.gov/eligibility.asp.

8. Unpacking PTSD

1. Marine Corps Association & Foundation, "The Warrior Ethos," accessed April 30, 2016, https://www.mca-marines.org/gazette/bookreview/warrior-ethos.

2. Jonathan Shay, *Achilles in Vietnam: Combat Trauma and the Undoing of Character* (New York: Scribner, 1994), 5.

3. Truth in advertising: I edited this book for our series at Cornell University Press.

4. Matthew Friedman, "The National Center for PTSD," in *The Praeger Handbook of Veterans Health: History, Challenges, Issues, and Developments*, vol. 4, *Future Directions in Veterans' Healthcare*, ed. Thomas Miller (Santa Barbara, CA: Praeger, 2012), 111–12.

5. Friedman, 102–3.

Profile: Karen Parko

1. US Department of Veterans Affairs, "Epilepsy Centers of Excellence," accessed August 25, 2016, http://www.epilepsy.va.gov/About_the_ECoEs.asp.

9. Returning to Civilian Life

1. National Conference of State Legislators, "Veterans and College: State and Community Roles in Supporting College Completion for Veterans," May 30, 2014, http://www.ncsl.org/research/education/veterans-and-college.aspx.

2. US Department of Veterans Affairs, "VA New York Harbor Health Care System," accessed March 31, 2016, http://www.nyharbor.va.gov/services/vital.asp.

3. VA Campus Toolkit, "What Is the VITAL Initiative?," http://www.mentalhealth.va.gov/studentveteran/vital.asp#sthash.zfBewf5h.dpuf.

10. Suicide Prevention

1. *Crisis Hotline: Veterans Press 1*, directed by Ellen Goosenberg Kent (Burbank, CA: HBO Documentaries, 2013), http://www.hbo.com/documentaries/crisis-hotline-veterans-press-1/synopsis.html.

2. "For Suicidal Veterans, a Frayed Lifeline," editorial, *New York Times*, July 16, 2016, http://www.nytimes.com/2016/07/17/opinion/sunday/for-suicidal-veterans-a-frayed-lifeline.html?_r=0.

3. US Department of Veterans Affairs, Office of Suicide Prevention, "Suicide among Veterans and Other Americans, 2001–2014," August 3, 2016, http://www.mentalhealth.va.gov/docs/2016suicidedatareport.pdf.

4. US Department of Veterans Affairs, "Suicide among Veterans."

5. E. A. Deisenhammer, C.-M. Ing, R. Strauss, G. Kemmler, H. Hinterhuber, and E. M. Weiss, "The Duration of the Suicidal Process: How Much Time Is Left for Intervention between Consideration and Accomplishment of a Suicide Attempt?," *Journal of Clinical Psychiatry* 70, no. 1 (2009): 19–24; T. R. Simon, A. C. Swann, K. E. Powell, L. B. Potter, M. Kresnow, and P. W. O'Carroll, "Characteristics of Impulsive Suicide Attempts and Attempters," *Suicide and Life-Threatening Behavior* 32 (2001): 49–59; C. L. Williams, J. A. Davidson, and I. Montgomery, "Impulsive Suicidal Behavior," *Journal of Clinical Psychology* 36, no. 1 (1980): 90–94.

6. S. B. Vyrostek, J. L. Annest, and G. W. Ryan, "Surveillance for Fatal and Nonfatal Injuries—United States, 2001," *MMWR Surveillance Summaries* 53 (2004): 1–57, http://www.cdc.gov/mmwR/preview/mmwrhtml/ss5307a1.htm.

7. D. A. Brent and J. Bridge, "Firearms Availability and Suicide: Evidence, Interventions, and Future Directions," *American Behavioral Scientist* 46 (2003): 1192–1210; D. A. Brent, J. A. Perper, C. J. Allman, G. M. Moritz, M. E. Wartella, and J. P. Zelenak, "The Presence and Accessibility of Firearms in the Homes of Adolescent Suicides: A Case-Control Study," *Journal of the American Medical Association* 266 (1991): 2989–95; A. Kellermann, F. Rivara, G. Somes, D. Reay, J. Francisco, J. G. Banton, J. Prodzinski, C. Fligner, and B. B. Hackman, "Suicide in the Home in Relation to Gun Ownership," *New England Journal of Medicine* 327 (1992): 467–72; D. C. Grossman, B. A. Mueller, C. Riedy, M. D. Dowd, A. Villaveces, J. Prodzinski, J. Nakagawara, J. Howard, N. Thiersch, and R. Harruff, "Gun Storage Practices and Risk of Youth Suicide and Unintentional Firearm Injuries," *Journal of the American Medical Association* 293 (2005): 707–14; M. Miller, D. Azrael, and C. Barber, "Suicide Mortality in the U.S.: The Importance of Attending to Method in Understanding Population-Level Disparities in the Burden of Suicide," *Annual Review of Public Health* 33 (2012): 393–408; M. Miller, A. Swanson, and D. Azrael, "Are We Missing Something Pertinent? A Bias Analysis of Unmeasured Confounding in the Firearm-Suicide Literature," *Epidemiologic Reviews* 38, no. 1 (2016): 62–69; A. Anglemyer, T. Horvath, and G. Rutherford, "The Accessibility of Firearms and Risk for Suicide and Homicide Victimization among Household Members: A Systematic Review and Meta-Analysis," *Annals of Internal Medicine* 160, no. 2 (2014): 101–10.

11. Overcoming Disability

1. US Department of Veterans Affairs, VA Palo Alto Health Care System, "Polytrauma System of Care," 7.

2. US Department of Veterans Affairs, "Spinal Cord Injuries and Disorders System of Care," https://www.sci.va.gov/VAs_SCID_System_of_Care.asp.

3. US Department of Veterans Affairs, "Spinal Cord Injuries."

4. National Institutes of Health, "Study Finds Most Americans Are in Good Visual Health but 14 Million Are Visually Impaired," May 9, 2006, accessed August 28, 2017, https://www.nih.gov/news-events/news-releases/study-finds-most-americans-have-good-vision-14-million-are-visually-impaired.

5. Centers for Disease Control and Prevention, "Improving the Nation's Vision Health: A Coordinated Public Health Approach," April 20, 2009.

13. Off the Streets

1. Point-in-time counts, required by the Department of Housing and Urban Development, take place annually on a single night in January when various groups go out to estimate how many homeless people there are in shelters of some kind as well as unsheltered in American cities and towns. HUD Exchange, "PIT and HIC Guides, Tools, and Webinars," 2017, https://www.hudexchange.info/programs/hdx/guides/pit-hic/#general-pit-guides-and-tools.

2. National Alliance to End Homelessness, "Fact Sheet: Veteran Homelessness," last modified April 2015, http://www.endhomelessness.org/library/entry/fact-sheet-veteran-homelessness.

3. National Coalition for Homeless Veterans, "Background and Statistics," http://nchv.org/index.php/news/media/background_and_statistics.

4. Stefan G. Kertesz, Travis P. Baggett, James J. O'Connell, David S. Buck, and Margot B. Kushel, "Permanent Supportive Housing for Homeless People—Reframing the Debate," *New England Journal of Medicine* 375 (2016): 2115–17, doi:10.1056/NEJMp1608326, http://www.nejm.org/doi/full/10.1056/NEJMp1608326.

5. US Department of Veterans Affairs, "HUD-VASH Resource Guide for Permanent Housing and Clinical Care," https://www.va.gov/HOMELESS/docs/Center/144_HUD-VASH_Book_WEB_High_Res_final.pdf.

6. US Department of Veterans Affairs, "Homeless Veterans," https://www.va.gov/homeless/housing.asp.

7. Juneau Economic Development Council, "Vulnerability Index: Prioritizing the Street Homeless Population by Mortality Risk," http://www.jedc.org/forms/Vulnerability%20Index.pdf.

8. US Department of Veterans Affairs, "Homeless Veterans."

9. World Health Organization, "Social Determinants of Health," http://www.who.int/social_determinants/en/.

10. Uchenna S. Ucendu, "Institutional Journey in Pursuit of Health Equity: Veterans Health Administration's Office of Health Equity," *American Journal of Public Health* 104, no. S4 (2014): S511–S513, doi:10.2105/AJPH.2014.302183.

11. D. K. McInnes, B. A. Petrakis, A. L. Gifford, S. R. Rao, T. K. Houston, S. M. Asch, and T. P. O'Toole, "Retaining Homeless Veterans in Outpatient Care: A Pilot Study of Mobile Phone Text Message Appointment Reminders," *American Journal of Public Health* 104, no. S4 (2014): S588–94, doi:10.2105/AJPH.2014.302061.

12. US Department of Veterans Affairs, "Homeless Veterans."

13. Suzanne Gordon, *The Battle for Veterans' Healthcare: Dispatches from the Frontlines of Policy-Making and Patient Care* (Ithaca, NY: Cornell Publishing, 2017), 48–50.

14. US Department of Veterans Affairs, "National Call Center for Homeless Veterans," https://www.va.gov/HOMELESS/NationalCallCenter.asp.

14. Alternatives to Jail

1. Justice for Vets, "What Is a Veterans Treatment Court?," accessed June 1, 2017, http://justiceforvets.org/what-is-a-veterans-treatment-court/.

2. A. K. Finlay, M. Stimmel, J. Blue-Howells, J. Rosenthal, J. McGuire, I. Binswanger, D. Smelson, et al., "Use of Veterans Health Administration Mental Health and Substance Use Disorder Treatment after Exiting Prison: The Health Care for Reentry Veterans Program," *Administration and Policy in Mental Health* 44, no. 2 (2017): 177–87, doi:10.1007/s10488-015-0708-z, https://www.ncbi.nlm.nih.gov/pubmed/26687114.

3. US Department of Veterans Affairs, "Fact Sheet. VA Services for Veterans Involved in the Justice System: VA's Veterans Justice Outreach Program," last modified October 2011.

4. Finlay et al., "Use of Veterans."

5. US Department of Veterans Affairs, "Fact Sheet."

6. US Department of Veterans Affairs, "Fact Sheet."

7. Finlay et al., "Use of Veterans."

8. Ellen Lawton, "A History of the Medical Legal Partnership Movement," Community Health Forum, Fall/Winter 2014, accessed May 3, 2017, http://medical-legalpartnership.org/wp-content/uploads/2015/01/NACHC-Magazine-A-History-of-the-Medical-Legal-Partnership-Movement.pdf.

9. Vet Centers are unique because they provide mental health treatment to veterans who have served in combat or are survivors of military sexual trauma regardless of discharge status.

10. US Department of Veterans Affairs, "Fact Sheet."

11. US Department of Veterans Affairs, "Fact Sheet. Veterans Court Inventory 2014 Update," last modified February 2016, https://www.va.gov/HOMELESS/docs/VTC-Inventory-FactSheet-0216.pdf.

12. Justice for Vets, "The History," accessed May 24, 2017, http://www.justiceforvets.org/vtc-history.

13. California Courts, "Collaborative Justice Courts," accessed April 25, 2017, http://www.courts.ca.gov/programs-collabjustice.htm.

14. Collaborative Justice, "What Is Collaborative Justice?," http://www.collaborativejustice.org/what.htm.

15. California Courts, "Collaborative Justice Courts."

16. Hannah Albarazi, "SF Veterans Get Expanded Path to Justice," *SF Bay*, December 29, 2014, https://sfbay.ca/2014/12/29/sf-veterans-get-expanded-path-to-justice/.

17. Superior Court of California, County of San Francisco, "Veterans Justice Court," http://www.sfsuperiorcourt.org/divisions/collaborative/veterans-justice.

18. Hawaii State Judiciary, "Hawaii Veterans Treatment Court Celebrates More Successful Graduates," last modified May 13, 2016, http://www.courts.state.hi.us/news_and_reports/featured_news/2016/05/hawaii-veterans-treatment-court-celebrates-15-successful-graduates.

19. It Takes an Ohana, "Veterans Treatment Court," 2014, http://ittakesanohana.org/wp-content/uploads/2014/08/Veterans.Court-Brochure.pdf.

15. Specializing in Elder Care

1. Linda O. Nichols, Jennifer Martindale-Adams, Carolyn W. Zhu, Erin K. Kaplan, Jeffrey K. Zuber, and Teresa M. Waters, "Impact of REACH II and REACH VA Dementia Caregiver Interventions on Healthcare Costs," *Journal of the American Geriatrics Society* 65 (2017): 931.

2. Nichols et al., "Impact of REACH II."

3. Institute of Medicine, *Retooling for an Aging America: Building a Health Care Workforce* (Washington, DC: National Academies, 2008), 5, https://eldercareworkforce.org/research/iom-report/research:retooling-for-an-aging-america-building-the-health-care-workforce/.

4. Howard Gleckman, "Who Will Care for the Elderly and Disabled?," *Kaiser Health News*, July 20, 2009, https://khn.org/news/072009gleckman/.

5. American Geriatrics Society, "Projected Future Need for Geriatricians," accessed November 23, 2017, https://www.americangeriatrics.org/sites/default/files/inline-files/Projected%20Future%20Need%20for%20Geriatricians.pdf.

6. James S. Powers, "U.S. Geriatrics, an Historical Perspective," in *Creating a Value Proposition for Geriatric Care: The Transformation of American Healthcare* (New York: Springer, 2017), 5–10.

7. US Department of Veterans Affairs, "Geriatric Research Education and Clinical Center (GRECC)," https://www.va.gov/grecc/.

8. Truth in advertising: Andrew Budson is my cousin.

9. Andrew E. Budson and Maureen K. O'Connor, *Seven Steps to Managing Your Memory: What's Normal, What's Not, and What to Do about It* (New York: Oxford University Press, 2017).

10. US Department of Veterans Affairs, Office of Academic Affiliations, "VA Fellowships in Advanced Geriatrics," https://www.va.gov/oaa/specialfellows/programs/SF_AdvGeriatric.asp.

11. Negar Golchin, Scott H. Frank, April Vince, Lisa Isham, and Sharon B. Meropol, "Polypharmacy in the Elderly," *Journal of Research in Pharmacy Practice* 4, no. 2 (2015): 85–88, https://www.ncbi.nlm.nih.gov/pmc/articles/PMC4418141/.

12. Katie Hafner and Griffin Palmer, "Skin Cancers Rise, along with Questionable Treatments," *New York Times*, November 20, 2017, https://www.nytimes.com/2017/11/20/health/dermatology-skin-cancer.html.

13. Powers, *Creating a Value Proposition*.

14. Powers, *Creating a Value Proposition*.

15. US Department of Veterans Affairs, Center for Healthcare Organization and Implementation Research, "Hartmann Promotes Resident-Centered Care in CLCs," https://www.choir.research.va.gov/features/Interview_Hartmann_Promotes_Resident_Centered_CLCs.asp.

16. VA Illiana Health Care System, video highlighting Green House Homes, http://www.thegreenhouseproject.org/solutions/green-house-projects-veterans.

16. Knocking on Heaven's Door

1. Frontline, "Facing Death. Facts & Figures," accessed June 24, 2017, http://www.pbs.org/wgbh/pages/frontline/facing-death/facts-and-figures/.

2. Mary Ersek, Susan C. Miller, Todd H. Wagner, Joshua M. Thorpe, Dawn Smith, Cari R. Levy, Risha Gidwani, et al., "Association between Aggressive Care and Bereaved Families' Evaluation of End-of-Life Care for Veterans with Non-Small Cell Lung Cancer Who Died in Veterans Affairs Facilities," *Cancer*, April 1, 2017.

3. Mary Ersek, Joshua M. Thorpe, Hyejin Kim, and Dawn Smith, "Exploring End-of-Life Care in Veterans Affairs Community Living Centers," *Journal of the American Geriatrics Society* 63 (2015): 644–50, doi:10.1111/jgs.13348.

4. Ersek et al., "Association between Aggressive Care," 2.

5. Ersek et al., "Exploring End-of-Life Care," 4–5.

6. I use the term "treatment" rather than "care" deliberately here because what many patients receive when they are seriously or terminally ill is the former rather than the latter. Indeed, one could argue that the focus on narrow treatment drives out any possibility of delivering genuine care.

7. Diane Meier, "Increased Access to Palliative Care and Hospice Services: Opportunities to Improve Value in Health Care," *Milbank Quarterly*, September 2011, 343, https://www.milbank.org/quarterly/articles/increased-access-to-palliative-care-and-hospice-services-opportunities-to-improve-value-in-health-care/.

8. Meier, 350.

9. Meier, 349.

10. Meier, 356.

11. Meier, 354.

12. US Department of Veterans Affairs, Health Services Research & Development, "Improving End of Life Care for Veterans: PROMISE," https://www.hsrd.research.va.gov/for_managers/stories/promise.cfm.

13. We Honor Veterans, https://www.wehonorveterans.org/.

14. Vincent Mor, Nina R. Joyce, Danielle L. Coté, Risha A. Gidwani, Mary Ersek, Cari R. Levy, Katherine E. Faricy-Anderson, et al., "The Rise of Concurrent Care for Veterans with Advanced Cancer at the End of Life," *Cancer*, December 15, 2015, http://onlinelibrary.wiley.com/doi/10.1002/cncr.29827/abstract.

15. US Department of Veterans Affairs, "Improving End of Life Care."

16. US Department of Veterans Affairs, "Bereaved Family Survey, English with Female Pronouns," https://www.cherp.research.va.gov/PROMISE/PROMISE%20Website%20files/ENG_FEMALE_2013_Survey_Bereavement_Veterans_Affair_HR_May3.pdf.

17. Ersek et al., "Exploring End-of-Life Care," 4–5.

18. Melissa W. Wachterman, Corey Pilver, Dawn Smith, Mary Ersek, Stuart R. Lipsitz, and Nancy L. Keating, "Quality of End-of-Life Care Provided to Patients with Different Serious Illnesses," *JAMA Internal Medicine* 176, no. 8 (2016): 1095–1102, http://jamanetwork.com/journals/jamainternalmedicine/article-abstract/2529496.

19. Ann Kutney-Lee, Caitlin W. Brennan, Mark Meterko, and Mary Ersek, "Organization of Nursing and Quality Care for Veterans at the End of Life," *Journal of Pain Symptom Management* 49, no. 3 (2015): 570–77, http://www.jpsmjournal.com/article/S0885-3924%2814%2900397-2/abstract.

17. Better Care Where?

1. Merritt Hawkins, "Survey: Physician Appointment Wait Times up 30% from 2014," https://www.merritthawkins.com/clients/BlogPostDetail.aspx?PostId=40867.

2. Elisabeth Rosenthal, "The Health Care Waiting Game: Long Waits for Doctors' Appointments Have Become the Norm," *New York Times*, July 5, 2014, https://www.nytimes.com/2014/07/06/sunday-review/long-waits-for-doctors-appointments-have-become-the-norm.html?mcubz=0&_r=0.

3. Robin Osborn and Cathy Schoen, "The Commonwealth Fund 2013 International Health Policy Survey in Eleven Countries," http://www.commonwealthfund.org/~/media/files/publications/in-the-literature/2013/nov/pdf_schoen_2013_ihp_survey_chartpack_final.pdf.

4. Osborn and Schoen, 11.

5. Phillip Longman and Suzanne Gordon, "VA Health Care: A System Worth Saving," American Legion, May 2017, https://www.legion.org/sites/legion.org/files/legion/publications/59VAR0817%20Longman%20Gordon%20Report.pdf.

6. Veterans Health Administration, "Pending Appointment and Electronic Wait List Summary—National, Facility, and Division Level Summaries: Wait Time Calculated from Preferred Date for the Period Ending: 5/15/2017," https://www.va.gov/HEALTH/docs/DR70_052017_Pending_and_EWL_Biweekly_Desired_Date_Division.pdf.

7. US Department of Veterans Affairs, Office of Public Affairs, "State of the VA Fact Sheet," May 31, 2017, http://w w w.blogs.va.gov/VAntage/wp-content/uploads/2017/05/StateofVA_FactSheet_5-31-2017.pdf.

8. RAND Corporation, Assessment B (Health Care Capabilities), September 1, 2015, https://www.va.gov/opa/choiceact/documents/assessments/Assessment_B_Health_Care_Capabilities.pdf.

9. North Carolina Rural Health Research Program, "82 Rural Hospital Closures: January 2010–Present," http://www.shepscenter.unc.edu/programs-projects/rural-health/rural-hospital-closures/.

10. Lauren Weber and Andy Miller, "A Hospital Crisis Is Killing Rural Communities: This State Is Ground Zero," *Huffington Post*, September 22, 2017, https://www.huffingtonpost.com/entry/rural-hospitals-closure-georgia_us_59c02bf4e4b087fdf5075e38.

11. Veterans Health Administration, Office of the Inspector General, "Review of Alleged Patient Deaths, Patient Wait Times and Scheduling Practices at the Phoenix VA Health Care System," August 26, 2014, https://www.va.gov/oig/pubs/VAOIG-14-02603-267.pdf.

12. Alicia A. Mundy, "The VA Isn't Broken, Yet," *Washington Monthly*, March–May 2016.

13. Institute of Medicine, *To Err Is Human: Building a Safer Health System* (Washington, DC: National Academies, 1999).

14. Martin A. Makary and Michael Daniel, "Medical Error—the Third Leading Cause of Death in the US," *BMJ* 353 (2016): i2139, doi: 10.1136/bmj.i2139.

15. As for the idea that the private sector would never tolerate reckless practice, consider the cases of Vyant Patel, a surgeon who killed dozens of patients and moved from state to state in the United States and was finally stopped in Australia. Or there is nurse Charles Cullen, reputed to be the most dangerous serial killer in the United States, who was passed from hospital to hospital like a pedophile priest. Just Google Cullen and Patel to discover the horrifying details.

16. Dr. Thomas Insel interview, National Public Radio, October 7, 2015, hetakeaway.org/story/dr-thomas-insel-mental-health-system-badly-broken/.

17. Mental Illness Policy, "About 50% of Individuals with Severe Psychiatric Disorders (3.5. Million People) Are Receiving No Treatment," n.d., http://mentalillnesspolicy.org/consequences/percentage-mentally-ill-untreated.html.

18. Treatment Advocacy Center, "Consequences of Non Treatment," accessed October 13, 2015, http://www.treatmentadvocacycenter.org/problem/consequences-of-non-treatment.

19. US Department of Health and Human Services, SAMHSA, "Report to Congress on the Nation's Substance Abuse and Mental Health Workforce Issues," January 24, 2013, https://store.samhsa.gov/shin/content/PEP13-RTC-BHWORK/PEP13-RTC-BHWORK.pdf.

20. Treatment Advocacy Center, "Consequences"; Mental Illness Policy, "About 50%."

21*Shrink Rap* (blog), "Why Shrinks Don't Take Your Insurance," November 14, 2007, http://psychiatrist-blog.blogspot.com/2007/11/why-shrinks-dont-take-your-insurance.html.

22. Dinah Miller, "Why Psychiatrists Don't Take Insurance," Kevin MD, January 25, 2014, http://www.kevinmd.com/blog/2014/01/psychiatrists-insurance.html.

23. T. F. Bishop, M. J. Press, S. Keyhani, and H. A. Pincus, "Acceptance of Insurance by Psychiatrists and the Implications for Access to Mental Health Care," *Journal of the American Medical Association* 71, no. 2 (2014), http://archpsyc.jamanetwork.com/article.aspx?articleid=1785174.

24. D. Mechanic, "More People Than Ever Before Are Receiving Behavioral Health Care in the United States, but Gaps and Challenges Remain," *Health Affairs* 33, no. 8 (2014): 1416–24. See also Bishop et al., "Acceptance of Insurance."

25. American Psychological Association, "Does Your Insurance Cover Mental Health Services? What You Need to Know about Mental Health Coverage," http://www.apa.org/helpcenter/parity-guide.aspx.

26. Barry B. Cepelewicz, "Firing a Patient: When It's Needed and How Physicians Can Handle It Correctly," *Medical Economics*, January 23, 2014, http://medicaleconomics.modernmedicine.com/medical-economics/content/tags/malpractice/firing-patient-when-its-needed-and-how-physicians-can-han?page=full.

27. Treatment Advocacy Center, "No Room at the Inn: Trends and Consequences of Closing Public Psychiatric Hospitals," accessed August 9, 2016, http://tacreports.org/bed-study.

28. Treatment Advocacy Center, "Trends in Hospital Bed Availability," accessed August 11, 2016, http://www.tacreports.org/trends-in-availability.

29. Eurostat Statistics Explained, "Health Care Resource Statistics—Beds," accessed August, 11, 2016, http://ec.europa.eu/eurostat/statistics-explained/index.php/Healthcare_resource_statistics_-_beds.

30. Organisation for Economic Co-operation and Development, "Health Statistics 2014—Frequently Requested Data," accessed August, 10, 2016, http://www.oecd.org/els/health-systems/oecd-health-statistics-2014-frequently-requested-data.htm.

31. April Dembosky, "Kaiser Agrees to Pay $4 Million Fine over Mental Health Care," KQED News, September 9, 2014, http://ww2.kqed.org/stateofhealth/2014/09/09/kaiser-agrees-to-pay-4-million-fine-over-mental-health-care-drops-lawsuit/.

32. Stuart Pfeifer, "His 83-Year-Old Wife Jumped to Her Death from a Kaiser Clinic. Why?," *Los Angeles Times*, September 26, 2015, http://www.latimes.com/business/la-fi-kaiser-mental-health-20150926-story.html.

33. Katherine E. Watkins, Brad Smith, Ayse Akincigil, Melony E. Sorbero, Susan Paddock, Abigail Woodroffe, Cecilia Huang, Stephen Crystal, and Harold Alan Pincus, "The Quality of Medication Treatment for Mental Disorders in the Department of Veterans Affairs and in Private-Sector Plans," *Psychiatric Services* 67, no. 4 (2016): 391–96. See also C. N. Barry, T. R. Bowe, and A. Suneja, "An Update on the Quality of Medication Treatment for Mental Disorders in the VA," *Psychiatric Services* 67, no. 8 (2016): 930.

34. Claire A. Hoffmire, Janet E. Kemp, and Robert M. Bossarte, "Changes in Suicide Mortality for Veterans and Nonveterans by Gender and History of VHA Service Use, 2000–2010," *Psychiatric Services* 66, no. 9 (2015): 959–65, http://ps.psychiatryonline.org/doi/abs/10.1176/appi.ps.201400031?trendmd-shared=0&journalCode=ps.

35. A. M. Kilbourne, R. V. Ignacio, H. M. Kim, and F. C. Blow, "Datapoints: Are VA Patients with Serious Mental Illness Dying Younger?," *Psychiatric Services* 60, no. 5 (2009): 589.

36. Terri Tanielian, Coreen Farris, Caroline Batka, Carrie M. Farmer, Eric Robinson, Charles C. Engel, Michael Robbins, and Lisa H. Jaycox, *Ready to Serve: Community-Based Provider Capacity to Deliver Culturally Competent, Quality Mental Health Care to Veterans and Their Families*, RAND Corporation, 2014, https://www.rand.org/pubs/research_reports/RR806.html.

37. Terri Tanielian, Carrie M. Farmer, Rachel M. Burns, Erin L. Duffy, and Claude Messan Setodji, *Ready or Not? Assessing the Capacity of New York State Health Care Providers to Meet the Needs of Veterans*, Rand Corporation, 2018, https://nyshealthfoundation.org/wp-content/uploads/2018/02/RAND-Ready-or-Not-Veterans-Care-March-2018.pdf.

38. Dean G. Kilpatrick, Connie L. Best, Daniel W. Smith, Harold Kudler, and Vickey Cornelison-Grant, *Serving Those Who Have Served: Educational Needs of Health Care Providers Working with Military Members, Veterans, and Their Families*, December 1, 2011, https://www.mirecc.va.gov/docs/visn6/Serving_Those_Who_Have_Served.pdf.

39. Russell Lemle, "Choice Program Expansion Jeopardizes High-Quality VHA Mental Health Services," *Federal Practitioner*, March 2018, https://www.mdedge.com/fedprac/article/159219/mental-health/choice-program-expansion-jeopardizes-high-quality-vha-mental.

40. National Academies of Sciences, Engineering, and Medicine, *A Consensus Study Report: Evaluation of the Department of Veterans Affairs Mental Health Services*, 2018, https://www.nap.edu/read/24915/chapter/1#ii.

41. Michael Blecker, "Letter of Dissent," June 29, 2016, https://www.swords-to-plowshares.org/wp-content/uploads/Dissent-Letter-from-Commissioner-Michael-Blecker-06-29-2016.pdf.

42. A. K. Jha, J. B. Perlin, K. W. Kizer, and R. A. Dudley, "Effect of the Transformation of the Veterans Affairs Health Care System on the Quality of Care," *New England Journal of Medicine* 348, no. 22 (2003): 2218–27.

43. S. Woolhandler and D. U. Himmelstein, "Competition in a Publicly Funded Healthcare System," *BMJ* 335 (2007): 1126–29.

44. P. G. Shekelle, S. Asch, P. Glassman, S. Matula, A. Trivedi, and I. Miake-Lye, "Comparison of Quality of Care in VA and Non-VA Settings: A Systematic Review," VA-ESP Project #05-226, September 2010, https://www.hsrd.research.va.gov/publications/esp/quality.cfm. For a full bibliography of peer-reviewed studies comparing VA and non-VA care see Association

of VA Psychologist Leaders, "Comparison of VA to Community Healthcare; Summary of Research 2000–2016," March 23, 2016, http://advocacy.avapl.org/pubs/FACT%20sheet%20 literature%20review%20of%20VA%20vs%20Community%20Heath%20Care%2003 %2023-16.pdf.

45. American Customer Satisfaction Index (ASCI), Selected years, http://www.theacsi. org/index.php?option=com_content&view=article&id=63&Itemid=101/.

46. Association of VA Psychologist Leaders, "Comparison."

47. RAND Corporation, Assessment B.

48. R. Edayathumangalam, "Veterans Health Administration Compared to Private Sector for Older Cancer Patients," *Focus*, August 14, 2011, http://www.focushms.com/features/ veterans-health-administration-compared-to-private-sector-for-older-cancer-patients/.

49. A. Parikh-Patel, C. R. Morris, R. Martinsen, and K. W. Kizer, *Disparities in Stage at Diagnosis, Survival, and Quality of Cancer Care in California by Source of Health Insurance*, UC Davis Institute for Population Health Improvement, https://www.ucdmc.ucdavis.edu/iphi/ resources/1117737_CancerHI_100615.pdf.

50. Department of Veterans Affairs, "VA Research on Diabetes," https://www.research. va.gov/topics/diabetes.cfm.

51. Eve Kerr, "VA System Superior for Diabetes Care," *Issues in Diabetes*, http://www. diabeticmctoday.com/HtmlPages/DMC1004/PDF%20FILES/dmc1004_Kerr.pdf; Association of VA Psychologist Leaders, "Comparison."

52. Association of VA Psychologist Leaders, "VA Medical Innovations and Discoveries," http://advocacy.avapl.org/pubs/VA%20Medical%20Innovations%20and%20Discoveries %20Fact%20Sheet%20June%202016.pdf.

53. Longman and Gordon, "VA Healthcare."

54. Joe Manchin, press release, "Manchin, Heller Introduce Legislation following Shocking Report That VA Buried Medical Mistakes," November 13, 2017, https://www.manchin. senate.gov/newsroom/press-releases/manchin-heller-introduce-legislation-following-shocking- report-that-va-buried-medical-mistakes.

55. Joe Carlson, "Cleveland Clinic Cases Highlight Flaws in Oversight," *Modern Healthcare*, June 7, 2014, http://www.modernhealthcare.com/article/20140607/MAGAZINE/306079939.

56. Suzanne Gordon, *The Battle for Veterans' Healthcare: Dispatches from the Frontlines of Policy Making and Patient Care* (Ithaca, NY: Cornell Publishing, 2017), 33.

57. Daniel P. Kessler, "Evaluating the Medical Malpractice System and Options for Reform," *Journal of Economic Perspectives* 25, no. 2 (2011): 93–110, https://www.ncbi.nlm. nih.gov/pmc/articles/PMC3195420/.

58. Kessler, "Evaluating the Medical."

59. Michelle M. Mello and Jeffrey N. Catalano, "Should Medical Malpractice Settlements Be Secret?," *JAMA Internal Medicine* 175, no. 7 (2015): 1135–37, doi:10.1001/jamaint ernmed.2015.1038, https://jamanetwork.com/journals/jamainternalmedicine/article-abstract/ 2293075.

60. Lisa Rappaport, "In Malpractice Settlements, Injured Parties Often Agree to Keep Mum," Reuters, May 11, 2013, https://www.reuters.com/article/us-malpractice- nondisclosure/in-malpractice-settlements-injured-parties-often-agree-to-keep-mum- idUSKBN0NW21H20150511.

Conclusion

1. Peter S. Hussey, Jeanne S. Ringel, Sangeeta Ahluwalia, Rebecca Anhang Price, Christine Buttorff, Thomas Concannon, Susan L. Lovejoy, et al., "Resources and Capabilities of the Department of Veterans Affairs to Provide Timely and Accessible Care to Veterans," RAND Corporation, 2015, https://www.rand.org/pubs/research_reports/RR1165z2.html.

2. Suzanne Gordon, "Yes, Trump Is Privatizing the VA," *Hill*, June 16, 2017, http://thehill.com/blogs/pundits-blog/the-military/338172-yes-trump-is-privatizing-the-va.

3. American Federation of Government Employees, "Staff the VA News," accessed December 10, 2017, https://www.afge.org/about-us/agencies/department-of-veterans-affairs-va/staff-the-va/staff-the-va-news/.

4. Suzanne Gordon, "Veterans Health Administration Needs Stronger Recruitment Methods," *Hill*, February 23, 2018, http://thehill.com/opinion/healthcare/375346-veterans-health-administration-needs-stronger-recruitment-methods.

5. Gordon, "Veterans Health Administration."

6. Centers for Medicare and Medicaid Services Alliance to Modernize Healthcare Federally Funded Research and Development Center, "Independent Assessment of the Health Care Delivery Systems and Management Processes of the Department of Veterans Affairs," September 1, 2015, xvi, https://www.va.gov/opa/choiceact/documents/assessments/Integrated_Report.pdf.

7. Stephen K. Trynosky, "Beyond the Iron Triangle: Implications for the Veterans Health Administration in an Uncertain Policy Environment," School of Advanced Military Studies, United States Army Command and General Staff College, 2014, 60.

8. Trynosky, "Beyond the Iron Triangle."

9. Daniel Zwerdling, "At VA Hospitals, Training and Technology Reduce Nurses' Injuries," February 25, 2015, https://www.npr.org/2015/02/25/387298633/at-va-hospitals-training-and-technology-reduce-nurses-injuries.

10. David Shulkin, Shereef Elnahal, Ellen Maddock, and Megan Shaheen, *Best Care Everywhere* (Washington, DC: US Department of Veterans Affairs, 2017).

11. Shulkin et al., *Best Care Everywhere*.

12. Suzanne Gordon, "Why Is the VA Hiding a PR Goldmine?," *Washington Monthly*, December 8, 2017, https://washingtonmonthly.com/2017/12/08/why-is-the-va-hiding-a-pr-goldmine/.

13. Kenneth W. Kizer, foreword to *The Battle for Veterans' Healthcare: Dispatches from the Frontlines of Policy Making and Patient Care*, by Suzanne Gordon (Ithaca, NY: Cornell Publishing, 2017), 13.

14. Conservative Coalition: Support Veterans Health Care Choice and Protect Taxpayers, "Letter to Senators and Congressional Representatives," October 23, 2017.

15. "Steven A. Cohen among the Million-Dollar Donors to Trump Inauguration," Market Watch, April 19, 2017, http://www.sec.marketwatch.com/story/steven-a-cohen-among-the-million-dollar-donors-to-trump-inauguration-2017-04-19.

16. Cohen failed to supervise portfolio manager Mathew Martoma, who was indicted and is now serving nine years in prison for insider trading. Illegal insider trades avoided losses and netted profits of approximately $275 million for Cohen's hedge fund. Cohen himself narrowly escaped being indicted. Wikipedia, s.v. "Mathew Martoma," https://en.wikipedia.org/wiki/Mathew_Martoma.

17. Memorandum of Agreement between United States Department of Veterans Affairs and Cohen Veterans Network Inc., October 17, 2017, 4–5.

18. Cohen Veterans Network, "VA Partners with Cohen Veterans Network to Increase Access to Mental Health Resources," press release, February 27, 2018, https://www.cohenveteransnetwork.org/wp-content/uploads/2018/02/CVN-VA-Feb-2018.pdf.

19. Phil Roe, "VA Care in the Community Act," accessed December 10, 2017, https://veterans.house.gov/communitycare/.

20. US Department of Veterans Affairs, "VA Announces Veterans Coordinated Access & Rewarding Experiences Act," accessed December 10, 2017, https://www.blogs.va.gov/VAntage/42270/va-announces-veterans-coordinated-access-rewarding-experiences-act/.

21. Jon Tester, "Tester: Replace Veterans Choice Program with Bipartisan Community Care Plan," November 29, 2017, https://www.tester.senate.gov/?p=press_release&id=5645.

22. John McCain, "Senators McCain & Moran Introduce Legislation to Reform VA into 21st Century Health Care System," December 4, 2017, https://www.mccain.senate.gov/public/index.cfm/press-releases?ID=5D9B8429-6F94-46AF-AAEB-DA470617D64D.

23. House Committee on Veterans Affairs, "VA Asset and Infrastructure Review (AIR) Act of 2017," Chairman Phil Roe, MD, accessed December 10, 2017, https://veterans.house.gov/uploadedfiles/va_air_act_one_pager.pdf.

24. Doug Lamborn, "Veterans Empowerment Act," press release, November 21, 2017, https://lamborn.house.gov/news/documentsingle.aspx?DocumentID=2175.

25. Avik Roy, "Achieving Health Care Independence for Veterans," FREOPP, November 11, 2016, https://freopp.org/achieving-health-care-independence-for-veterans-62e0bd7c8947.

26. Reid Abelson and Katie Thomas, "CVS and Aetna Say Merger Will Improve Your Health Care. Can They Deliver?," *New York Times*, December 5, 2017, https://www.nytimes.com/2017/12/04/health/cvs-aetna-merger.html.

27. Donald M. Berwick, *Escape Fire: Lessons for the Future of Health Care* (Commonwealth Fund, 2002), http://www.commonwealthfund.org/usr_doc/berwick_escapefire_563.pdf.

28 Fighting for Veterans Healthcare, "FFVHC Policy Analyses," https://ffvhc.org/resources/.

29. Suzanne Gordon, "VHA Budget Cuts Threaten Veteran Safety," *Tapped* (blog), *American Prospect*, September 15, 2017, http://prospect.org/blog/tapped/vha-budget-cuts-threaten-veteran-safety.

30. Suzanne Gordon, "Veterans Face Another Round of Threats to Health-Care Networks, *Tapped* (blog), *American Prospect*, October 16, 2017, http://prospect.org/blog/tapped/veterans-face-another-round-threats-health-care-networks.

31. Emily Wax-Thibodeaux, "VA Tried to Reallocate $460 Million Earmarked for Homeless Veterans. Now It Says That Won't Happen," *Washington Post*, December 6, 2017, Thihttps://www.washingtonpost.com/news/checkpoint/wp/2017/12/06/va-tried-to-reallocate-460-million-earmarked-for-homeless-veterans-now-it-says-that-wont-happen/?utm_term=.f3471ce06f32.

32. Dave Philipps and Nicholas Fandos, "New Veterans Affairs Chief: A Hands-On, Risk-Taking 'Standout,'" *New York Times*, May 9, 2017, https://www.nytimes.com/2017/05/09/us/politics/new-veterans-affairs-chief-a-hands-on-risk-taking-standout.html.

33. US Department of Veterans Affairs, Inspector General, "Accuracy and Timeliness of Payments Made under the Choice Program Authorized by the Veterans Access, Choice, and Accountability Act," September 12, 2017.

34. Dennis Wagner, "Arizona-Based VA Contractor Collected 'Tens of Millions' in Over Payments, Federal Audit Says," Azcentral, November 13, 2017, https://www.azcentral.com/story/news/local/arizona-investigations/2017/11/13/va-inspectors-question-millions-dollars-paid-triwest-veterans-healthcare-contract/737341001/.

35. Suzanne Gordon, "VA Officials Continue to Discuss Proposed Health-Care Changes out of Public View," *Tapped* (blog), *American Prospect*, November 22, 2017, http://prospect.org/blog/tapped/va-officials-continue-discuss-proposed-health-care-changes-out-public-view?.

36. Veterans of Foreign Wars, "VFW Survey: Veterans Want VA Fixed, Not Dismantled," March 29, 2017, https://www.vfw.org/news-and-publications/press-room/archives/2017/3/vfw-survey-veterans-want-va-fixed-not-dismantled.

37. Veterans Healthcare Action Campaign, https://www.vhcac.org/.

38. American Federation of Government Employees, "A Pocket Guide to Political Activities by Federal Employees," 2016 edition, https://www.afge.org/globalassets/documents/manuals/afgepocketguide.pdf.

39. Trynosky, "Beyond the Iron Triangle."

Epilogue

1. Maggie Haberman and Nicholas Fandos, "Trump Signs Bill Meant to Restore Trust in VA," *New York Times*, June 23, 2017, https://www.nytimes.com/2017/06/23/us/politics/trump-veterans-accountability-bill.html.

2. Jasper Craven, "At the VA, a Law Meant to Discipline Executives Is Being Used to Fire Low-Level Workers," *The Nation*, May 10, 2018, https://www.thenation.com/article/at-the-va-a-law-meant-to-discipline-executives-is-being-used-to-fire-low-level-workers/.

3. The Editorial Board, "A Coup at Veterans Affairs," *New York Times*, March 30, 2018, https://www.nytimes.com/2018/03/29/opinion/shulkin-out-veterans-affairs-koch.html.

4. Department of Veterans Affairs, Office of the Inspector General, Administrative Investigation VA Secretary and Delegation Travel to Europe, February 14, 2018, https://www.va.gov/oig/pubs/VAOIG-17-05909-106.pdf.

5. David J. Shulkin, "Privatizing the VA Will Hurt Veterans," *New York Times*, March 28, 2018, https://www.nytimes.com/2018/03/28/opinion/shulkin-veterans-affairs-privatization.html.

6. Dan Merica, "Dr. Ronny Jackson's glowing bill of health for Trump," CNN, January 16, 2018, https://www.cnn.com/2018/01/16/politics/dr-ronny-jackson-donald-trump-clean-bill-of-health/index.html.

7. Aaron Blake, "Lengthy List of Allegations against Ronny Jackson Annotated," *Washington Post*, April 25, 2018, https://www.washingtonpost.com/news/the-fix/wp/2018/04/25/the-list-of-allegations-against-ronny-jackson-annotated/?utm_term=.6ff52592b526.

8. US Department of Veterans Affairs, Office of Public and Intergovernmental Affairs, "Debunking the VA Privatization Myth," April 5, 2018, https://www.va.gov/opa/pressrel/pressrelease.cfm?id=4034.

9. US Department of Veterans Affairs, Office of Public and Intergovernmental Affairs, "Statement by Acting VA Secretary Robert Wilkie—Chris Wilson Fox and Friends Interview," May 1, 2018, https://www.va.gov/opa/pressrel/pressrelease.cfm?id=4047.

10. Dave Phillips and Nicholas Fandos, "VA Medical System Staggers as Chaos Engulfs Its Leadership," *New York Times*, May 6, 2018, https://www.nytimes.com/2018/05/04/us/politics/va-medical-system-chaos.html.

11. Nicholas Fandos, "Senate Approval Is Last Hurdle for an Overhaul of Veterans Health Care," *New York Times*, May 24, 2018, https://www.nytimes.com/2018/05/23/us/politics/veterans-health-care.html.

12. Suzanne Gordon and Jasper Craven, "Congress Is Poised to Push Veterans' Health Care Closer to Privatization," *Washington Monthly*, May 22, 2018, https://www.washingtonpost.com/news/the-fix/wp/2018/04/25/the-list-of-allegations-against-ronny-jackson-annotated/?utm_term=.6ff52592b526.

13. Nancy Pelosi, "Pelosi Statement on Passage of VA Mission Act," May 16, 2018, https://pelosi.house.gov/news/press-releases/pelosi-statement-on-passage-of-va-mission-act.

14. Bernie Sanders, "Sanders to Vote No on Mission Act," May 23, 2018, https://www.commondreams.org/newswire/2018/05/23/sanders-vote-no-va-mission-act.

15. Leo Shane, "Trump Disavows Parts of New VA Reform Law Hours after Praising It," *Military Times*, June 7, 2018, https://www.militarytimes.com/veterans/2018/06/07/trump-disavows-parts-of-new-va-reform-law-hours-after-praising-it/.

16. Erica Werner and Lisa Rein, "Trump Signs Veterans Health Bill as White House Works against Bi-Partisan Plan to Fund It," *Washington Post*, June 6, 2018, https://www.washingtonpost.com/business/economy/trump-to-sign-veterans-heath-bill-as-white-house-works-against-plan-to-fund-it/2018/06/06/1763ac70-68d9-11e8-bf8c-f9ed2e672adf_story.html?noredirect=on&utm_term=.44c4e048a069.

INDEX

have appeared in *Harper's*, the *Atlantic*, the *New York Times Magazine*, the *Boston Globe*, the *New York Times*, the *Los Angeles Times*, the *American Prospect*, the *Washington Monthly*, the *Nation*, *JAMA*, the *Annals of Internal Medicine*, *British Medical Journal*, and in numerous other publications.

She lives in the San Francisco Bay Area with her husband.

About the Author

Suzanne Gordon is an award-winning journalist and author who writes about health care delivery and health care systems and patient safety. Her latest book, *The Battle for Veterans' Healthcare: Dispatches from the Front Lines of Policy Making and Patient Care* was published by Cornell University Press in May 2017. She received the Disabled American Veterans (DAV) Special Recognition Award for her work covering veterans' health care. She is the Senior Policy Fellow at the Veterans' Healthcare Policy Institute.

Suzanne Gordon's other twenty books include *First, Do Less Harm: Confronting the Inconvenient Problems of Patient Safety* and *Beyond the Checklist: What Else Health Care Can Learn from Aviation Teamwork and Safety.*

She is the coeditor of the Culture and Politics of Health Care Work series at Cornell University Press. She has been a radio commentator for US CBS Radio and National Public Radio's Marketplace. Her articles